Acta Neurochirurgica Supplement

Volume 133

Series Editor

Hans-Jakob Steiger, Department of Neurosurgery, Heinrich Heine University, Düsseldorf, Germany

ACTA NEUROCHIRURGICA's Supplement Volumes provide a unique opportunity to publish the content of special meetings in the form of a Proceedings Volume. Proceedings of international meetings concerning a special topic of interest to a large group of the neuroscience community are suitable for publication in ACTA NEUROCHIRURGICA. Links to ACTA NEUROCHIRURGICA's distribution network guarantee wide dissemination at a comparably low cost. The individual volumes should comprise between 120 and max. 250 printed pages, corresponding to 20-50 papers. It is recommended that you get in contact with us as early as possible during the preparatory stage of a meeting. Please supply a preliminary program for the planned meeting. The papers of the volumes represent original publications. They pass a peer review process and are listed in PubMed and other scientific databases. Publication can be effected within 6 months. Hans-Jakob Steiger is the Editor of ACTA NEUROCHIRURGICA's Supplement Volumes. Springer Verlag International is responsible for the technical aspects and calculation of the costs. If you decide to publish your proceedings in the Supplements of ACTA NEUROCHIRURGICA, you can expect the following: • An editing process with editors both from the neurosurgical community and professional language editing. After your book is accepted, you will be assigned a developmental editor who will work with you as well as with the entire editing group to bring your book to the highest quality possible. • Effective text and illustration layout for your book. • Worldwide distribution through Springer-Verlag International's distribution channels.

Keki Turel • Ekkehard M. Kasper
Editors

Complications in Neurosurgery II

Springer

Editors
Keki Turel
Department of Neurosurgery
Bombay Hospital Institute of Medical Sciences
Mumbai, Maharashtra, India

Ekkehard M. Kasper
McMaster University Faculty of Health Sciences
and Hamilton General Hospital
Hamilton, ON, Canada

Department of Neurosurgery
Boston University, Chobanian and Avedisian
School of Medicine and Boston Medical Center
Boston, MA, USA

ISSN 0065-1419 ISSN 2197-8395 (electronic)
Acta Neurochirurgica Supplement
ISBN 978-3-031-61600-6 ISBN 978-3-031-61601-3 (eBook)
https://doi.org/10.1007/978-3-031-61601-3

This Springer imprint is published by the registered company Springer Nature Switzerland AG
The registered company address is: Gewerbestrasse 11, 6330 Cham, Switzerland

Dr. Turel and I wish to say thanks to the people involved in getting this book done.

To our patients

With this work, we hope to create and continue an open forum for honest discussions of one's complications in neurosurgery and what can be learned from each of them. This should result in improvements in care for the next patients, but this process rests on the courage and willingness of our colleagues to share with others the pitfalls, management errors, and surgical failure that can occur.

We hope this is more than an exercise in reflection and humility, but an opportunity that allows us to transmit a lesson to the next generation of health care professionals, should a similar situation occur in the future. We firmly believe that learning from failure and appropriate management in the face of adverse events is the best strategy for prevention.

Preface to Complications in Neurosurgery II

Complications can be unfortunate parts of surgery, making the consequences of treatment at times worse than the original disease, possibly bringing great suffering to the patient and their family, and tarnishing the reputation of the surgeon, the hospital, and the specialty at large.

Neurosurgery is an intricate field of medicine, demanding not only exemplary surgical skills with many years of diligent training but also pre-, intra-, and postoperative decision-making, all of which can have profound impacts on patients' lives. It is a vast specialty with a myriad of subspecialties, and it often features the early application of rapidly evolving technology. Though the fundamentals of anatomy, physiology, pathology, and meticulous microsurgery remain the same, the modes of modern imaging and surgical treatment paradigms are ever changing and becoming progressively more sophisticated and minimalistic.

Complications may arise from numerous factors, such as inadequate preoperative clinical and radiological assessment, case setup, or an error in execution; they may be related to the technology, the tools employed, or simply an insurmountable or dangerously located disease. In the United States alone, an estimated 200,000 preventable medical deaths occur every year, which amount to the equivalent of almost three fatal airline crashes per day. In attempts to minimize the occurrence of such devastating events, the field of aviation has developed strict and elaborate safety guidelines, protocols, and checklists. Even in aviation, complications now occur more often because of human error than because of technical snags or "accidents," such as bird strikes or abrupt and adverse changes in weather.

Medicine and surgery are "uncertain" fields of practice, and complications may occur because of a variety of avoidable and unavoidable factors. Surgery is risky and dangerous, and it carries a 6–12% overall complication rate. As surgeons, we too would have significantly better outcomes if we promulgated and assiduously followed rigorous guidelines. Dr Atul Gawande, the author of *The Checklist Manifesto*, emphasized that "checklists, when followed appropriately, have helped reduce complications by 36%, deaths by 47% and infections by 50%."

All this makes deliberating on the subject of complications very encompassing. While most medical conferences deal with staid and conventional discussion of diseases, both common and uncommon, with speakers extolling their superb management and results and with a slide on complications occasionally rushed in toward the end, only very few have shown the fortitude to highlight only the pitfalls of management or the confessions of errors and mistakes. As was said earlier, medicine is an uncertain field, and errors in judgement (besides ability and skill) are inevitable. Having encountered or committed a "mistake," we have a moral obligation to not forget it and to pass the lessons learned on to our colleagues and to the next generation of learners, lest they go through them again, at great and repetitive cost to humanity.

With this ideology and hope of having an open forum of unabashed declaration of one's failures and what one has learned and is willing to share with others on level ground, the first International Conference on Complications in Neurosurgery (ICCN) was held on 3–5 March 2017 in Mumbai, India. The speakers were clearly instructed to present only those complications experienced at their own hands or in their own facility. One had to refrain from presenting complications encountered by a surgeon at another service that one eventually happened to correct or salvage. That would be putting our colleagues down and would leave a bad taste behind. In fact, no one needed to talk about their own success, except for how they were able to achieve it, having encountered an unexpected disaster in their own patient. Such deliberations on complications proved to be far more humbling and enriching than those indulging in boastful competition.

Attended by 383 delegates from across the globe, and with 218 presentations made by 139 speakers from 24 countries, the first ICCN was a thumping success and vindicated our belief in discussing complications on an open platform. For the first time, the barrier was broken, and the image of complications was transformed from being the ghost that haunted to an experience that would make one wiser (and humble). Each case encounter was accepted as a teacher that would give out the most important career lessons. Subsequent conferences, national, continental, and international, have now begun dedicating a session or two to the discussion of complications. I was invited by most organizers to prepare such sessions with participation from colleagues from across the world. Indeed, we have inadvertently sown the seeds of a new concept—of a new era in neurosurgery.

The selected papers of first ICCN were edited and compiled in the first book of a series, *Complications in Neurosurgery*, and published by Springer. Simultaneously, appreciating the concept and acknowledging the worldwide response, the then president of the World Federation of Neurosurgical Societies (WFNS), Prof. Franco Servadei introduced, for the first time in the history of WFNS, a committee on complications in neurosurgery, appointing me as its chair.

Bolstered by the success of first ICCN and supported by various International Societies, the second ICCN was held in Mumbai 2 years later, in January 2019. This 3-day conclave was attended again with great enthusiasm, as we coursed through one neurosurgical subspecialty after another, discussing the prevention and management of common and uncommon complications. As at the first ICCN, we had all the presentations in a single grand ballroom because running parallel sessions would have denied the delegates the opportunity to participate in the entire proceedings of all the subspecialties of neurosurgery. The conference was inaugurated by the legendary and internationally revered guru of meditation and founder of "Art of Living," Sri Sri Ravi Shankar, who extolled the virtues of meditation in the avoidance of complications and conducted a mass meditation. An equally fascinating talk was given by Commander Rustom Palia of Air India, who spoke on how simulation exercises are regularly conducted for pilots and who narrated an extraordinary real-life experience of how the crew salvaged their aircraft carrying 350 passengers, when at the end of their 15-hour nonstop Delhi–JFK flight, they encountered the most unforeseen combination of bad weather, extremely poor visibility, the total malfunction of all three landing instruments, and the near total consumption of fuel. Presence of mind, quick thinking, and experience with manual landing in the face of failed electronics saved hundreds of lives.

The second ICCN was attended by nearly four hundred neurosurgeons and spine surgeons from more than 35 countries and received a warm reception. Like the first ICCN, this conference too ended with loads of lessons to carry home and with a pledge not only to continue with such conferences but also to create a platform for regular communication on complications in neurosurgery, on which one can chronicle the confounding or complicated cases that one has encountered and share with peers and other colleagues and thus learn on a regular basis.

This book, the second on the same theme—i.e. complications in neurosurgery—is a tribute to the concept and the incredible contributors who were brave enough to share their complications for colleagues to learn from and future patients to benefit from. Again, the emphasis of such an undertaking is on the anticipation/avoidance of complications and being prepared to anticipate and manage them. Equally illuminating are the presentations on allied issues such as ethics, morals, and the legal implications of complications, which are seldom discussed. We are confident that the selected chapters of the second ICCN, presented herein, are absorbing and true sources of education.

Mumbai, India — Keki Turel
Boston, MA, USA — Ekkehard M. Kasper

Acknowledgement

We would like to extend our gratitude to everyone who has assisted Professor Keki Turel and me in the preparation of this significant volume, which represents the selected proceedings from the Second International Conference on Complications in Neurosurgery held in Mumbai.

Most importantly, we would like to extend our gratitude to all authors for their outstanding contributions, and we admire their insight and specialized expertise. We were able to select only a small number of the thoughtful presentations, which were turned into articles representing the wide spectrum of subspecialty cases presented at ICCN 2; however, we appreciate all the input we have received from many of our conference attendees, as well as co-workers and colleagues.

The editorial staff at Springer and in particular my office staff, Mrs. Brenda Paine from Hamilton, Ontario, Canada, have done an exceptional and most diligent job in helping me to collect and edit these works. For that, I am most grateful. Due to the pandemic, we had some delays in collecting the works during my tenure as Academic Head of Neurosurgery at McMaster University in Hamilton, Ontario; however, we continued this work later from Boston University and have now successfully compiled a comprehensive volume.

Finally, I would like to express deepest gratitude to my wife Ines and my family for their never-ending support and tolerance during the many hours needed to bring this undertaking over the finish line.

Prof. Ekkehard M. Kasper MD PhD—Boston, on behalf of Prof. Keki Turel—Mumbai

Contents

Preventing Wrong-Level Spine Surgery

James Paul Agolia, Scott Robertson, Keki Turel, and Ekkehard M. Kasper

Abstract

Importance: Wrong-level spine surgery (WLSS), a medical error in which a surgeon operates at an unintended vertebral level, is considered a "never event." However, it continues to be a problem in spine surgery today despite the implementation of preventive measures such as the Universal Protocol. The consequences of this event are severe for both the afflicted patient and the treating physician and may result not only in physical harm but also in costly medicolegal proceedings.

Observations: While WLSS incidence varies with the patient population and practice setting, large studies generally report rates below 1%. Given the ubiquity of spine surgery, this remains a concerning number. Risk factors for WLSS can be categorized into three domains: patient factors, imaging issues, and technical issues. Awareness of risk factors allows surgeons to plan for difficulties in level localization. Many techniques for preventing WLSS have been developed, including invasive preoperative marking strategies. Intraoperative radiography or fluoroscopy is necessary but not sufficient for WLSS prevention, in that many errors occur after imaging. The evidence for prevention methods remains of low quality, necessitating future prospective comparison studies.

Conclusions and relevance: Consensus has been reached in professional societies: All spine surgeons should implement WLSS prevention protocols. We assess the reported techniques for safer surgery and emphasize one crucial time-out element: the time-out for level localization (TOLL). Addressing WLSS as a problem specific to spine surgery, we show that by using specially tailored prevention strategies, such measures will allow WLSS to become a true never event.

Keywords

Wrong-level spine surgery · Wrong-site spine surgery Localization · Level error · Wrong-site surgery

Abbreviations

CT	Computed tomography
IRACE	Intraoperative radiography and confirming exclamation
LSTV	Lumbosacral transitional vertebrae
MRI	Magnetic resonance imaging
TOLL	Time-out for level localization
UP	Universal protocol
WLE	Wrong-level exposure
WLSS	Wrong-level spine surgery
WSS	Wrong-site surgery
WSSS	Wrong-site spine surgery

Supplementary Information The online version contains supplementary material available at https://doi.org/10.1007/978-3-031-61601-3_1.

J. P. Agolia
Harvard Medical School, Boston, MA, USA

S. Robertson
Department of Neurosurgery, Laredo Medical Center, Laredo, TX, USA

K. Turel
Department of Neurosurgery, Bombay Hospital Institute of Medical Sciences, Mumbai, Maharashtra, India

E. M. Kasper (✉)
McMaster University, Faculty of Health Sciences, Hamilton, ON, Canada

Department of Neurosurgery, Boston University, Chobanian and Avedisian School of Medicine, Boston, MA, USA
e-mail: kaspere@mcmaster.ca

K. Turel, E. M. Kasper (eds.), *Complications in Neurosurgery II*, Acta Neurochirurgica Supplement 133,
https://doi.org/10.1007/978-3-031-61601-3_1

Introduction

Mistakes in healthcare do happen, but certain medical errors are considered preventable and should rarely, if ever, occur. The National Quality Forum has developed a list of 29 such "never events" or "serious reportable events," and the first of those listed is "surgery or other invasive procedure performed on the wrong site" [1]. This category includes wrong-level spine surgery (WLSS), a "never event" specific to spine surgery [2] that has been particularly refractory to prevention methods.

WLSS occurs when the surgeon operates at a vertebral level that was not the intended surgical target. It is a rare but serious scenario with negative consequences for the patient and physician [2–7]. WLSS fails to alleviate the patient's symptoms and causes additional surgical trauma to the patient at an unintended level, which may have detrimental effects on the biomechanical or neural elements of the vertebral column, particularly in cases of fusion surgery. If the mistake is not detected and corrected in the operating room, it often requires further surgery. In addition to physical harm, the patient may suffer emotional trauma and lose trust in the medical system. The surgeon may experience guilt and shame, ostracization among peers, and a stained reputation, leading to decreased referrals. Furthermore, WLSS may lead to medicolegal action (Appendix 3) [5, 7].

The aims of this study were to assess the reported incidence of WLSS, to define contributing factors, and to evaluate preventive methods. Because WLSS is a unique problem related to localizing a vertebral level of the spine, this review focuses specifically on WLSS, excluding other types of wrong-site surgery or wrong-patient surgery. WLSS is distinguished from wrong-level exposure (WLE), which denotes a surgical approach that is unintentionally executed to the wrong level of the spine and yet recognized before significant instrumentation and corrected intraoperatively [8]. Best thought of as a "near miss" of WLSS, WLE is comparatively common and likely does not affect patient outcomes [4, 5, 9–11]. (However, WLE with the introduction of a marking needle into the wrong disc may be associated with degenerative changes [12].) While broader reviews of wrong-site spine surgery (WSSS, which may include wrong-side or wrong-level spine surgery) [4, 5, 13] and wrong-site surgery (WSS, which can take place at any anatomical site in the body) [14] have been conducted, only two reviews have focused specifically on WLSS [2, 15], and neither has been comprehensive in scope.

The authors undertook this review as part of a growing international focus on complications in neurosurgery, for which the World Federation of Neurosurgical Societies (WFNS) decided to establish a committee on complications and national organizations host courses on complications. Short conference presentations on the topic were given at the first International Conference on Complications in Neurosurgery in Mumbai in 2017 and 2019 by the senior author, which will appear in published form as part of the conference proceedings [16].

Discussion/Observations

Incidence

The reported incidence of WLSS varies considerably (Supplementary Table 1). In large studies with a general patient population, the rate of WLSS is generally less than 1%, with more recent studies reporting lower rates. In national surveys of spine surgeons, the estimated rate of WLSS varies between 0.11% and 0.032% [7, 9, 17, 18]. While these estimates have the advantage of being obtained from a larger sample size, they can be skewed by response rates. Rather than estimating the incidence of WLSS as a fraction of total surgeries performed, researchers may estimate the proportion of spine surgeons who have performed it. For example, two surveys reported that about 50% of spine surgeons have performed at least one WLSS during their career [7, 19]. Another survey reported that 36% of spine surgeons had performed at least one WLSS that was not recognized intraoperatively [20]. According to raw incidence rates, WLSS may seem rare, but surveys show that the experience of WLSS is rather common among spine surgeons.

Estimating the incidence of WLSS is difficult for several reasons [2, 4, 5, 13, 15, 21]. First, the low incidence of WLSS requires a large denominator of fully assessed surgical cases. Second, there may be a bias toward underreporting in that surgeons may be ashamed to publish "failures" or may be advised not to publish them for fear of litigation. Third, the incidence of WLSS may vary with procedure type, patient characteristics, and practice setting. Fourth, studies may have been conducted to determine the incidence of WLE, WSSS, or WSS in general, instead of focusing on WLSS. Different definitions of the problem compromise study interpretation.

Contributing Factors

Though the quality of available evidence is low, many studies have described the risk factors contributing to WLSS (Supplementary Table 2), and many of these factors have been reviewed elsewhere [2, 4, 5, 15]. Predisposing factors can generally be grouped into three categories: [1] patient-specific risk factors, [2] issues with intraoperative imaging, and [3] problems related to surgical technique.

Patient Characteristics

While some risk factors are inherent to the patient or pathology, identifying them allows for tailored prevention. These risk factors include anomalous or variant anatomy and the characteristics of a patient's pathology.

Many authors have suggested that anatomical variants such as lumbosacral transitional vertebrae (LSTV) may be precipitating factors for WLSS [10, 22–25]. Kwaan et al. found that LSTV was present in 5/10 cases of WLSS [26]. In a national survey, spine surgeons indicated that anomalous anatomy could be a factor in 38% of WLSS events [17], while in a more recent but smaller survey, 15% of surgeons stated that anatomical variants contributed to WLSS events [20]. If LSTV or other anatomical variants are not recognized, vertebral numbering may vary when counting cranially versus caudally [20, 25].

Studies have consistently shown a higher incidence of WLSS in lumbar than in cervical procedures. Jhawar et al. found that WLSS occurred in 0.13% of lumbar cases but 0.076% of cervical cases [17]. Marquez-Lara et al. found that WLSS occurred at a rate of 0.026% in lumbar cases but only 0.010% in cervical cases [27, 28]. In a prospective study, the two variables independently associated with WLE were older age (age >55) and levels above L5-S1 [29]. Furthermore, the rate of WLE appears to increase as one ascends the lumbar spine; in one study, the rates of WLE at L5-S1, L4-L5, and L3-L4 were 0.04%, 4.0%, and 6.9%, respectively [30].

Intraoperative Imaging Issues

This category includes the lack of any intraoperative imaging, poor image quality, misinterpretations of the images, or failure to reconfirm the level with intraoperative imaging after exposure has occurred. Older studies have noted that intraoperative radiography or fluoroscopy was not performed in some cases of WLSS [7, 26], and authors have identified the lack of WLSS as a major contributor to WLSS occurrence [17, 31].

When intraoperative imaging has been performed, poor image quality may hinder proper level identification [10, 20, 22, 32, 33]. Errors in interpretation include inconsistent numbering, the use of different anatomical landmarks in different images, and confusion due to LSTV and other anatomical variants [9, 20, 31, 32]. In some cases of WLSS, radiography was performed at the start of the case to determine the location of the incision, but the level was not radiographically confirmed after exposure. This was identified in a national survey as the foremost reason for WLSS [20].

Technical Contributors

Even when intraoperative radiographs are taken, the retractors or another radiopaque marker can be moved without permanently marking the intended level, allowing WLSS to occur [9, 31, 32]. In microsurgical approaches, movement of the tubular retractor can contribute to WLSS [9], and when one group implemented a protocol to prevent the movement of the tubular retractor, they saw a decrease in WLSS incidence [34].

A posterior approach is associated with an increased incidence of WLSS [27, 28]. McCulloch asserts that the "laminar trap," in which surgeons are guided by an overhanging lamina toward the wrong disc space, is a major technical cause of WLSS [35]. Increasing surgeon experience appears to be associated with a decreased incidence of WLSS, suggesting that more-experienced surgeons may be more skilled at level localization [7, 30].

Prevention

While techniques to prevent WLSS are abundant, evidence to support these interventions is generally of low quality, and how disparate interventions can be integrated into a unified approach remains unclear. Prevention measures include site verification checklists, intraoperative imaging, preoperative marking procedures, and more-advanced interventions (Supplementary Table 3).

Preoperative Checklists and System Approaches

Integrating initiatives from the Canadian Orthopedic Association, the American Academy of Orthopedic Surgeons, and the North American Spine Society (please see Supplementary Table 3 for references and reviews of this topic), the Joint Commission for the Accreditation of Healthcare Organizations promulgated the Universal Protocol (UP) in 2004. The UP requires (1) preoperative verifications of the patient, site, and procedure; (2) preoperative site marking; and (3) a pre-incision time-out [36].

Despite these advances in patient safety, only very limited evidence indicates that the UP has reduced WLSS incidence [4, 13, 15]. Two systematic reviews found no evidence that the UP was effective in preventing WLSS [4, 15]. In a retrospective review of wrong surgery events in the Veterans Health Administration between 2004 and 2013, 10 WLSS events would have occurred despite flawless implementations of the UP [31]. One single-center retrospective study did find a significant decrease in WLSS events after the UP was instituted [37]. However, a reanalysis of the data showed that the decrease in WLSS began before UP implementation, making it less likely that the introduction of the UP was the sole contributor to the decline [13, 38]. While the effectiveness of the UP in preventing WLSS remains unclear at best [2], the UP in its current form is clearly insufficient as a sole prevention strategy [13, 39] given that WLSS continue to occur.

The UP aims to reduce WSS in general through preprocedure verification, site marking, and a time-out, but it does not do enough to address the unique anatomical challenges of the spine [21] that can lead to WLSS [4, 5, 13, 40]. While James et al. found no significant difference in WSS incidence after UP promulgation, they did find a nonsignificant decrease when spine cases were excluded, suggesting that WLSS is uniquely intractable to the UP [2, 9]. Unlike other types of WSS, many errors leading to WLSS are made after the incision—that is, after the required elements of the UP have been completed. Thus, WLSS might be a problem more with intraoperative level localization than with preoperative preparation [37]. The UP does suggest that "special intraoperative imaging techniques may be used for locating and marking the exact vertebral level"; however, intraoperative imaging is not specifically mandated [36].

As WLSS differs from other types of WSS, it requires unique solutions that should be bundled into one coherent process. For example, two hospitals audited their respective experiences of WLSS, conducted root-cause analyses, and developed their own WLSS prevention checklists, both of which included intraoperative radiography with a fixed level marker [41, 42]. One hospital was able to strengthen its WLSS prevention protocol by analyzing each WLSS event, instituting a protocol change, and tracking the outcomes after each change [43]. Another example is the intraoperative radiography and confirming exclamation (IRACE) method, in which a wire is preoperatively inserted into a spinous process, fluoroscopy is performed to plan the incision, and the circulating nurse confirms the procedure and side. Fluoroscopy is repeated intraoperatively. In 818 such cases, only one instance of WLE was corrected with intraoperative fluoroscopy [44].

Intraoperative Radiography or Fluoroscopy

Intraoperative imaging is the most critical part of any WLSS prevention protocol, and multiple convergent lines of evidence support its efficacy. Large surveys have shown that most spine surgeons perform intraoperative radiography or fluoroscopy. Mody et al. found that 80% of spine surgeons performed intraoperative radiography [7], and Jhawar et al. found that 64% of spine surgeons believed that intraoperative radiography should be the standard of care [17]. More recently, 100% of spine surgery fellows performed intraoperative radiography routinely and planned to do so in their future practices [45]. Mayer et al. found that 86–89% of surgeons perform intraoperative fluoroscopy to localize the level, while 54–58% use intraoperative radiography [20]. A focus group of spine-deformity surgeons put forth intraoperative radiography or fluoroscopy with a radiopaque marker in the disc space as a consensus recommendation [46]. Intraoperative imaging for level localization thus appears to be a widespread practice, as expected according to North American Spine Society recommendations [3].

While a randomized controlled trial of intraoperative radiography for WLSS prevention is not feasible [4], several lesser-quality studies have shown its benefit. The strongest of these is a prospective study that attempted to expose the intended level via the palpation of anatomical landmarks alone, with subsequent intraoperative fluoroscopy to correct any WLE. A 15% rate of WLE was observed; all instances were corrected after intraoperative fluoroscopy revealed the error [29]. One retrospective study noted that intraoperative radiography or fluoroscopy was instituted after the failure of the UP to prevent WLSS [31], and two retrospective studies noted a decrease in the rate of or the elimination of WLSS after intraoperative radiography or fluoroscopy was adopted [34, 47]. While these nonrandomized studies could be limited by unknown confounders or confirmation bias for a widely used technique, they support the routine use of intraoperative radiography or fluoroscopy for level localization.

However, WLSS has occurred even in cases in which intraoperative radiography or fluoroscopy was performed [7, 9, 15, 22, 26, 32, 37, 48]. For example, in a retrospective analysis of neurosurgical malpractice cases, 16 cases of lumbar WLSS had "localizing X-rays in the operating room" [49]. The definitions in the literature on what constitutes an intraoperative localizing image may be inconsistent; true confirmatory intraoperative imaging occurs after exposure—not before incision—with a marker at the level to be operated on [4]. Instead of a single instance of intraoperative imaging, perhaps a sequence of intraoperative radiographs should be performed, with one before incision, one after exposure but before discectomy or decompression, and one after instrumentation [50], as supported by the results of two retrospective studies of the "British protocol" [51, 52]. Having intraoperative radiography or fluoroscopy available at all points of the operation, to minimize uncertainly in level at any point intraoperatively, might be necessary [50]. However, the literature also points to problems in interpreting and communicating the results of intraoperative imaging.

Image Interpretation and the Communication of Imaging Results

Interpreting intraoperative radiographs may be difficult in cases of LSTV or other variant anatomy. Implementing a standardized method of counting vertebrae, with a consistent reference point that is defined preoperatively, would be the best way to prevent confusion [23, 25]. Recognizing this, a focus group of spine surgeons recommended using an established method of vertebral counting, which includes using C2 as the reference point [46]. In difficult cases, such as in patients with LSTV, surgeons should seek the assistance of a radiologist [32]. Though 98% of spine surgery fellows do not ask for assistance in interpreting intraoperative films [45], spine surgeons agree that a radiologist should be involved in image interpretation in cases where level localization is unclear [46]. Communication about the surgical level among all members of the surgical team is critical, and an intraoperative time-out may facilitate this [43].

Invasive Preoperative Marking

Under fluoroscopic or CT guidance, the percutaneous placement of a marker (e.g., needle, wire, fiducial, or coil) at the intended spinal level can be performed preoperatively, making localization with intraoperative fluoroscopy or radiography a simple task. While more-promising techniques have been described than can be cited here (Supplementary Table 3), evidence that they prevent WLSS is generally of low quality.

Inserting a needle or wire preoperatively under CT or fluoroscopic guidance into the bone or adjacent soft tissue has been a relatively successful and well-studied technique to mark the spinal level [53–57]. One version of this technique was used in a large case series, consisting of 1986 patients, which demonstrated only six WLE events and no WLSS events; notably, intraoperative fluoroscopy with one or two needles in facet joint capsules was performed to correct any exposure errors [8]. Other case series have suggested that preoperative needle or wire insertion is an accurate localization strategy [44, 58–60]. This technique may have the beneficial side effect of decreasing radiation exposure to operating room personnel [55, 57, 60]. However, the needle or wire can be inserted nonperpendicularly, which could lead the surgeon into the incorrect level [58, 60]. Thus, this technique is best used in conjunction with intraoperative imaging after exposure [54, 58].

The percutaneous image-guided placement of coils at the surgical level is another successful technique. While coils can be inserted endovascularly in cases of dural arteriovenous fistulae [61, 62], coils can also be placed into the pedicle of the surgical level [63–67]. In an excellent retrospective controlled study, Marquardt and colleagues showed that the insertion of a coil into a dural arteriovenous fistula decreased the incidence of WLE, decreased operative time, and decreased radiation exposure in the coil marking group compared to the control group [61].

Like coil insertion, the percutaneous placement of fiducials has also been described as a successful technique for level localization, particularly in difficult cases [68–71]. Upadhyaya and colleagues conducted a retrospective study showing that fiducial placement into the pedicle at the appropriate level could reduce intraoperative fluoroscopy time, though no WLSS occurred in either the experimental group or the historical control group [72].

As noted by many authors, invasive preoperative marking may be most useful for patients in whom intraoperative localization is anticipated to be difficult, including in patients who have aberrant anatomy [55, 64, 66–70, 72]. Many of these methods were developed for use in the thoracic spine, where localization may be particularly challenging [56, 57, 59, 60, 63, 64, 68–72].

Other Methods

Automated image processing may help reduce human error in image interpretation. The LevelCheck algorithm was designed to label an intraoperative radiograph with spinal levels, using a preoperative CT or MRI scan as input [73, 74]. Lab studies have shown that LevelCheck performed as well as manual level numbering, and initial clinical studies have been promising, with accurate localization in all subjects and no WLSS [75, 76]. In a retrospective study of 20 patients, LevelCheck identified spinal levels with 100% accuracy [77]. This algorithm could be a valuable decision support tool for preventing WLSS.

Intraoperative spinal navigation, intraoperative CT, intraoperative MRI, and intraoperative ultrasound could be effective means of preventing WLSS, though they may not be available in low-resource settings. These methods and associated references are discussed further in Supplementary Table 3.

Education

The education of spine surgeons on WLSS is lacking. A survey of spine surgery fellows found that only 33% of trainees had formal didactics on WSS prevention, though 61% were interested in having them. The 30% of respondents who had experienced WSS were significantly more likely to be interested in formal education on preventing it [45]. Particularly because of this substantial interest in WLSS prevention among trainees, specific didactics should be included in spine surgeon training [13, 45].

Conclusion

When proper precautions are taken, nearly all WLSS is preventable. For the sake of patient safety, the medical community should not rest until WLSS has been eliminated. In addition to following the UP, each institution should have a process to prevent WLSS that should be followed in every spine case.

Recommendations

1. There must be a consistent and specific definition for the problem to be eliminated. We echo DeVine and colleagues' [13] recommendation that WLSS be considered a unique type of WSS, as its causes and prevention strategies differ from those of other types of WSS. We believe

that the term *WLSS* should be used because it points to the unique anatomical issue in spine surgery [2]. In reporting WSS data, the Joint Commission and other monitoring organizations should report separate data for WLSS. This will help to evaluate prevention strategies by comparing WLSS incidence before and after implementation. Rates of WLE and other near misses could aid research and should be reported separately.

2. Intraoperative radiography or fluoroscopy following exposure, with a radiopaque marker at the level of interest, should be mandatory in all cases of spine surgery, and image quality should be optimized by using the strategies mentioned above. Every hospital policy should require this step, and it should be documented in the medical record. However, intraoperative imaging is insufficient as the sole prevention strategy.
3. To prevent the misinterpretation of intraoperative imaging, a second time-out, the time-out for level localization (TOLL), should be jointly performed by the entire operating room team after intraoperative imaging. This time-out would be similar to that in WLSS prevention protocols described previously [16, 41–43, 78]. TOLL should include confirmation that the images are of the correct patient and date, the imaging quality is sufficient, and the intended surgical level is reliably and clearly marked with a radiopaque marker. Automated level identification could be performed to verify manual counting. Preoperative images should be available on-screen for direct comparison to intraoperative imaging. TOLL should be documented in the medical record. In particular, the reference point for counting should be documented and must be consistent between preoperative and intraoperative images. Postinstrumentation intraoperative imaging should be performed, followed by a third time-out to confirm that surgery was performed at the correct level.
4. When the anatomy is abnormal or difficult to visualize, a radiologist should be called for an intraoperative consultation, and imaging repeated if necessary. A two-part confirmation—counting from cranial to caudal and then from caudal to cranial—can be employed to reduce miscounting. Most importantly, the visible reference points used to determine the level in preoperative imaging and intraoperative imaging must be consistent [23, 39].
5. Invasive marking or more-advanced intraoperative navigation should not be a routine WLSS prevention approach, as these methods are likely less cost-effective and may not be available in some settings [66]. However, they should be used in patients with multiple risk factors for WLSS [39, 66, 67, 72].

Declarations of Interest This research did not receive any specific grant from funding agencies in the public, commercial, or not-for-profit sectors.

References

1. National Quality Forum (NQF). Serious reportable events in healthcare—2011 update: a consensus report. NQF. 2011. https://www.qualityforum.org/Publications/2011/12/Serious_Reportable_Events_in_Healthcare_2011.aspx. Accessed 29 February 2020.
2. Grimm BD, Laxer EB, Blessinger BJ, Rhyne AL, Darden BV. Wrong-level spine surgery. JBJS Rev. 2014;2(3):e2. https://doi.org/10.2106/JBJS.RVW.M.00052.
3. North American Spine Society. Sign, mark & X-ray: prevention of wrong-site spinal surgery; 2014. https://www.spine.org/Portals/0/Assets/Downloads/ResearchClinicalCare/SMAX2014Revision.pdf. Accessed 5 January 2021.
4. Devine J, Chutkan N, Norvell DC, Dettori JR. Avoiding wrong site surgery: a systematic review. Spine. 2010;35(9):28–36. https://doi.org/10.1097/BRS.0b013e3181d833ac.
5. Palumbo MA, Bianco AJ, Esmende S, Daniels AH. Wrong-site spine surgery. J Am Acad Orthop Surg. 2013;21(5):312–20. https://doi.org/10.5435/JAAOS-21-05-312.
6. Author. Patient safety first alert–implementing a correct site surgery policy and procedure. AORN J. 2002;76(5):785–8. https://doi.org/10.1016/s0001-2092(06)61031-4.
7. Mody MG, Nourbakhsh A, Stahl DL, Gibbs M, Alfawareh M, Garges KJ. The prevalence of wrong level surgery among spine surgeons. Spine. 2008;33(2):194–8. https://doi.org/10.1097/BRS.0b013e31816043d1.
8. Patel A, Runner RP, Bellamy JT, Rhee JM. A reproducible and reliable localization technique for lumbar spine surgery that minimizes unintended-level exposure and wrong-level surgery. Spine J. 2019;19(5):773–80. https://doi.org/10.1016/j.spinee.2018.12.005.
9. James MA, Seiler JG, Harrast JJ, Emery SE, Hurwitz S. The occurrence of wrong-site surgery self-reported by candidates for certification by the American Board of Orthopaedic Surgery. J Bone Joint Surg Am. 2012;94(1):e2. https://doi.org/10.2106/JBJS.K.00524.
10. Hadjipavlou AG, Marshall RW. Wrong site surgery. Bone Jt J. 2013;95(4):434–5. https://doi.org/10.1302/0301-620X.95B4.31235.
11. Hudgins WR. Exposure of two interspaces for lumbar disc surgery. J Neurosurg. 1975;42(1):59–60. https://doi.org/10.3171/jns.1975.42.1.0059.
12. Nassr A, Lee JY, Bashir RS, et al. Does incorrect level needle localization during anterior cervical discectomy and fusion lead to accelerated disc degeneration? Spine. 2009;34(2):189–92. https://doi.org/10.1097/BRS.0b013e3181913872.
13. DeVine JG, Chutkan N, Gloystein D, Jackson K. An update on wrong-site spine surgery. Glob Spine J. 2020;10(1):41S–4S. https://doi.org/10.1177/2192568219846911.
14. Hempel S, Maggard-Gibbons M, Nguyen DK, et al. Wrong-site surgery, retained surgical items, and surgical fires: a systematic review of surgical never events. JAMA Surg. 2015;150(8):796–805. https://doi.org/10.1001/jamasurg.2015.0301.
15. Longo UG, Loppini M, Romeo G, Maffulli N, Denaro V. Errors of level in spinal surgery: an evidence-based systematic review. J Bone Joint Surg Br. 2012;94(11):1546–50. https://doi.org/10.1302/0301-620X.94B11.29553.
16. Agolia JP, Kasper EM. Wrong level spine surgery. In: Turel K, Chernov MF, Sarkar H, editors. Complications in neurosurgery. Cham: Springer; 2021. https://www.springer.com/gp/book/9783030128869. Accessed 16 November 2020.
17. Jhawar BS, Mitsis D, Duggal N. Wrong-sided and wrong-level neurosurgery: a national survey. J Neurosurg Spine. 2007;7(5):467–72. https://doi.org/10.3171/SPI-07/11/467.
18. Matsumoto M, Hasegawa T, Ito M, et al. Incidence of complications associated with spinal endoscopic surgery: nationwide survey in 2007 by the Committee on Spinal Endoscopic Surgical Skill

Qualification of Japanese Orthopaedic Association. J Orthop Sci. 2010;15(1):92–6. https://doi.org/10.1007/s00776-009-1428-6.
19. Groff MW, Heller JE, Potts EA, Mummaneni PV, Shaffrey CI, Smith JS. A survey-based study of wrong-level lumbar spine surgery: the scope of the problem and current practices in place to help avoid these errors. World Neurosurg. 2013;79(3-4):585–92. https://doi.org/10.1016/j.wneu.2012.03.017.
20. Mayer JE, Dang RP, Duarte Prieto GF, Cho SK, Qureshi SA, Hecht AC. Analysis of the techniques for thoracic- and lumbar-level localization during posterior spine surgery and the occurrence of wrong-level surgery: results from a national survey. Spine J. 2014;14(5):741–8. https://doi.org/10.1016/j.spinee.2013.06.068.
21. Francis T, Benzel E. Wrong level spine surgery: a perspective. World Neurosurg. 2013;79(3):451–2. https://doi.org/10.1016/j.wneu.2012.07.020.
22. Hsiang J. Wrong-level surgery: a unique problem in spine surgery. Surg Neurol Int. 2011;2:79769. https://doi.org/10.4103/2152-7806.79769.
23. Lindley EM, Botolin S, Burger EL, Patel VV. Unusual spine anatomy contributing to wrong level spine surgery: a case report and recommendations for decreasing the risk of preventable "never events". Patient Saf Surg. 2011;5:33. https://doi.org/10.1186/1754-9493-5-33.
24. Malanga GA, Cooke PM. Segmental anomaly leading to wrong level disc surgery in cauda equina syndrome. Pain Physician. 2004;7(1):107–10.
25. Dubois JLC, Nissen J. Potential wrong-level surgery for an intradural thoracic spinal tumour: the importance of optimum imaging and consistency in the direction in which the level is determined. Br J Neurosurg. 2016;30(2):202–3. https://doi.org/10.3109/02688697.2016.1153040.
26. Kwaan MR, Studdert DM, Zinner MJ, Gawande AA. Incidence, patterns, and prevention of wrong-site surgery. Arch Surg. 2006;141(4):353–8. https://doi.org/10.1001/archsurg.141.4.353.
27. Marquez-Lara A, Nandyala SV, Hassanzadeh H, Noureldin M, Sankaranarayanan S, Singh K. Sentinel events in cervical spine surgery. Spine. 2014;39(9):715–20. https://doi.org/10.1097/BRS.0000000000000228.
28. Marquez-Lara A, Nandyala SV, Hassanzadeh H, Sundberg E, Jorgensen A, Singh K. Sentinel events in lumbar spine surgery. Spine. 2014;39(11):900–5. https://doi.org/10.1097/BRS.0000000000000247.
29. Ammerman JM, Ammerman MD, Dambrosia J, Ammerman BJ. A prospective evaluation of the role for intraoperative X-ray in lumbar discectomy. Predictors of incorrect level exposure. Surg Neurol. 2006;66(5):470–3. https://doi.org/10.1016/j.surneu.2006.05.069.
30. Wiese M, Krämer J, Bernsmann K, Ernst WR. The related outcome and complication rate in primary lumbar microscopic disc surgery depending on the surgeon's experience: comparative studies. Spine J. 2004;4(5):550–6. https://doi.org/10.1016/j.spinee.2004.02.007.
31. Paull DE, Mazzia LM, Neily J, et al. Errors upstream and downstream to the universal protocol associated with wrong surgery events in the Veterans Health Administration. Am J Surg. 2015;210(1):6–13. https://doi.org/10.1016/j.amjsurg.2014.10.030.
32. Watts BV, Rachlin JR, Gunnar W, et al. Wrong site spine surgery in the veterans administration. Clin Spine Surg. 2019;32(10):454–7. https://doi.org/10.1097/BSD.0000000000000771.
33. Mannoji C, Koda M, Furuya T, et al. Radiograms obtained during anterior cervical decompression and fusion can mislead surgeons into performing surgery at the wrong level. Case Rep Orthop. 2014;2014:398457. https://doi.org/10.1155/2014/398457.
34. Ebata S, Sato H, Orii H, Sasaki S, Ohba T, Haro H. Risk management in posterior spinal endoscopic surgery in lumbar diseases. J Orthop Sci. 2013;18(3):369–73. https://doi.org/10.1007/s00776-013-0360-y.
35. McCulloch JA. Complications (adverse effects). In: Principles of microsurgery for lumbar disc disease. New York: Raven Press; 1989. p. 225–38.
36. The Joint Commission. National patient safety goals effective July 2020 for the hospital program. 2020. https://www.jointcommission.org/-/media/tjc/documents/standards/national-patient-safety-goals/2020/npsg_chapter_hap_jul2020.pdf. Accessed 13 September 2020.
37. Vachhani JA, Klopfenstein JD. Incidence of neurosurgical wrong-site surgery before and after implementation of the universal protocol. Neurosurgery. 2013;72(4):590–5. https://doi.org/10.1227/NEU.0b013e318283c9ea.
38. Algie CM, Mahar RK, Wasiak J, Batty L, Gruen RL, Mahar PD. Interventions for reducing wrong-site surgery and invasive clinical procedures. Cochrane Database Syst Rev. 2015;3:CD009404. https://doi.org/10.1002/14651858.CD009404.pub3.
39. Hsu W, Kretzer RM, Dorsi MJ, Gokaslan ZL. Strategies to avoid wrong-site surgery during spinal procedures. Neurosurg Focus. 2011;31(4):E5. https://doi.org/10.3171/2011.7.FOCUS1166.
40. Stahel PF, Mehler PS, Clarke TJ, Varnell J. The 5th anniversary of the "universal protocol": pitfalls and pearls revisited. Patient Saf Surg. 2009;3(1):14. https://doi.org/10.1186/1754-9493-3-14.
41. Sebet G, Broms M. Preventative measures to minimize the risk of wrong level spine surgery. First do no harm. Quality and patient safety division, Massachusetts Board of Registration in Medicine. 2012. https://www.mass.gov/doc/91217-0/download. Accessed 27 January 2021.
42. Folcarelli PH, Gugliemi C. Spinal surgery protocol—an aid in the identification of the correct spine level. First do no harm. Quality and patient safety division, Massachusetts Board of Registration in Medicine. 2012. https://www.mass.gov/doc/91217-0/download. Accessed 27 January 2021.
43. Srivatsa S, Vira S, Schils J, Shook S, Gill A, Krishnaney AA. Reducing wrong level spinal surgeries through root cause analyses: a 10-year longitudinal analysis of a single tertiary institution's iterative policy improvements. Spine. 2020;46(11):E648–54. https://doi.org/10.1097/BRS.0000000000003864.
44. Irace C, Corona C. How to avoid wrong-level and wrong-side errors in lumbar microdiscectomy. J Neurosurg Spine. 2010;12(6):660–5. https://doi.org/10.3171/2009.12.SPINE09627.
45. Mesfin A, Canham C, Okafor L. Prevention training of wrong-site spine surgery. J Surg Educ. 2015;72(4):680–4. https://doi.org/10.1016/j.jsurg.2015.01.010.
46. Vitale M, Minkara A, Matsumoto H, et al. Building consensus: development of best practice guidelines on wrong level surgery in spinal deformity. Spine Deform. 2018;6(2):121–9. https://doi.org/10.1016/j.jspd.2017.08.005.
47. Williams RW. Microdiskectomy–myth, mania, or milestone? An 18-year surgical adventure. Mt Sinai J Med. 1991;58(2):139–45.
48. Goodkin R, Laska LL. Wrong disc space level surgery: medicolegal implications. Surg Neurol. 2004;61(4):323–41. https://doi.org/10.1016/j.surneu.2003.08.022.
49. Fager CA. Malpractice issues in neurological surgery. Surg Neurol. 2006;65(4):416–21. https://doi.org/10.1016/j.surneu.2005.09.026.
50. Pao J-L, Chen W-C, Chen P-Q. Clinical outcomes of microendoscopic decompressive laminotomy for degenerative lumbar spinal stenosis. Eur Spine J. 2009;18(5):672–8. https://doi.org/10.1007/s00586-009-0903-2.
51. Asopa V, Ellis G, Shetty R. Three ways to avoid incorrect-level lumbar spine surgery. Ann R Coll Surg. 2012;94(5):359. https://doi.org/10.1308/003588412x13373405385214a.
52. Dablouk MO, Sajjad J, Lim C, Kaar G, O'Sullivan MGJ. Intraoperative imaging for spinal level localisation in lumbar surgery. Br J Neurosurg. 2019;33(3):352–6. https://doi.org/10.1080/02688697.2018.1562030.

53. Krämer J, Wittenberg RH. Microdiscectomy for lumbar disc herniation. Orthop Traumatol. 1993;2(1):10–8. https://doi.org/10.1007/BF02620531.
54. Chin KR, Seale J, Cumming V. Avoidance of wrong-level thoracic spine surgery using sterile spinal needles: a technical report. Clin Spine Surg. 2017;30(1):E54–8. https://doi.org/10.1097/BSD.0b013e3182a35762.
55. Slotty P, Kröpil P, Klingenhöfer M, Steiger H-J, Hänggi D, Stummer W. Preoperative localization of spinal and peripheral pathologies for surgery by computed tomography-guided placement of a specialized needle system. Neurosurgery. 2010;66(4):784–7. https://doi.org/10.1227/01.NEU.0000367450.79418.5B.
56. Thambiraj S, Quraishi NA. Intra-operative localisation of thoracic spine level: a simple "'K'-wire in pedicle" technique. Eur Spine J. 2012;21(2):221–4. https://doi.org/10.1007/s00586-012-2193-3.
57. Sammon PM, Gibson R, Fouyas I, Hughes MA. Intra-operative localisation of spinal level using pre-operative CT-guided placement of a flexible hook-wire marker. Br J Neurosurg. 2011;25(6):778–9. https://doi.org/10.3109/02688697.2011.584987.
58. Mohanlal P, Pal D, Timothy J. Localisation of spinal level in lumbar microdiscectomy. Eur J Orthop Surg Traumatol. 2006;16(3):207–9. https://doi.org/10.1007/s00590-005-0059-7.
59. Cornips E, Beuls E, Geskes G, Janssens M, van Aalst J, Hofman P. Preoperative localization of herniated thoracic discs using myelo-CT guided transpleural puncture: technical note. Childs Nerv Syst. 2007;23(1):21–6. https://doi.org/10.1007/s00381-006-0223-3.
60. Ahmadi SA, Slotty PJ, Schröter C, Kröpil P, Steiger H-J, Eicker SO. Marking wire placement for improved accuracy in thoracic spinal surgery. Clin Neurol Neurosurg. 2014;119:100–5. https://doi.org/10.1016/j.clineuro.2014.01.025.
61. Marquardt G, Berkefeld J, Seifert V, Gerlach R. Preoperative coil marking to facilitate intraoperative localization of spinal dural arteriovenous fistulas. Eur Spine J. 2009;18(8):1117–20. https://doi.org/10.1007/s00586-009-0946-4.
62. Britz GW, Lazar D, Eskridge J, Winn HR. Accurate intraoperative localization of spinal dural arteriovenous fistulae with embolization coil: technical note. Neurosurgery. 2004;55(1):252–4. https://doi.org/10.1227/01.neu.0000127883.26964.81.
63. Binning MJ, Schmidt MH. Percutaneous placement of radiopaque markers at the pedicle of interest for preoperative localization of thoracic spine level. Spine. 2010;35(19):1821–5. https://doi.org/10.1097/BRS.0b013e3181c90bdf.
64. Castle-Kirszbaum M, Maingard J, Goldschlager T, Chandra RV. Preoperative coil localization for spinal surgery: technical note. J Neurosurg Spine. 2019;32(3):483–7. https://doi.org/10.3171/2019.8.SPINE19762.
65. Maduri R, Starnoni D, Barges-Coll J, David Hajdu S, Michael DJ. Bone cylinder plug and coil technique for accurate pedicle localization in thoracic spine surgery: a technical note. Surg Neurol Int. 2019;10:104. https://doi.org/10.25259/SNI-258-2019.
66. Young RM, Prasad V, Wind JJ, Olan W, Caputy AJ. Novel technique for preoperative pedicle localization in spinal surgery with challenging anatomy. J Neurosurg Spine. 2014;20(4):400–3. https://doi.org/10.3171/2013.12.SPINE13477.
67. Reitman CA. Pearls: wrong-level surgery prevention. Clin Orthop. 2016;474(3):636–9. https://doi.org/10.1007/s11999-015-4627-9.
68. Madaelil TP, Long JR, Wallace AN, et al. Preoperative fiducial marker placement in the thoracic spine: a technical report. Spine. 2017;42(10):E624–8. https://doi.org/10.1097/BRS.0000000000001890.
69. Marichal DA, Barnett DW, Meler JD, Layton KF. Fiducial marker placement for intraoperative spine localization. J Vasc Interv Radiol. 2011;22(1):95–7. https://doi.org/10.1016/j.jvir.2010.09.017.
70. Anaizi AN, Kalhorn C, McCullough M, Voyadzis J-M, Sandhu FA. Thoracic spine localization using preoperative placement of fiducial markers and subsequent CT. A technical report. J Neurol Surg Part Cent Eur Neurosurg. 2015;76(1):66–71. https://doi.org/10.1055/s-0034-1371512.
71. Macki M, Bydon M, McGovern K, et al. Gold fiducials are a unique marker for localization in the thoracic spine: a cost comparison with percutaneous vertebroplasty. Neurol Res. 2014;36(10):925–7. https://doi.org/10.1179/1743132814Y.0000000413.
72. Upadhyaya CD, Wu J-C, Chin CT, Balamurali G, Mummaneni PV. Avoidance of wrong-level thoracic spine surgery: intraoperative localization with preoperative percutaneous fiducial screw placement. J Neurosurg Spine. 2012;16(3):280–4. https://doi.org/10.3171/2011.3.SPINE10445.
73. De Silva T, Uneri A, Ketcha MD, et al. 3D–2D image registration for target localization in spine surgery: investigation of similarity metrics providing robustness to content mismatch. Phys Med Biol. 2016;61(8):3009–25. https://doi.org/10.1088/0031-9155/61/8/3009.
74. Otake Y, Schafer S, Stayman JW, et al. Automatic localization of vertebral levels in X-ray fluoroscopy using 3D-2D registration: a tool to reduce wrong-site surgery. Phys Med Biol. 2012;57(17):5485–508. https://doi.org/10.1088/0031-9155/57/17/5485.
75. Manbachi A, De Silva T, Uneri A, et al. Clinical translation of the levelcheck decision support algorithm for target localization in spine surgery. Ann Biomed Eng. 2018;46(10):1548–57. https://doi.org/10.1007/s10439-018-2099-2.
76. De Silva T, Uneri A, Ketcha MD, et al. Registration of MRI to intraoperative radiographs for target localization in spinal interventions. Phys Med Biol. 2017;62(2):684–701. https://doi.org/10.1088/1361-6560/62/2/684.
77. Lo S-FL, Otake Y, Puvanesarajah V, et al. Automatic localization of target vertebrae in spine surgery: clinical evaluation of the LevelCheck registration algorithm. Spine. 2015;40(8):476–83. https://doi.org/10.1097/BRS.0000000000000814.
78. Ladak A, Spinner RJ. Redefining "wrong site surgery" and refining the surgical pause and checklist: taking surgical safety to another level. World Neurosurg. 2014;81(5):e33–5. https://doi.org/10.1016/j.wneu.2013.02.055.

Carotid Complications in Skull Base Surgery

Miguel A. Arraez, Cinta Arraez, Angela Ros, Antonio Selfa, and Bienvenido Ros

Abstract

Carotid artery rupture is a worrisome complication that sometimes occurs during microsurgical or endoscopic skull base procedures. Many identifiable aspects are related to prevention, intraoperative management, and immediate postoperative endovascular treatment. This article deals with microsurgical and endoscopic cases in which the carotid artery or its branches have been damaged in the context of a resection of skull base lesions. Factors related to the anatomy of the skull base and the arteries and their variations are considered, along with intraoperative measures to control the bleeding. Finally, depending on the case, recommendations for immediate postoperative endovascular management are made.

Keywords

Skull base surgery · Carotid rupture

Introduction

Surgery on the skull base carries a comparatively high risk of potential complications. About one in every three publications about skull base surgery is related to complications and one in 15 skull base publications is related to major vascular injury. Among them, carotid injury is one of the most worrisome complications that may lead to disastrous consequences from either open microsurgical operations or endoscopic approaches [1–5]. In this article, four cases of intraoperative carotid artery rupture are presented, along with special considerations related to prevention and intraoperative management, which differ depending on the individual scenario.

Case 1

A 45-year-old male patient complained of a progressive loss of vision in their right eye that was due to a meningioma's invading the optic canal. A previous left side clinoidal meningioma had been treated with surgery & radiosurgery due to recurrence 5 years ago. A right pterional approach was performed to achieve optic nerve decompression (Fig. 1). Anterior clinoidectomy was carried out with an ultrasonic drill, and the perioptic infiltrated dura was cut and progressively removed with microscissors. When the lateral aspect of the dural sleeve was cut, brisk bleeding from the lateral aspect of carotid artery emanated because an aberrant ophthalmic artery coming from the duramater had been damaged. The tear was, fortunately, small enough to be coagulated with bipolar after it had been substantially reduced and almost stopped with cottonoids and suction.

M. A. Arraez (✉) · C. Arraez · A. Ros · A. Selfa · B. Ros
Malaga Regional University Hospital, University of Malaga, Malaga, Spain
e-mail: marraezs@uma.es

K. Turel, E. M. Kasper (eds.), *Complications in Neurosurgery II*, Acta Neurochirurgica Supplement 133,
https://doi.org/10.1007/978-3-031-61601-3_2

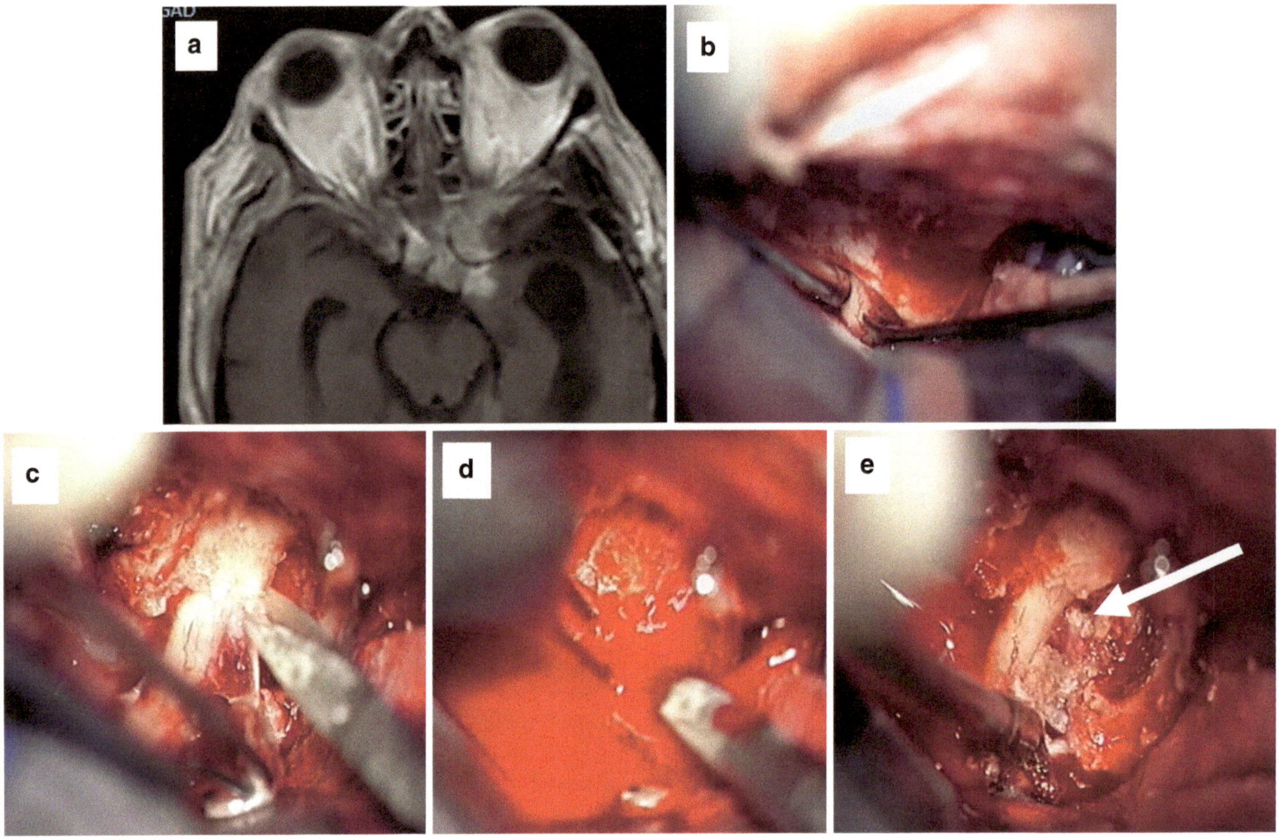

Fig. 1 Right optic nerve invasion via meningioma (**a**). Right pterional approach with clinoidectomy and optic sheath exposure (**b**). A resection of infiltrated dura: cutting with scissors immediately before the damage of the ophthalmic artery, with anomalous origin arising from infiltrated dura (**c**). Bleeding (**d**) and the bipolar coagulation of the bleeding point (white arrow, **e**)

Case 2

A 24-year-old female patient underwent two skull base procedures in 2004 at the age of 14 for the resection of a clival chordoma (via an extended transmaxillary approach and a right far-lateral approach). These surgeries were followed by Sterotactic Radiosurgery. In 2014—i.e., 10 years later—a recurrent chordoma located at the left petroclival and retro-parapharyngeal space was diagnosed (Fig. 2). The tumor encased the carotid artery in three segments, including the petrous region. A transnasal transmaxillary-transpterygoid-transclival endoscopic approach was undertaken. During the drilling of the involved petrous bone, the carotid artery was damaged. Initial hemorrhage control attempts via tamponade were not effective, as the artery had not been exposed enough at that point of the operation, and a Foley catheter balloon was inflated inside the resection cavity in an attempt to stop the bleeding. The patient was then expeditiously transferred to the angiography room. Conventional digital subtraction angiography showed leakage at the injured point and some small distortion in the artery, which were effectively controlled by the balloon. The arteriogram showed good collateral circulation through the posterior communicating (PCom) artery, which allowed the internal carotid artery to be sacrificed. The patient was successfully treated by the interventional neuroradiologists (INR) team and awoke without neurological deficit.

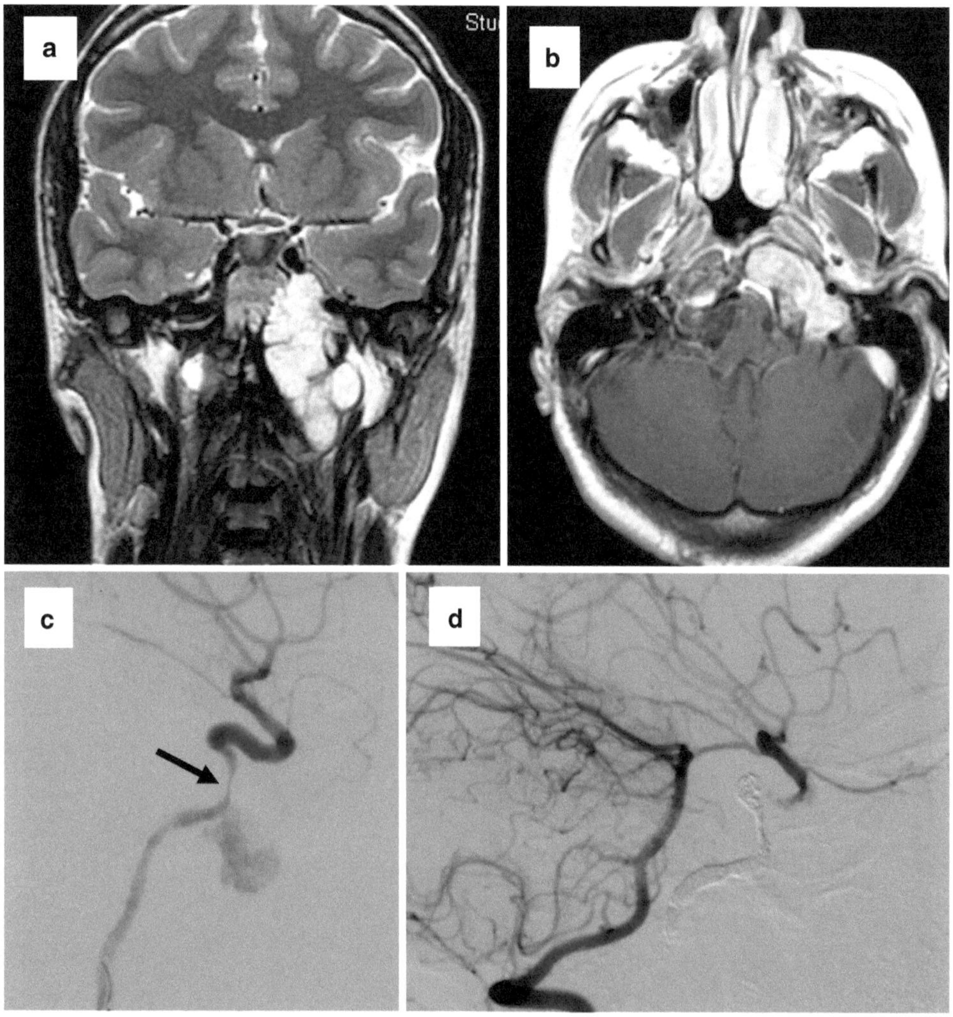

Fig. 2 Recurrent chordoma at the left parapharyngeal space and petrous apex (**a**, **b**). Angiography after the laceration of the internal carotid artery at the petrous segment and intraoperative tamponade with Foley ballon, showing blood leakage and a slight distortion (arrow) in the carotid wall (**c**). Carotid sacrifice without neurological deficit as flow from left PCom did fill the anterior circulation (**d**)

Case 3

A 19-year-old female patient was diagnosed with a pituitary lesion that grew under magnetic resonance imaging (MRI) surveillance. One of the remarkable findings on preoperative MRI was a flat sella, as illustrated on the sagittal and coronal views (Fig. 3). An endoscopic endonasal approach was taken. After drilling the sellar floor, the dura was opened with the aid of a sharp hook, and brisk bleeding gushed from the left carotid artery. Floseal and compression were applied, and afterwards, the bleeding stopped. A Foley balloon was inflated inside the sphenoid sinus, and surgery was aborted. The patient underwent emergent angiographic exploration, which revealed a small intraluminal hematoma. Subsequent MRI showed the narrowing of the carotid artery and small ischemic lesions scattered in the white matter. The patient recuperated well and was discharged neurologically intact. A follow-up MRA done 1 year later showed patency in the intracranial vessels and no change in the caliber of the left.

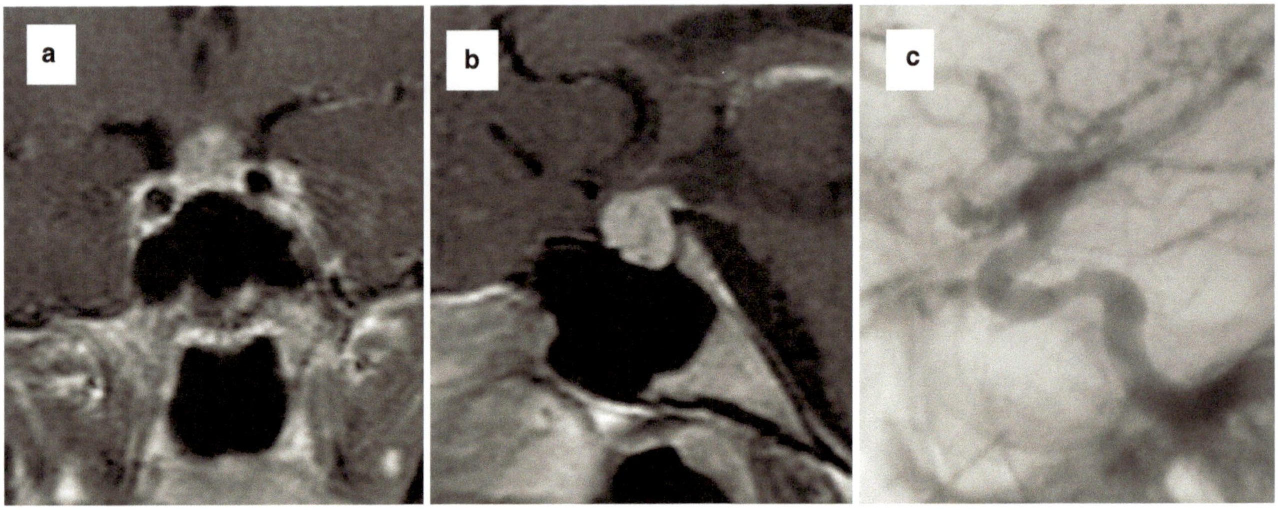

Fig. 3 In case 3, a 19-year-old patient with pituitary lesion and flat sella. MRI with coronal view (**a**) and sagittal view (**b**). After left intraoperative carotid tear, angiography showing a reduction in the lumen due to wall hematoma (**c**). No postoperative neurological deficit

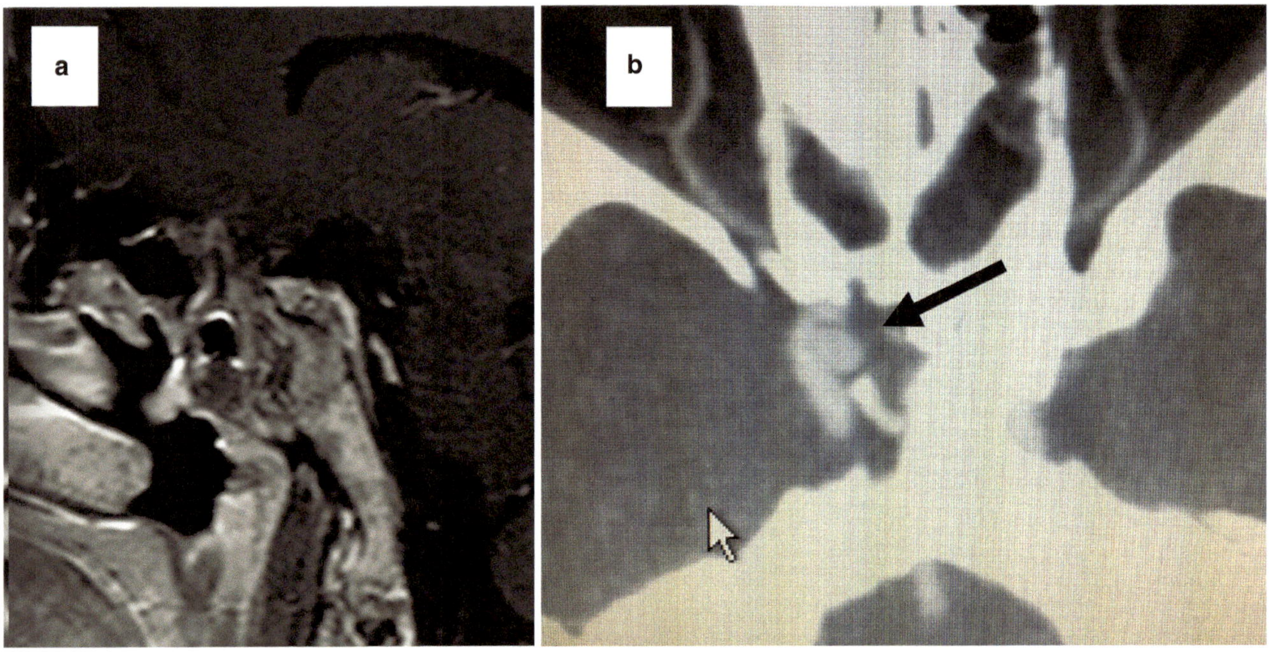

Fig. 4 In case 4, sagittal section through the right cavernous sinus in a recurrent GH invasive macroadenoma showing intense scarring and tumor (**a**). Angio-CT (**b**). after intraoperative carotid bleeding showing pseudoaneurysm formation (arrow) at the cavernous segment of the carotid artery

Case 4

A 42-year-old female with acromegaly was operated on because of a recurrent pituitary tumor adjacent to the right cavernous sinus. The procedure was carried out without neuronavigation as originally planned, because of technical problems. Very firm scar tissue from the previous pituitary surgery, which had been performed 6 years prior, was encountered. The resection was carried out with ring curettes and included blindly scraping the paracavernous aspect of the tumor. At this point, arterial bleeding was encountered, which could be controlled with Floseal and Surgicel. A postoperative angio-CT was urgently performed, revealing a traumatic carotid intracavernous aneurysm, which could be uneventfully coiled during the same hospital admittance. There were no neurological sequelae from this incident (Fig. 4).

Discussion

Major vascular injury is one of the most problematic situations during skull base surgeries, irrespective of the modality of approach (microsurgical or endoscopic). This complication may lead to the death of the patient or severe disability. This worrisome scenario presents important considerations for prevention, intraoperative management, and immediate postoperative management [5].

The first important aspect that needs to be considered in this setting is related to the topographic anatomy of the carotid artery and its branches. Case 1 illustrates a traumatically ruptured ophthalmic artery at some unexpected site at the lateral aspect of the right carotid artery, which was encased in a tumor. Many publications are available on the anatomical variations of the intracranial ICA and the respective developmental aspects, which are related to three embryological arterial branch systems (phylogenetically called the branchial arteries): the carotid system, the stapedial system, and the ventral pharyngeal system [6–8]. These may appear as only two branches [9]. The concomitant embryologic development of the ophthalmic artery and middle meningeal artery explains important variant anastomosis seen between these two arteries and also explains the presence of various dural branches arising from the ophthalmic artery [7], which likely represents the condition found in case 1. The ophthalmic artery can separate from the carotid at different positions along the optic canal interior: 40% leave the carotid from the upper internal part, 30% arise from the internal part, 20% arise from the upper central part, and 10% emerge at the end of the cavernous segment of the middle of the carotid artery at a steep angle (according to Ganiusmen; 7). In our case, no full postoperative angiographic examination was carried out, might may have helped to clarify the exact nature of the anatomical variation, but dura mater was in proximity to the origin of the afflicted vessel.

Regarding the enormous relevance of the anatomy in cases of major vascular injuries, we must not only consider the anatomy of the vessels themselves and all their variants but also assess the anatomy of the skull base proper. In case 3, a flat sella (as depicted on the coronal and axial views) contributed to the inappropriate opening that led to left carotid laceration. This unfortunate complication could most likely have been avoided with the use of intraoperative neuronavigation because the lack of three-dimensional viewing is well known in endoscopy. This is usually not a problem, but in this setting, it may have led to the misperceived spatial relationship between bone and vessels, and if that is the case, then it resulted in carotid or cavernous sinus bleeding. In the past, we have not been using neuronavigation in "de novo" pituitary cases. Normally, we advocate for the use of this intraoperative technology only in the setting of reoperations—but from this case, we learned that a radiographically flat sella is a morphological indicator of complex anatomical relationships, which warrant the use of this technology.

Case 4 is a good example of how recurrent pituitary tumors benefit from neuronavigation when trying to avoid complications. The scarred and distorted anatomy in such recurrent cases may lead to carotid injury, especially when the tumor is involving the cavernous sinus and encasing the respective carotid artery segment. The combination of technical failure from the neuronavigation system and a scared surgical field created a complex setting, and our maneuvers provoked marked bleeding from the right cavernous sinus. With some luck, that was easily controlled. Despite this successful intraoperative management, a postoperative angio-CT showed a traumatic pseudoaneurysm that needed to be coiled.

Case 2 illustrates the risk of carotid damage from a combination of factors: the involvement of two or more segments of the internal carotid artery because of a tumor, previous radiation therapy, and the carotid's being encircled with tumor tissue by more than 120° [10]. The carotid laceration was caused during the drilling of an infiltrated petrous bone portion, so the artery had not been exposed enough yet. Possibilities for effective surgical maneuverability in such acute situations are very limited in endoscopic skull base surgery, and the placement of a Foley balloon seems to be a very good choice as an effective temporary tamponade when classical local hemostatic agents fail to control the bleeding, as was the case in our patient. Also, in these moments, considering what the best agent could be to repair the affected vessel is important if the opportunity arises. Macerated muscle appears to be the most effective way to patch a hole, according to many [11]. Bipolar coagulation, on the other hand, must be restricted to the tear of a very small vessels or a small laceration [1, 3, 12].

A crucial aspect of postoperative management in carotid artery damage at the skull base is the role of angiography and endovascular therapy. The availability of a biplane 24 h/day is paramount when taking on complex skull base cases with the potential of vascular complications. Cases 2 and 3 were taken immediately to the INR suite after we had realized that the carotid was seriously injured. In case 2, the initial angiographic study showed leakage at the petrous bone segment of the ICA, and it also showed the effect of the Foley balloon's supporting the wall adjacent to the tear. Good collateral flow from the posterior circulation through the PCom artery was seen, so the carotid artery could be sacrificed (via coiling), fortunately without neurological deficit. Current endovascular techniques of stenting (flow diverters) may avoid needing to sacrifice an injured vessel [4], depending on the site of damage and the characteristics of the vessels involved. However, this was not possible in our patient, because the technology was not yet available at that time. Some authors have tried to avoid sacrificing the carotid artery by means of emergency bypass surgery or even in other settings by practicing prophylactic bypass placements (e.g., ECA to MCA) in case of high-risk lesions [5].

In case 3, angiography showed an intraluminal hematoma without compromising the carotid flow. However, some of the ischemic or embolic event had happened intraoperatively: Postoperative MRI displayed an altered FLAIR signal in the ipsilateral hemisphere, which was not expected in a 19-year-old patient. Again, endovascular procedures/stenting can be helpful in such cases—that is, when a risk of occlusion follows the luminal compromise. Our patient was under antiplatelet therapy, and 1 year later, angio-MRI showed patency at the point of previous vessel damage without a marked reduction in the caliber of the artery.

Conclusions

Major vascular injury is a potentially life-threatening complication of microsurgical and endoscopic approaches to the skull base. Many factors increase the risk of its occurring: alterations in the anatomy of the vessels and/or skull base, previous treatments (surgery, radiation) for tumoral lesions, the length of involvement and/or the needed exposure of the carotid artery segment, and a lack of appropriate intraoperative technology. Intraoperative steps to control the bleeding include applications of classic and modern hemostatic agents, and a muscle patch is considered the best biological repair tissue for a damaged vessel wall. Bipolar coagulation must be restricted to small vessels and/or small tears. Endovascular management is crucial for the accurate assessment of vascular damage and allows for immediate treatment (coiling, stenting) when needed.

References

1. Chin OY, Ghosh R, Fang CH, Baredes S, Liu JK, Eloy JA. Internal carotid artery injury in endoscopic endonasal surgery: a systematic review. Laryngoscope. 2016;126(3):582–90.
2. Ganiusmen O, Citak G, Samancioglu A, Korkmaz H, Binatli AO. Anatomic evaluation of the ophthalmic artery in optic canal decompression: a cadaver study of 20 optic canals. Turk Neurosurg. 2017;27(1):31–6.
3. Gardner PA, Tormenti MJ, Pant H, Fernandez-Miranda JC, Snyderman CH, Horowitz MB. Carotid artery injury during endoscopic endonasal skull base surgery: incidence and outcomes. Neurosurgery. 2013;73(2):261–9.
4. Martinakis VG, Dalainas I, Katsikas VC, Xiromeritis K. Endovascular treatment of carotid injury. Eur Rev Med Pharmacol Sci. 2013;17(5):673–88.
5. Rangel-Castilla L, McDougall CG, Spetzler RF, Nakaji P. Urgent cerebral revascularization bypass surgery for iatrogenic skull base internal carotid artery injury. Neurosurgery. 2014;10(4):640–7.
6. Bonasia S, Bojanowski M, Robert T. Embryology and anatomical variations of the ophthalmic artery. Neuroradiology. 2020;62(2):139–52.
7. Bonasia S, Smajda S, Ciccio G, Robert T. Anatomic and embryologic analysis of the dural branches of the ophthalmic artery. AJNR Am J Neuroradiol. 2021;42(3):414–21.
8. Toma N. Anatomy of the ophthalmic artery: embryological consideration. Neurol Med Chir. 2016;56(10):585–91.
9. Bracard S, Liao L, Zhu F, Gory B, Anxionnat R, Braun M. The ophthalmic artery: a new variant involving two branches from the supracavernous internal carotid artery. Surg Radiol Anat. 2020;42(2):201–5.
10. AlQahtani A, London NR, Castelnuovo P, et al. Assessment of factors associated with internal carotid injury in expanded endoscopic endonasal skull base surgery. JAMA Otolaryngol Head Neck Surg. 2020;146(4):364–72.
11. Wang WH, Lieber S, Lan MY, Wang EW, Fernandez-Miranda JC, Snyderman CH, Gardner PA. Nasopharyngeal muscle patch for the management of internal carotid artery injury in endoscopic endonasal surgery. J Neurosurg. 2019;133:1382–7.
12. AlQahtani A, Castelnuovo P, Nicolai P, Prevedello DM, Locatelli D, Carrau RL. Injury of the internal carotid artery during endoscopic skull base surgery: prevention and management protocol. Otolaryngol Clin N Am. 2016;49(1):237–52.

Cerebral Venous Infarction After AVM Resection: Pictorial

Vladimír Beneš

Abstract

A case report of a 68-year-old otherwise-healthy female patient with Spetzler-Martin (SM) grade I arteriovenous malformation (AVM) in her left frontal region is presented. After an uneventful surgery, cerebral venous infarction developed, and the patient was rendered hemiparetic with motor aphasia. After bony decompression, slow improvement was seen, and 3 months after surgery, the patient was neurologically intact. Six months after AVM resection, cranioplasty was performed. Infarction was caused by the thrombosis of a long primary draining vein, which finished its course in the normal cortical venous system. The case supports the venous origin of postoperative bleeding after AVM resection instead of the normal perfusion pressure phenomenon.

Keywords

Cerebral arteriovenous malformation · venous occlusive disease

Case Report

The patient was a 68-year-old healthy right-handed woman. She was treated and well compensated for arterial hypertension, and dyslipidemia was also well compensated by diet. One month before admission, she collapsed without convulsions on several occasions. Magnetic resonance (MR) performed elsewhere showed a Spetzler-Martin (SM) grade I arteriovenous malformation (AVM) in her left frontal lobe (Fig. 1). Angiography performed at our hospital confirmed the diagnosis (Figs. 2, 3, and 4). The AVM was drained via a long draining vein running laterally and terminating in the

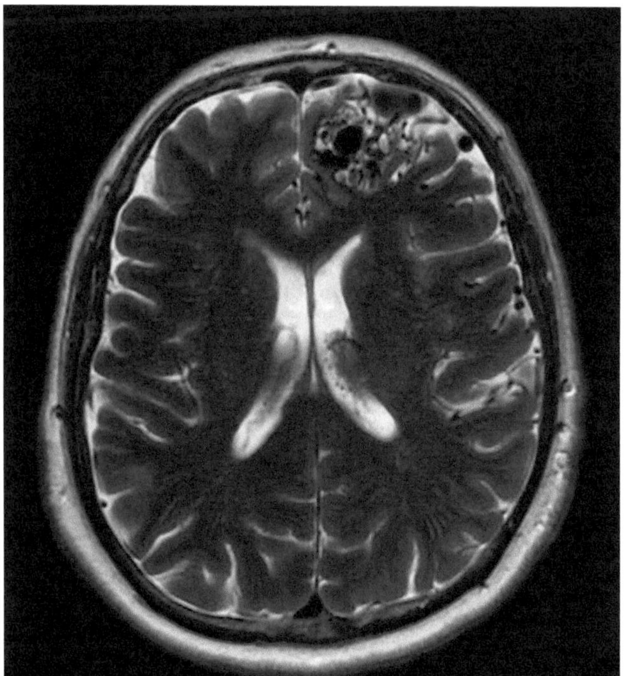

Fig. 1 Left frontal AVM

V. Beneš (✉)
Department of Neurosurgery and Neurooncology, 1st Medical Faculty, Institute of Clinical Neurodisciplines, Charles University and University Military Hospital, Prague, Czech Republic
e-mail: vladimir.benes@uvn.cz

K. Turel, E. M. Kasper (eds.), *Complications in Neurosurgery II*, Acta Neurochirurgica Supplement 133,
https://doi.org/10.1007/978-3-031-61601-3_3

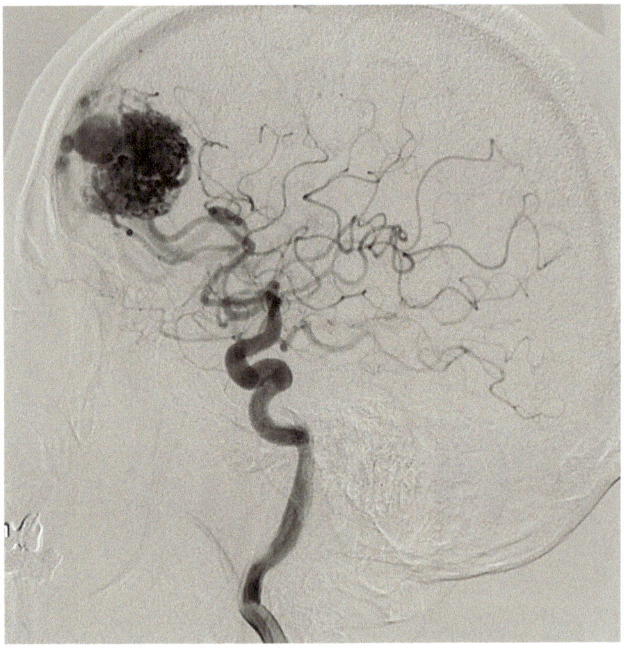

Fig. 2 SM grade I AVM fed by middle cerebral artery branches

cortical veins of the left hemisphere. A short minor vein drained the nidus into the superior sagittal sinus, and another small vein drained anteriorly. The therapeutic options were explained to the patient, and she opted for surgery.

Uneventful surgery (Figs. 5 and 6) was followed by angiography under anesthesia in the same instance (Fig. 7), and the patient was transferred to the intensive care unit (ICU). The patient awoke with hemiparesis and complete motor aphasia. Computed tomography (CT) performed before awakening showed bleeding in the vicinity of the resection cavity consistent with venous infarction (Fig. 8). Over the next 3 days, the patient became sleepy but remained arousable and oriented. CT was performed, showing the enlargement of the infarcted hemorrhagic area, resulting in a marked cerebral shift (Fig. 9). Bony decompression was performed (Fig. 10). After the decompression, the patient's status improved, and she was fully awake, yet with persistent hemiparesis and with motor aphasia. Early rehabilitation and logopedic therapy and re-education were initiated. Over the next 3 months, the patient fully recovered from her neurological deficits, and at about 5 months after the initial sur-

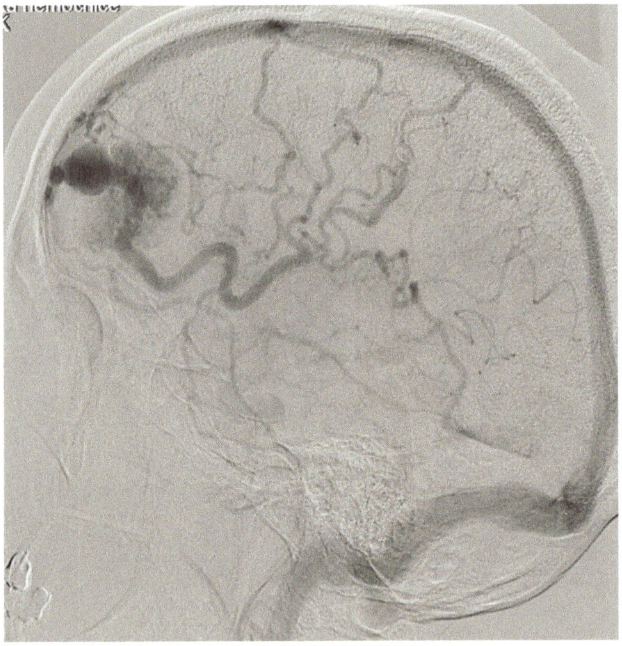

Fig. 3 Long main AVM vein draining into the normal cortical venous system

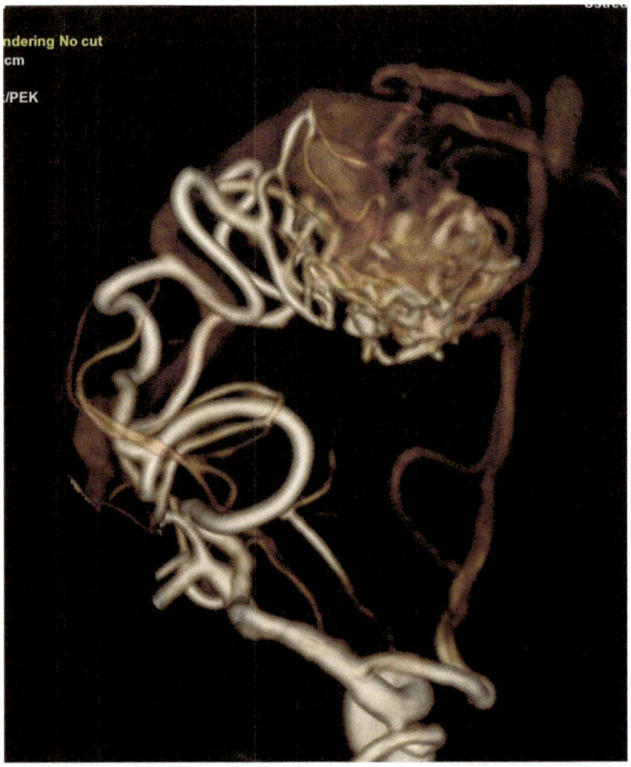

Fig. 4 3D angiogram shows main draining vein, secondary vein entering the superior sagittal sinus, and another vein running anterosuperiorly

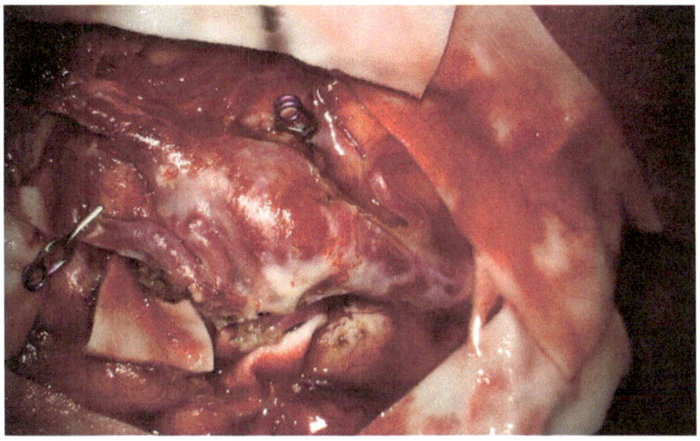

Fig. 5 AVM. Venous varix in the middle. To the left runs the secondary vein into the superior sagittal vein, and the main draining vein runs to the right

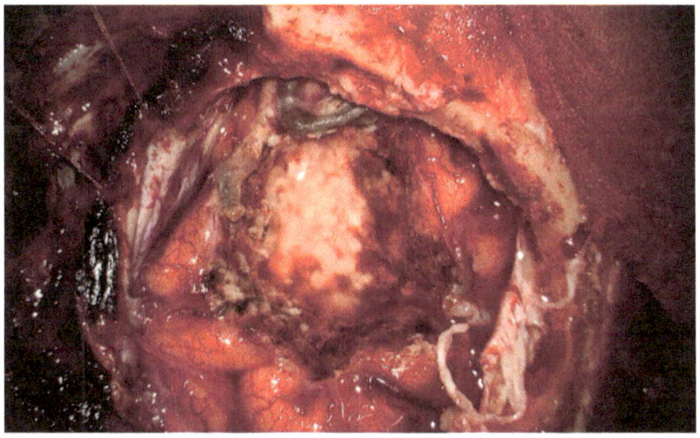

Fig. 6 Resection cavity and the stumps of the veins. At the anterior aspect of the cavity, already thrombosed secondary AVM vein

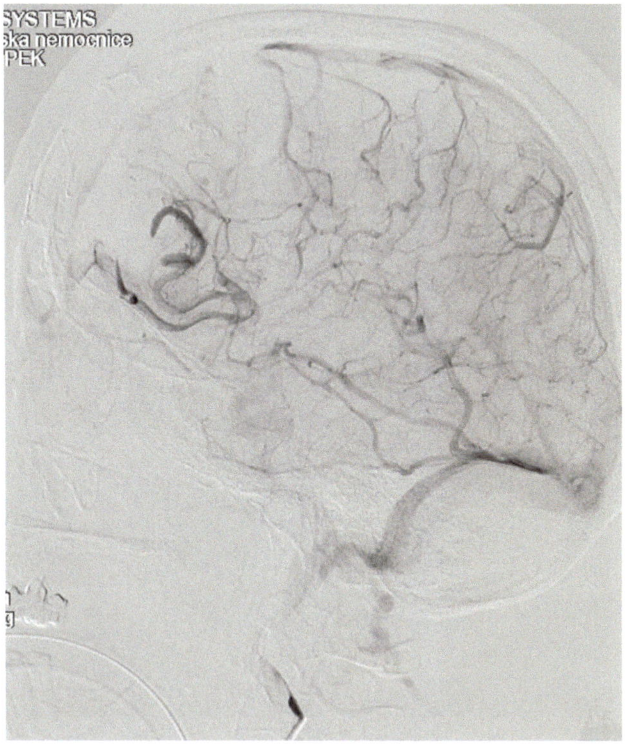

Fig. 7 Angiography 20 min after resection. The original vein is missing (thrombosed?), engorged veins are in the vicinity of the resection cavity. Superior sagittal sinus purely opacified

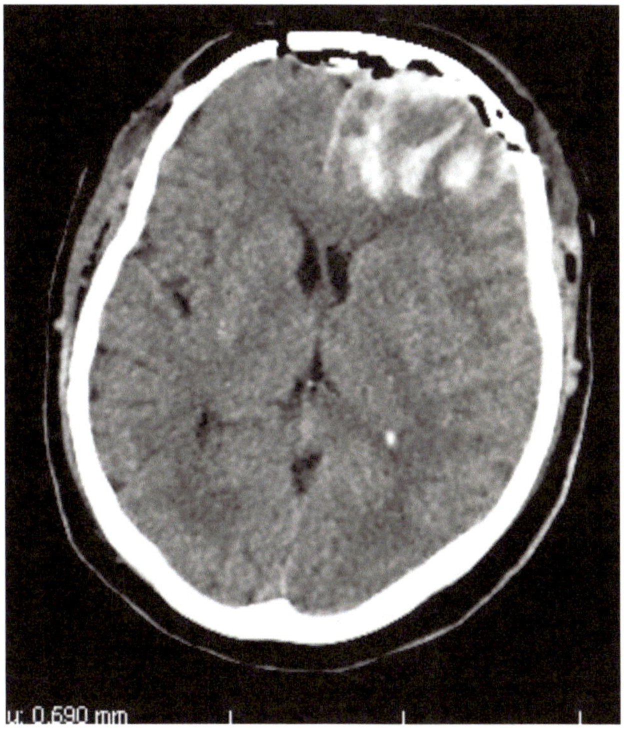

Fig. 8 CT 3 h after surgery. Venous infarction in the left frontal lobe

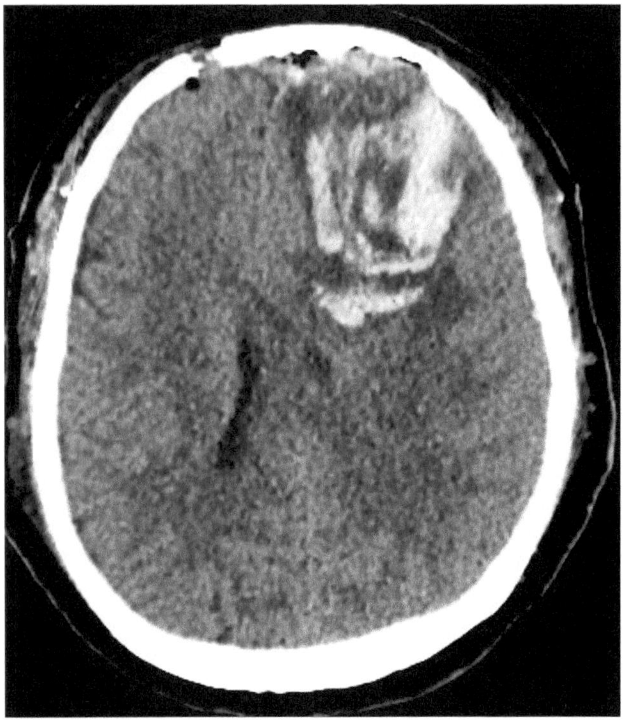

Fig. 9 CT 4 days after surgery. Enlargement of the venous infarction and pronounced brain shift

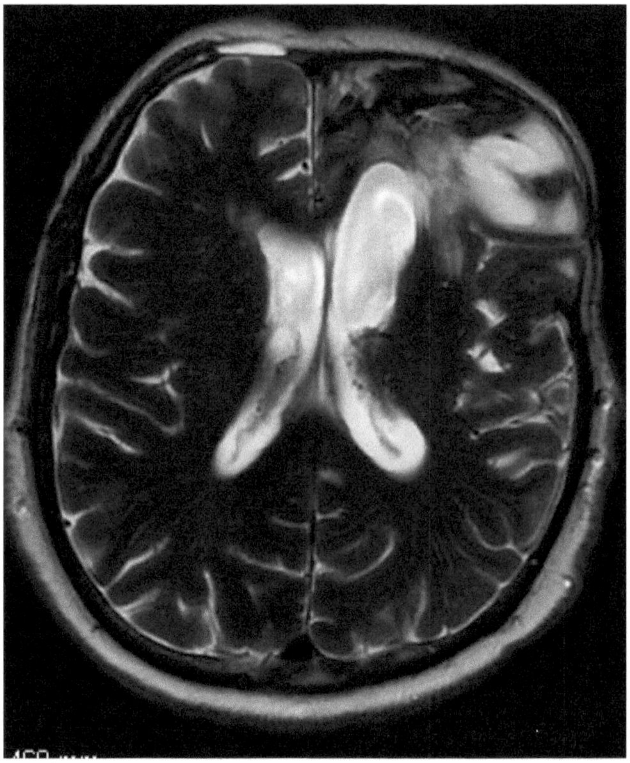

Fig. 11 Final MR 6 months after surgery and cranioplasty

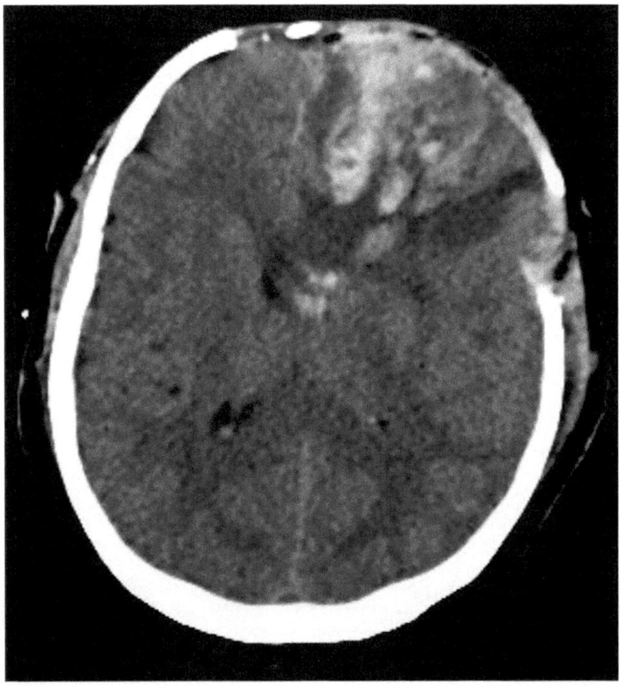

Fig. 10 CT after decompression

gery, cranioplasty was performed (Fig. 11). After the cranioplasty, the patient returned to all her original activities without any restrictions.

Discussion

Four possible causes of postoperative bleeding in AVM surgery are known: postsurgical insufficient hemostasis, bleeding from an AVM remnant, normal perfusion pressure breakthrough (NPPB), and the venous occlusive phenomenon. The first is insufficient hemostasis at the end of the procedure. The second is bleeding from any overlooked AVM remnant. These causes are considered common surgical complications, both nonspecific and specific to AVM surgery. Two further causes are still subject to some debate. One cause is a phenomenon described by Spetzler as "normal perfusion pressure breakthrough" (NPPB) [1]. Briefly, the arteries in the AVM vicinity are paralyzed in the vasodilated state by the long-standing steal caused by the AVM shunts. After AVM resection, these vessels cannot contend with the sudden rush of blood under normal perfusion pressure, leading to edema and bleeding. In the 1990s, the author tried to develop a model of NPPB. Various shunts between the carotid artery and the jugular vein were constructed in rabbits. Even with the occlusion of the contralateral carotid artery and unilateral vertebral artery occlusion, the occlusion of the shunt did not produce any cerebral bleedings 6 months after the procedure. All experimental animals survived shunt occlusion without incident [2]. Lastly, Yasargil suggested the problem to be on the venous side of the AVM: The so-called venous occlusive phenomenon is enhanced by the length or stenoses of the veins and sinuses draining the AVM. Venous thrombosis is then the cause of regular venous infarction in the region of the given vein [3]. The presented case supports venous thrombosis as being the cause of postoperative bleeding.

Conflict of Interest Supported by AZV grant NV19-04-00270.

References

1. Spetzler RF, Wilson CB, Weinstein P, Mehdorn M, Townsend J, Telles D. Normal perfusion pressure breakthrough theory. Clin Neurosurg. 1978;25:651–72.
2. Beneš V. Arteriovenous malformations. NPPB modeling. Doctoral thesis. Charles University Prague, 1998, p. 312.
3. Yasargil MG. Microneurosurgery. IIIB. AVM of the brain, clinical considerations, general and special operative techniques, surgical results, nonoperated cases, cavernous and venous angiomas, neuroanesthesia. Stuttgart: Thieme; 1988. p. 479.

Pial Laceration from a Dural Suture Causing Devastating Neurological Deficits

Abhijit Goyal-Honavar, Edmond Jonathan Gandham, and Ari George Chacko

Abstract

A 39-year-old man received empiric treatment for pulmonary tuberculosis (TB). After developing sensory seizures he was restarted on anti-TB drugs when a brain MRI showed a 4.3 cm left parietal enhancing lesion with extensive edema. After TB treatment, imaging showed a reduction in size and edema. Later, he developed headache and seizures, and MRI showed recurrent edema and an enlarging lesion. Neurosurgery decided to biopsy the lesion to obtain a diagnosis. At craniotomy, a frozen section was reported as granulomatous inflammation. However, he returned postOP with a new right hemiparesis and MRI showed a cystic lesion under the motor cortex, with no enhancement. Craniotomy was performed and the lesion was excised and exploration revealed that one of the dural stitches had lacerated the brain as a cause of the cyst formation. The case differential and management is discussed in detail.

Keywords

Tuberculoma · Cyst · Pial laceration · Complication

Case Report

A 39-year-old man elsewhere received 9 months of empiric treatment for pulmonary tuberculosis (TB) in 2012. After developing sensory seizures in January 2016, he was restarted on three anti-TB drugs when a brain MRI showed a 4.3 cm left parietal enhancing conglomerate lesion with extensive cerebral edema (Fig. 1a, b). With anti-TB treatment, serial imaging showed a reduction in the lesion size and the brain edema (Fig. 1c–f). In April 2018, he went to our infectious disease unit with a headache and seizures, and the MRI showed increased perilesional edema and an enlarging lesion (Fig. 1g, h). Neurosurgery was called for a consultation, and we decided to biopsy the lesion to obtain a diagnosis because of the resurgence of symptoms and the progression of disease on anti-TB therapy. At craniotomy, we mapped the sensorimotor cortex with intraoperative monitoring (somatosensory evoked potentials), and we saw a yellow discoloration of the postsensory gyrus from where a frozen section was obtained. It was reported as granulomatous inflammation. No further dissection was performed, but because the brain was full, a duraplasty was performed and the bone replaced. He did well after surgery and was discharged on the third postoperative day (POD) without any deficits. On the fifth POD, he returned with a new right hemiparesis, but no drowsiness, headache, seizures, or fever. We considered cortical venous thrombosis, hematoma, cerebritis, or subclinical seizures as possible etiologies. No hematoma was found on plain computed tomography (CT), but a thin extradural collection (Fig. 2a) was found. The contrast CT showed a suspicious hypodensity anterior to the residual tuberculoma (Fig. 2b). He was treated with mannitol, steroids, intravenous hydration, and a higher dose of anticonvulsants. An emergent MRI showed no cortical/dural venous thrombosis but a definite 3.5 cm cystic lesion was under the motor cortex, anterior to the tuberculoma, with no enhancement of the wall (Fig. 2c). During emergency recraniotomy, we removed a thin extradural hematoma that was not very remarkable: no subdural hematoma. We saw the surface of the tuberculoma on the sensory gyrus and excised it completely at this time, but we did not find any communica-

A. Goyal-Honavar · E. J. Gandham · A. G. Chacko (✉)
Section of Neurosurgery, Department of Neurological Sciences, Christian Medical College Hospital, Vellore, Tamil Nadu, India

K. Turel, E. M. Kasper (eds.), *Complications in Neurosurgery II*, Acta Neurochirurgica Supplement 133,
https://doi.org/10.1007/978-3-031-61601-3_4

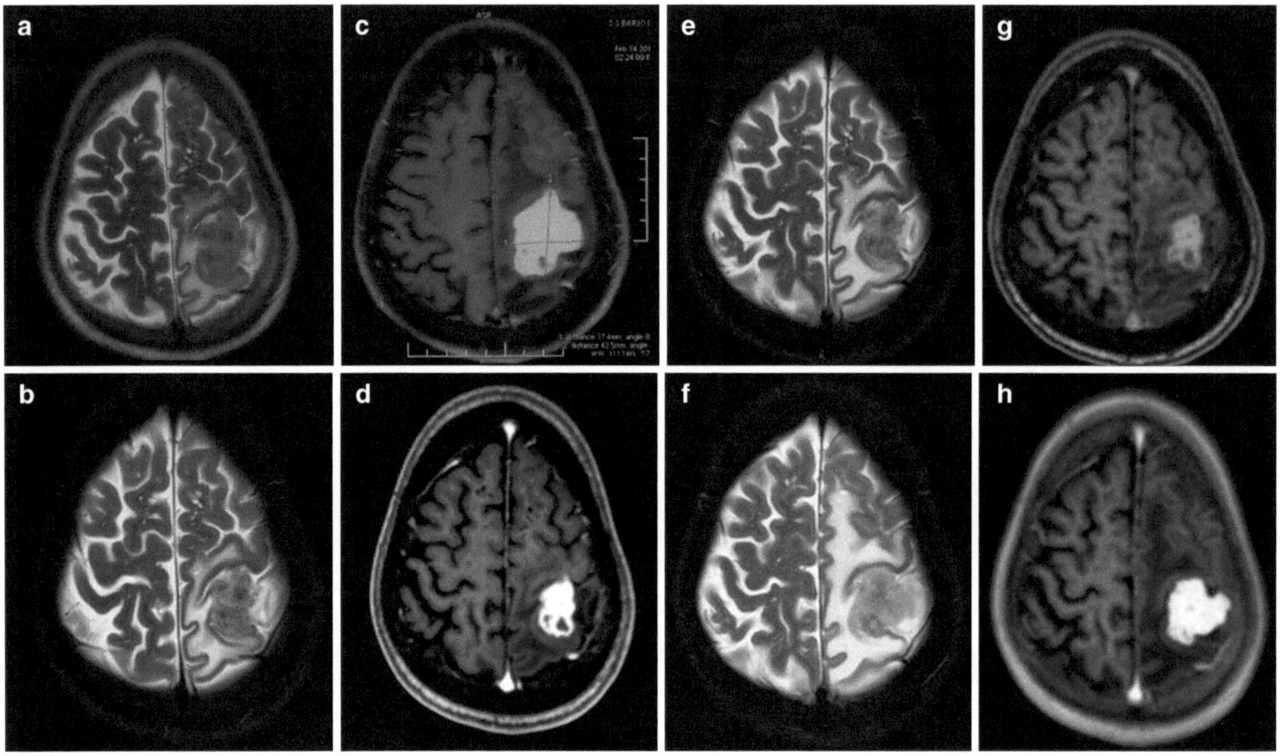

Fig. 1 Brain MRI in January 2016 showing (**a**) a 4.3 cm conglomerate lesion with significant perilesional edema in the left parietal lobe, enhancing brilliantly on the T1w contrast image (**b**). After 18 months of anti-TB treatment, the edema and the lesion size have decreased (**c**, **d**). The anti-TB treatment was continued, and at 24 months after treatment, the lesion had remained about the same size (**e**, **f**). At 27 months, the patient had a headache and seizures, and the T2w and contrast images showed an increase in edema and in the size of the lesion, to 3.1 cm (**g**, **h**)

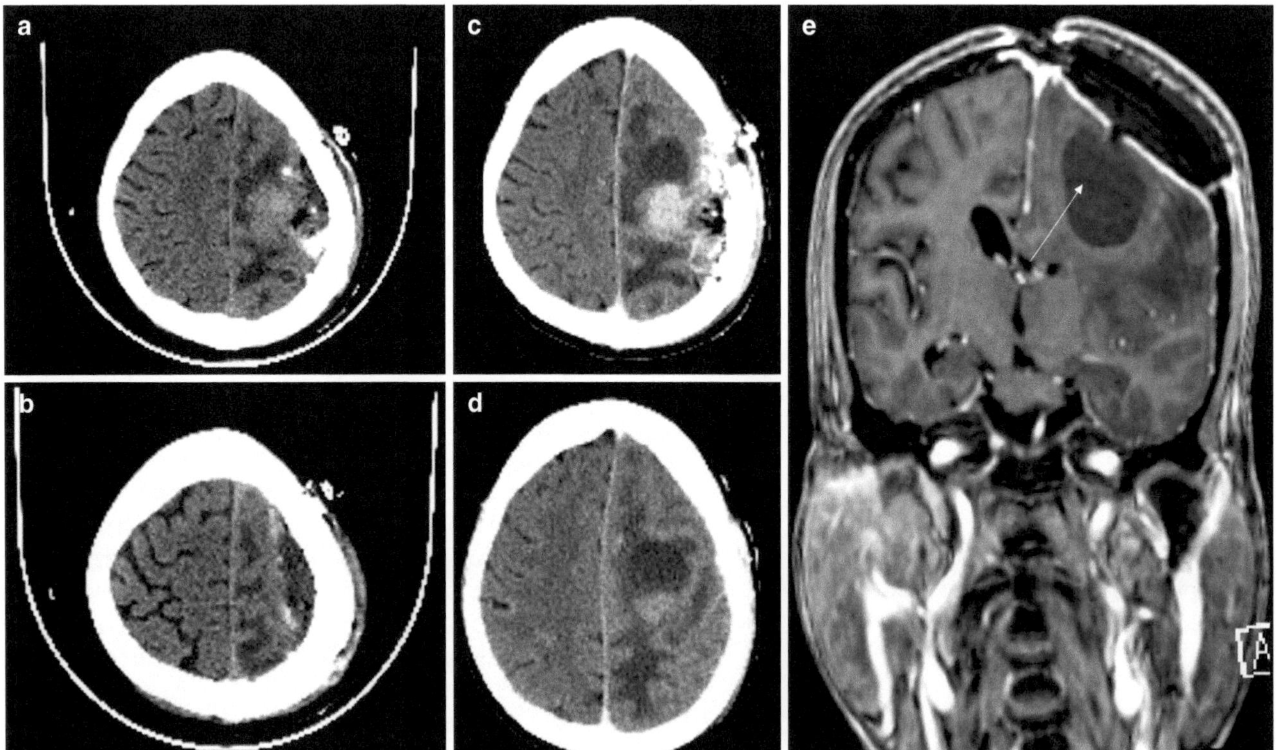

Fig. 2 The patient returned to us on postoperative day 6 with new onset right hemiparesis, at which time a plain CT revealed a thin extradural collection (**a**, **b**) and a contrast CT revealed a suspicious hypodensity anterior to the residual tuberculoma (**c**, **d**). This was characterized by the MRI (**e**) as a cystic lesion under the motor cortex (white arrow)

tion at the depths with the cyst. In fact, the sensory gyrus bulged into the cavity previously occupied by the tuberculoma. Upon extending the previous dural opening further anteriorly, we found that one of the Prolene dural stitches had lacerated the pia and cortex. From here, we entered the cyst through which we evacuated thin yellow fluid under pressure. Ten days after the re-exploration, significant function had been restored for the patient, they were walking, and they had regained some power in their upper limb. The biopsy was reported as "granulomatous inflammation suggestive of tuberculosis"; however, all cultures were negative. At follow-up 16 months later, he had recovered grade 5/5 power but continued to have mild difficulty with rapid finger tapping.

Discussion

Tuberculomas: Controversies in Diagnosis and Management

The diagnosis of intracranial tuberculoma is often presumptive, based most often on radiological features, coupled with evidence of TB elsewhere and a response to treatment [1]. In our case, the prior history of pulmonary tuberculosis and brain MRI features of a lobulated, T2w hyperintense, homogenous contrast-enhancing lesion was consistent with a solid noncaseating TB granuloma, and empiric anti-TB therapy was therefore started [2, 3]. Over the course of 18 months, a decrease in edema and a decrease in the size of the lesion were noted. A satisfactory radiological response of lesions occurs in 20–80% [4–7] of cases and is defined as a reduction in perilesional edema, lesion size, and calcification, supporting the presumptive diagnosis [1, 8]. The subsequent recurrence of symptoms and increase in the size of the lesion raised the possibility of drug resistance, a fungal granuloma, or a malignant lesion. Paradoxical response to anti-TB therapy is common, including an increase in the size of tuberculomas or the development of new tuberculomas [4, 5, 9, 10], and usually occurs within the first 3–6 months of initiating therapy. This phenomenon is best explained by inflammatory host reactions rather than a failure of treatment [11–13], an observation that is supported by the development in lesions with documented sensitivity to first-line drugs [12]. Despite the evidence of granulomatous inflammation in the excised tissue, no tuberculous bacilli were detected on acid-fast staining, cultures, or Gene Xpert PCR assay—a feature reported in 60% of cases [7, 14].

Surgery in Tuberculomas

Clear indications for surgical intervention include life-threatening mass effects and a pathological confirmation of the diagnosis when the clinicoradiological picture suggests other pathologies [10, 15]. In this case, we opted for a craniotomy and open biopsy with the use of cortical mapping, instead of a stereotactic biopsy, as the lesion was located very superficially. Because a frozen section from the excised tissue confirmed the presence of granulomatous inflammation and because it appeared in an eloquent area, we did not proceed with radical excision [10].

Pathogenesis of Early Postoperative Cysts

When our patient returned to us with hemiparesis on POD 5, we noted that the cause of his symptoms was an intraparenchymal cystic collection anterior to the original lesion just under the motor cortex. Tuberculomas are usually not associated with cysts, and the early radiographic appearance of the cystic lesion was unlike an abscess. We hypothesize that the inadvertent pial laceration from the dural suture created a channel for the ingress of cerebrospinal fluid (CSF) into the motor cortex, rapidly forming a cyst. The brain swelling, hemostatic material, blood, and inflammation from the surgery likely cordoned off the subdural and subarachnoid spaces around the laceration, inhibiting the free flow of CSF over the convexity and forcing it through the pial laceration into the parenchyma of the motor cortex proper. We were unable to reach the cyst after completely excising the tuberculoma and therefore drained the cyst of its clear fluid through the laceration and found no hematoma or xanthochromia. Symptomatic postoperative cystic lesions are rare occurrences indeed, and to our knowledge, this is the only reported case of an early parenchymal symptomatic cyst not connected to the resection cavity of the primary lesion. Prior reports of early postoperative symptomatic cysts describe clinical deterioration due to a cyst's forming in resection cavities of tumors as early as the third postoperative day [16, 17]. Authors have hypothesized that the pathogenesis of these cysts usually involves communication with the ventricles [18], the rapid decompression of intracranial pressure [19], or a flap-valve mechanism allowing the one-way ingress of CSF [17, 20]. In addition to a ball-valve mechanism, arising either from scar tissue or the roof of the resection cavity, CSF may be forced into such spaces because of the increased pressure of respiratory inspiration and cardiac systole [21]. In cases where additional factors come into play, such as the absence of bony counterpressure, these cysts have been shown to grow into extracranial compartments, as in one report of an iatrogenic cyst following the excision of a juvenile nasal angiofibroma that grew through the bony defect in the middle cranial fossa to form a pulsatile parapharyngeal swelling [22]. In lesions where the ventricles were opened at surgery, an endoscopic visualization of the cyst has revealed the presence of a slit-valve mechanism, representing an iatrogenic version of an arachnoid cyst [20]. In other cases, inflammation induced via adjuvant chemotherapeutic wafers containing 1,3-bis(2-chloroethyl)-1-

nitrosourea (BCNU) used in glioma surgery has been implicated in the formation of postoperative cysts, though they occur later in the postoperative period (6 days to 6 weeks) [23, 24]. All described cases have been shown to respond poorly to medical therapy (such as treatment with hyperosmolar agents) and ultimately required some form of surgical intervention, ranging from an external drain to craniotomy and evacuation. While the best modality to manage these cysts remains subject to debate, where some authors have recommended fenestration in favor of permanent CSF shunting devices [21], surgical intervention is acceptable in all symptomatic cases.

Avoidance of Complications

Attention to detail is vital during dural closure, ensuring that the tip of the needle is always within view, to avoid brain injury. The dogma regarding watertight dural closure has been questioned for supratentorial surgeries where the incidence of subdural and subgaleal effusions requiring surgical intervention was not different in a series comparing primary or secondary watertight closures and the mere approximation of the dura with a few interrupted sutures [25].

Conclusion

Acute changes in sensorium and the new recruitment of deficits following neurosurgery must be taken seriously and evaluated diligently, including the use of imaging. Acute postoperative cysts developing at or adjacent to the site of surgery are probably secondary to a ball-valve mechanism and must be managed operatively. This complication may have been avoided by performing careful dural suturing, by effecting a complete excision of the lesion at primary surgery, and by opting for dural approximation rather than watertight dural closure.

References

1. Marais S, Van Toorn R, Chow FC, Manesh A, Siddiqi OK, Figaji A, Schoeman JF, Meintjes G. Management of intracranial tuberculous mass lesions: how long should we treat for? Wellcome Open Res. 2020. https://doi.org/10.12688/wellcomeopenres.15501.3
2. Azeemuddin M, Alvi A, Sayani R, Khan MK, Farooq S, Beg MA, Awan S, Wasay M. Neuroimaging findings in tuberculosis: a single-center experience in 559 cases. J Neuroimaging. 2019;29(5):657–68.
3. Bernaerts A, Vanhoenacker FM, Parizel PM, Van Goethem JW, Van Altena R, Laridon A, De Roeck J, Coeman V, De Schepper AM. Tuberculosis of the central nervous system: overview of neuroradiological findings. Eur Radiol. 2003;13(8):1876–90.
4. Anuradha HK, Garg RK, Sinha MK, Agarwal A, Verma R, Singh MK, Shukla R. Intracranial tuberculomas in patients with tuberculous meningitis: predictors and prognostic significance. Int J Tuberc Lung Dis. 2011;15(2):234–9.
5. Gupta M, Bajaj BK, Khwaja G. Paradoxical response in patients with CNS tuberculosis. J Assoc Physicians India. 2003;51:257–60.
6. Harder E, Al-Kawi MZ, Carney P. Intracranial tuberculoma: conservative management. Am J Med. 1983;74(4):570–6.
7. Poonnoose SI, Rajshekhar V. Rate of resolution of histologically verified intracranial tuberculomas. Neurosurgery. 2003;53(4):873–8.
8. van Toorn R, du Plessis A-M, Schaaf HS, Buys H, Hewlett RH, Schoeman JF. Clinicoradiologic response of neurologic tuberculous mass lesions in children treated with thalidomide. Pediatr Infect Dis J. 2015;34(2):214–8.
9. Machida A, Ishihara T, Amano E, Otsu S. Late-onset paradoxical reactions 10 years after treatment for tuberculous meningitis in an HIV-negative patient: a case report. BMC Infect Dis. 2018;18(1):313.
10. Rajshekhar V. Surgery for brain tuberculosis: a review. Acta Neurochir. 2015;157(10):1665–78.
11. Nicolls DJ, King M, Holland D, Bala J, del Rio C. Intracranial tuberculomas developing while on therapy for pulmonary tuberculosis. Lancet Infect Dis. 2005;5(12):795–801.
12. Schoeman JF, Fieggen G, Seller N, Mendelson M, Hartzenberg B. Intractable intracranial tuberculous infection responsive to thalidomide: report of four cases. J Child Neurol. 2006;21(4):301–8.
13. Walker NF, Stek C, Wasserman S, Wilkinson RJ, Meintjes G. The tuberculosis-associated immune reconstitution inflammatory syndrome: recent advances in clinical and pathogenesis research. Curr Opin HIV AIDS. 2018;13(6):512–21.
14. Arseni C. Two hundred and one cases of intracranial tuberculoma treated surgically. J Neurol Neurosurg Psychiatry. 1958;21(4):308–11.
15. Akhaddar A. Surgical therapy. In: Turgut M, Akhaddar A, Turgut AT, Garg RK, editors. Tuberculosis of the central nervous system: pathogenesis, imaging, and management. Cham: Springer; 2017. p. 173–91.
16. Talacchi A, Corsini F, Gerosa M. Expanding cerebrospinal fluid cyst in the operative cavity: an unusual postoperative complication. Br J Neurosurg. 2011;25(5):641–3.
17. Yu J, Xiong W, Qu L, Huang H. Reoperation as a result of raised intracranial pressure associated with cyst formation in tumor cavity after intracranial tumor resection: a report of two cases. Case Rep Med. 2010. https://doi.org/10.1155/2010/634839.
18. Korinth MC, Weinzierl MR, Krings T, Gilsbach JM. Occurrence and therapy of space-occupying cystic lesions after brain tumor surgery. Zentralbl Neurochir. 2001;62(3):87–92.
19. Fujimori T, Shindo A, Ogawa D, Okada M, Hatakeyama T, Okauchi M, Kawanishi M, Miyake K, Tamiya T. A rare case of postoperative symptomatic cyst formation after resection of a large convexity meningioma. World Neurosurg. 2019;127:160–4.
20. Beez T, Remmel D, Steiger H-J. Endoscopic visualization of an iatrogenic valve mechanism: elucidating the pathogenesis of postoperative tumor bed cysts. World Neurosurg. 2018;115:213–5.
21. Bhaskara Rao M, Radhakrishnan K, Radhakrishnan VV, Gupta AK. Expanding cyst following temporal lobectomy: an unusual complication of epilepsy surgery. Clin Neurol Neurosurg. 1999;101(2):141–4.
22. Kutlay M, Colak A, Demircan N, Akin ON. Iatrogenic arachnoid cyst with distinct clinical picture as a result of bone defect in the floor of the middle cranial fossa: case report. Neurosurgery. 1998;43(5):1215–8.

23. Della Puppa A, Rossetto M, Ciccarino P, Del Moro G, Rotilio A, Manara R, Paola Gardiman M, Denaro L, d'Avella D, Scienza R. The first 3 months after BCNU wafers implantation in high-grade glioma patients: clinical and radiological considerations on a clinical series. Acta Neurochir. 2010;152(11):1923–31.
24. McGirt MJ, Villavicencio AT, Bulsara KR, Friedman HS, Friedman AH. Management of tumor bed cysts after chemotherapeutic wafer implantation: report of four cases. J Neurosurg. 2002;96(5):941–5.
25. Barth M, Tuettenberg J, Thomé C, Weiss C, Vajkoczy P, Schmiedek P. Watertight dural closure: is it necessary? A prospective randomized trial in patients with supratentorial craniotomies. Oper Neurosurg. 2008;63:352–8.

Venous Compromise/Deep Venous Thrombosis During Parasagittal Meningiomas Resection

Benedicto Oscar Colli, Carlos Gilberto Carlotti Junior, Ricardo Santos de Oliveira, and Guilherme Gozzoli Podolski Gondim

Abstract

We are reporting the case of JB, a 28-year-old male who presented to our hospital in 2009. The patient reported a progressive increase in a known mass that had been deforming their head since 2005. He had suffered from a first-time seizure four years later (in 2009). Neurological examination revealed a large tumor protruding in the parietal region, which was confirmed by CT. A subsequent MRI demonstrated a hyperostotic contrast-enhancing parasagittal tumor occluding the middle third of the superior sagittal sinus, with cortical veins joining the sinus adjacent to the tumor.

The patient was taken to the OR for a craniotomy and a resection of the tumor with cranioplasty in the same setting. The tumor was exposed by using a straight incision on the scalp. A craniotomy was performed around the tumor by using multiple burr holes; now the bone could be separated from the dura and removed. The intradural tumor was exposed, and a cortical vein draining into the tumor could not be preserved. Some residual tumor was left close to the anterior part of the superior sagittal sinus. The dura was reconstructed with pericranium, and the bony defect was closed with titanium mesh. The patient woke up initially paraplegic, but 7 days later, he started with proximal movements in both legs. Unfortunately, he died suddenly in the second postoperative week, due to pulmonary embolism. The case is reviewed in this manuscript to analyze the contributing factors of the complications that were observed and to suggest management strategies to avoid them.

Keywords

Venous compromising · Venous deep thrombosis · Parasagittal meningioma resection

Introduction

Meningiomas are the most common tumors among the central nervous system (CNS) tumors, accounting for 35.8% of primary cranial tumors [1]. Parasagittal meningiomas comprise between 21% and 31% of these intracranial meningiomas, and the distribution of meningiomas along the superior sagittal sinus (SSS) ranges from 14.8% to 33.9% in the anterior third, from 44.8% to 70.4% in the middle third, and from 9.2% to 29.6% in the posterior third of the sinus [2–5]. Surgical treatment is usually the method of choice for the management of most symptomatic meningiomas. Researchers have long noted [3, 4, 6, 7] that these tumors are associated with an increase in the incidence of deep venous thrombosis (DVT) and pulmonary embolism (PE) in bedridden postoperative patients [8–11]. Surgical treatment for parasagittal meningiomas is challenging because of the spatial proximity to motor areas and because the SSS and cortical veins drain into the sinus, especially for tumors in the middle third of the sinus [3, 4, 6, 11].

Here, we present the case of a 28-year-old patient who underwent the resection of a parasagittal hyperostotic meningioma. The patient sustained profound postoperative lower extremity paraplegia and developed DVT, which was followed by PE, which unfortunately resulted in death.

Case Report

A 28-year-old male patient presented to our department with a progressively enlarging tumor that had been noted for about four years. He had suffered a single seizure event fours

B. O. Colli (✉) · C. G. Carlotti Junior · R. S. de Oliveira · G. G. P. Gondim
Division of Neurosurgery, Department of Surgery, Ribeirão Preto Medical School, University of São Paulo, Ribeirão Preto, SP, Brazil
e-mail: bocolli@fmrp.usp.br; carlotti@fmrp.usp.br; podolski@usp.br

K. Turel, E. M. Kasper (eds.), *Complications in Neurosurgery II*, Acta Neurochirurgica Supplement 133,
https://doi.org/10.1007/978-3-031-61601-3_5

year prior to the current presentation. The physical examination at admission revealed a large tumor protruding from the central parietal region. Neurological examination was unremarkable. Computed tomography (CT) scans showed a central parietal, extra-axial hyperostotic tumor. Magnetic resonance imaging (MRI) showed contrast-enhancing bilateral parasagittal tumor components with a broad-based bilateral dural attachment and with a significant hyperostosis of the parietal bone, both suggestive of meningioma. The tumor occluded the blood flow in middle third of the superior sagittal sinus (SSS), and cortical veins were joining the sinus in the anterior part of the tumor (Fig. 1).

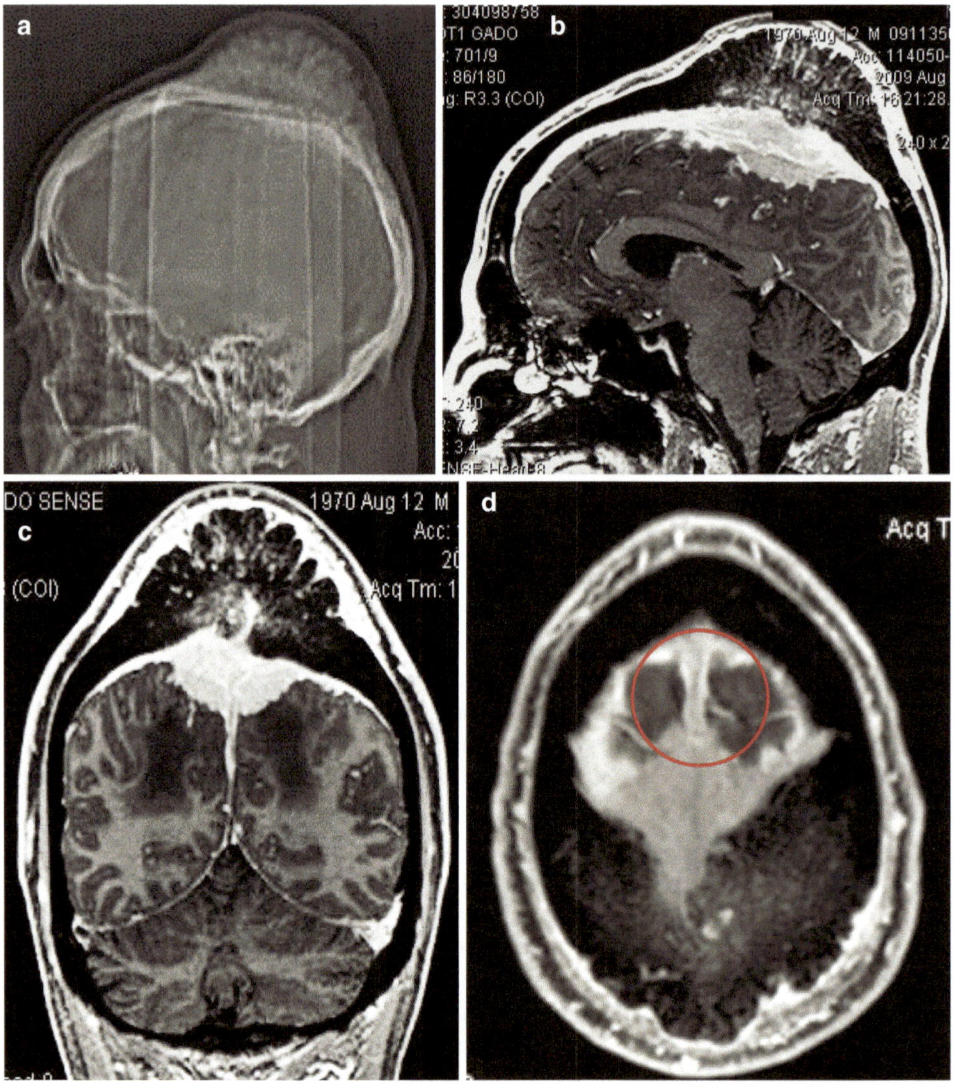

Fig. 1 (**a**) Preoperative computed tomography scout showing a huge parietal bone tumor protruding into the scalp. (**b–d**) Postcontrast T1-weighted MRI in sagittal (**b**), coronal (**c**), and axial (**d**) planes, showing a middle third hyperostotic parasagittal tentorial tumor occluding the superior sagittal sinus (**b**, **c**) and showing a posterior cortical vein draining into the sinus (**d**)

Surgery

The patient was extensively counseled, and he wished to proceed with resection. He was operated on in the supine position with his head partially flexed. A transverse straight scalp incision was carried out, which was centered on the midpoint of the osseous protrusion. The lesion was completely exposed by taking this approach (Fig. 2). A craniotomy was planned; it was performed around the tumor perimeter by using multiple burr holes; and the infiltrated bone could be separated from the dura and removed in toto. The intradural component of the tumor was now exposed for resection, during which a cortical vein draining posteriorly to the tumor could not be preserved. Some residual tumor was left close to the

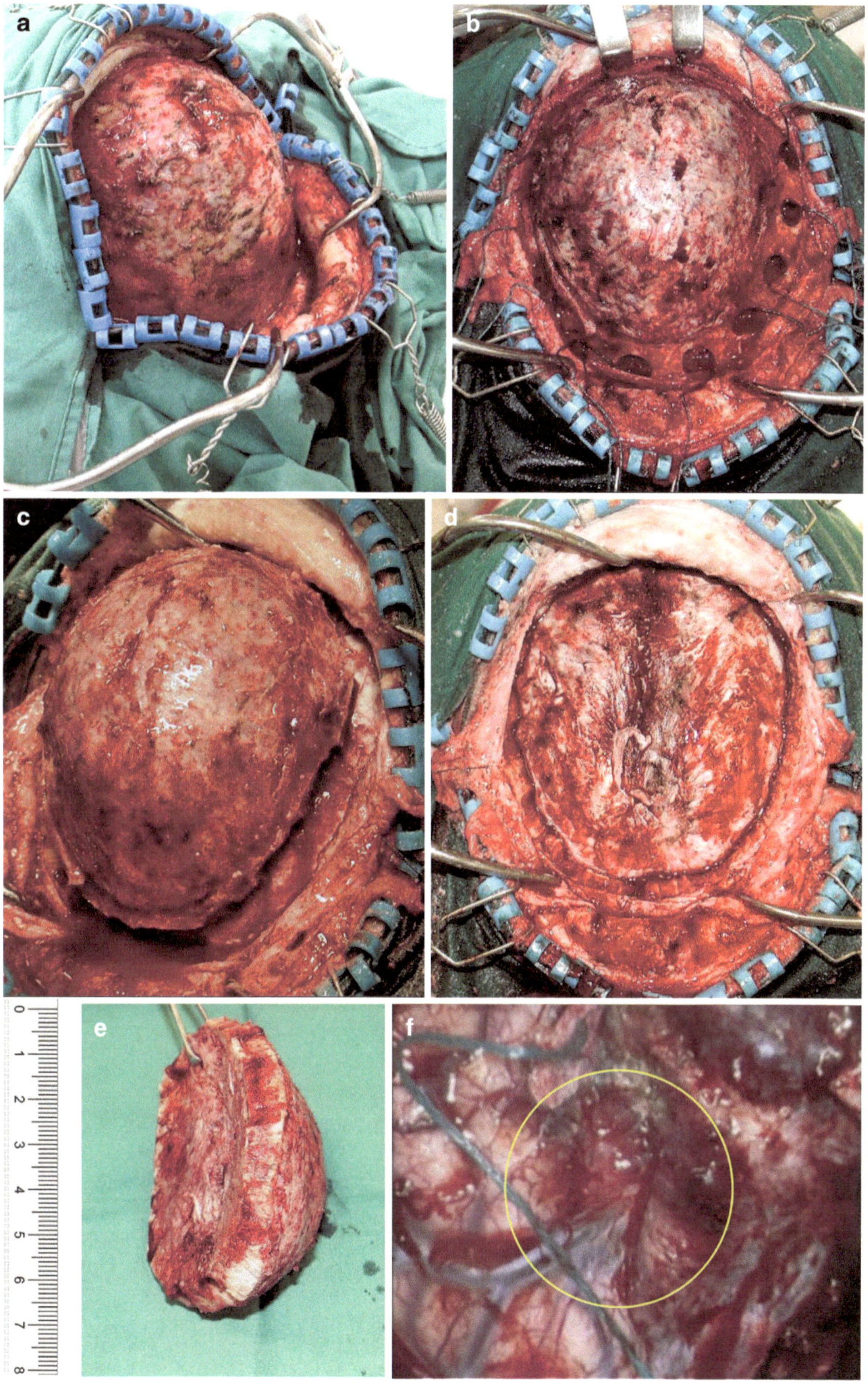

Fig. 2 Intraoperative views. (**a**) Exposure of the tumor through a transverse straight scalp incision centered in the tumor. (**b**) Multiple burr holes were made around the tumor. (**c**) Circular craniotomy done around the tumor. (**d**) Dural exposure after the removal of the bone flap. (**e**) Bone flap removed en bloc. (**f**) Parasagittal tumor exposed after bone flap removal, revealing a posterior cortical vein entering the tumor (*yellow circle*)

anterior part of the SSS. The dural defect was reconstructed with pericranium, and the missing bone was replaced with titanium mesh.

Postoperative Course

The patient woke up well, then the patient was extubated. However, upon neurological examination, the patient displayed bilateral lower extremity paraplegia. The immediate postoperative CT showed no surgical complication. He received standard postoperative care, and he was discharged on the fifth postoperative day to rehabilitation. As per the report from the rehabilitation facility, the patient began to show neurological recovery on the seventh postoperative day, with some proximal movements in both lower limbs. During the second postoperative week, however, the patient was readmitted in a nearby hospital after a period of acute respiratory distress. Unfortunately, the patient died suddenly in the hospital, and the probable diagnosis was a PE secondary to DVT.

Discussion

Planning surgery for parasagittal meningiomas requires a precise assessment of the main cortical veins around the tumor. These vessels are essential in draining normal brain parenchyma to the SSS, and the patency of the sinus is paramount. These veins are crucial when making a final decision about the extent of resection [3, 4, 6, 11]. Although the goal of most surgeries should be gross total tumor resection, sometimes leaving some residual tumor around draining veins or where they lead into the sinus is necessary to preserve normal venous drainage and outflow from adjacent eloquent brain areas. This is especially relevant for tumors in elderly patients, and it may be the best decision to avoid postoperative transient or permanent neurological deficits [4, 11, 12].

Our patient was a young male who presented with a hyperostotic meningioma with an occlusion of the middle third of the SSS and with a cortical vein draining to the SSS near the posterior margin of the tumor. We left a small residual tumor around a cortical vein that was found entering the tumor. Despite our best efforts to preserve the vessel, the patient presented with a dense postoperative paraplegia attributed to venous compromise at the surgical site. We consider this likely a technical problem that arose during tumor dissection, one that might be avoided with better skill or by deciding to resect even less tumor in this location. The dilemma of total vs. subtotal resection for these tumors thus remains unsolved for neurosurgeons.

The neurological deficit started to improve at the end of the first postoperative week. However, a second complication stopped the promising resolution of the neurological deficit: sudden respiratory distress and arrest, most likely from a fatal PE due to a DVT.

Preventing deep venous thrombosis in general neurosurgery can be accomplished intra- and postoperatively, by employing intermittent sequential pneumatic compression boots plus compression stockings and via early postoperative mobilization. In addition, the administration of low-molecular-weight heparin [8–10, 13–16] appears to effectively support these measures.

The incidence of deep venous thrombosis without the use of intermittent pneumatic compression boots was as high as almost 9.9%, which is significantly worse than the 3.5% seen in patients using intermittent pneumatic compression. This translates to a relative risk reduction in 64% and 52% of patients for DVT and PE, respectively, when using intermittent pneumatic compression [14]. African/Black genetic ancestry, older age, the location of the tumor in the skull base, overweight, inpatient status, impaired sensorium, nonelective cases, steroid use, ventilator use, and time from admission to surgery greater than 4 days are reported as preoperative risk factors for venous thromboembolism. Being in class 4 or higher among the American Society of Anesthesiologists (ASA) classes; cumulative, postoperative ventilation for longer than 48 h; returning to the operating room; and infection are also reported as additional intraoperative and postoperative risk factors for the development of thromboembolic complications [13, 17, 18].

Specifically for meningioma surgery, comparing the use of purely mechanical measures (compression stocking and intermittent pneumatic compression) and mechanical measures in combination with the application of heparin after surgery (unfractionated or low-molecular-weight heparin) has resulted in reduced DVT and PE rates for those patients in whom heparin was used, with better results from low-molecular-weight heparin [17–19]. Of note, this has not led to the introduction of pharmacological prophylaxis as a standard of care, because several studies have suggested that the use of prophylactic heparin increases the incidence of intracranial hemorrhage [8–10, 16]. Therefore, prophylactic heparin should be used with care, balancing the pros and cons individually for each patient.

In the patient in our case report, early mobilization was impossible because of his profound paraparesis, and the other mechanical measures for prophylaxis were used, but no low-molecular-weight heparin. Whether the addition of medical prophylaxis would have prevented this tragic complication remains an open question.

Conclusion

A preoperative assessment of the cortical veins around parasagittal tumors and the use of meticulous microsurgical techniques when operating at this site and when cortical veins are involved are essential for avoiding postoperative neurological deficits in patients with parasagittal meningiomas. Options for complication avoidance include the decision to leave a small residual tumor on parasagittal vessels or the habit of not employing rigid retractor systems during dissection. The intraoperative use of intraoperative corticogram (ICG) is also an option to monitor the patency of parasagittal vessels during microdissection.

The intra- and postoperative use of intermittent pneumatic compression, the use of compression stockings, and postoperative early mobilization are recommended as the most effective measures for preventing DVT and PE. Eventually, low-molecular-weight heparin may be used in certain cases after balancing the pros and cons for individual patients.

Conflict of Interest Statement The authors have no conflict of interest concerning the reported materials or methods.

References

1. Ostrom QT, Cioffi G, Gittleman H, Patil N, Waite K, Kruchko C, Barnholtz-Sloan JS. CBTRUS statistical report: primary brain and other central nervous system tumors diagnosed in the United States in 2012-2016. Neuro-Oncology. 2019;21(5):1–100.
2. Brodbelt AR, Barclay ME, Greenberg D, Williams M, Jenkinson MD, Karabatsou K. The outcome of patients with surgically treated meningioma in England: 1999–2013. A cancer registry data analysis. Br J Neurosurg. 2019;33:641–7. https://doi.org/10.1080/02688697.2019.1661965.
3. DiMeco F, Li KW, Casali C, Ciceri E, Giombini S, Filippini G, Broggi G. Meningiomas invading the superior sagittal sinus: surgical experience in 108 cases. Neurosurgery. 2004;55:1263–72. https://doi.org/10.1227/01.NEU.0000143373.74160.F2.
4. Mathiesen T. Parasagittal meningiomas. Meningiomas, part II (3rd series). Handb Clin Neurol. 2020;170:93–100. https://doi.org/10.1016/b978-0-12-822198-3.00031-8.
5. Mubeen B, Makhdoomi R, Nayil K, Rafiq D, Kirmani A, Salim O, Mustafa F, Aimen A, Khursheed A, Bashir S, Shafi S, Ramzan A. Clinicopathological characteristics of meningiomas: experience from a tertiary care hospital in the Kashmir Valley. Asian J Neurosurg. 2029;14:41–6. https://doi.org/10.4103/ajns.AJNS_228_16.
6. Eichberg DG, Casabella AM, Menaker SA, Shah AH, Komotar RJ. Parasagittal and parafalcine meningiomas: integral strategy for optimizing safety and retrospective review of a single surgeon series. Br J Neurosurg. 2020;34(5):559–64. https://doi.org/10.1080/02688697.2019.1635988.
7. Magill ST, Theodosopoulos PV, McDermott MW. Resection of falx and parasagittal meningioma: complication avoidance. J Neuro-Oncol. 2016;130(2):253–62. https://doi.org/10.1007/s11060-016-2283-x.
8. Chibbaro S, Cebula H, Todeschi J, Fricia M, Vigouroux D, Abid H, Kourbanhoussen H, Pop R, Nannavecchia B, Gubian A, Prisco L, Ligarotti GKI, Proust F, Ganau M. Evolution of prophylaxis protocols for venous thromboembolism in neurosurgery: results from a prospective comparative study on low-molecular-weight heparin, elastic stockings, and intermittent pneumatic compression devices. World Neurosurg. 2018;109:e510–6. https://doi.org/10.1016/j.wneu.2017.10.012.
9. Hamilton MG, Yee WH, Hull RD, Gali WA. Venous thromboembolism prophylaxis in patients undergoing cranial neurosurgery: a systematic review and meta-analysis. Neurosurgery. 2011;68:571–81. https://doi.org/10.1227/NEU.0b013e3182093145.
10. Salmaggi A, Simonetti G, Trevisan E, Beecher D, Carapella CM, DiMeco F, Conti L, Pace A, Filippini G. Perioperative thromboprophylaxis in patients with craniotomy for brain tumours: a systematic review. J Neuro-Oncol. 2013;2013(113):293–303. https://doi.org/10.1007/s11060-013-1115-5.
11. Wang X, Wang M-Y, Qian K, Chen L, Zhang F-C. Classification and protection of peritumoral draining veins of parasagittal and falcine meningiomas. World Neurosurg. 2018;117:e362–70. https://doi.org/10.1016/j.wneu.2018.06.037.
12. Munich SA, Eddelman D, Byrne RW. Retrospective review of a venous sparing approach to resection of parasagittal meningiomas. J Clin Neurosci. 2019;64:194–200. https://doi.org/10.1016/j.jocn.2019.02.013.
13. Algattas H, Kimmell KT, Vates GE, Jahromi BS. Analysis of venous thromboembolism risk in patients undergoing craniotomy. World Neurosurg. 2015;84(5):1372–9. https://doi.org/10.1016/j.wneu.2015.06.033.
14. Frisius J, Ebeling M, Karst M, Fahlbusch R, Schedel I, Gerganov V, Samii A, Lüdemann W. Prevention of venous thromboembolic complications with and without intermittent pneumatic compression in neurosurgical cranial procedures using intraoperative magnetic resonance imaging. A retrospective analysis. Clin Neurol Neurosurg. 2015;133:46–54. https://doi.org/10.1016/j.clineuro.2015.03.005.
15. Ganau M, Prisco L, Cebula H, Todeschi J, Abid H, Ligarotti G, Pop R, Proust F, Chibbaro S. Risk of deep vein thrombosis in neurosurgery: state of the art on prophylaxis protocols and best clinical practices. J Clin Neurosci. 2017;45:60–6. https://doi.org/10.1016/j.jocn.2017.08.008.
16. Wang X, Zhou YC, Zhu WD, Sun Y, Fu P, Lei DQ, Zhao HY. The risk of postoperative hemorrhage and efficacy of heparin for preventing deep vein thrombosis and pulmonary embolism in adult patients undergoing neurosurgery: a systematic review and meta-analysis. J Investig Med. 2017;65(8):1136–46. https://doi.org/10.1136/jim-2016-000235.
17. Eisenring CV, Neidert MC, Sabanés Bové D, Held L, Sarnthein J, Krayenbühl N. Reduction of thromboembolic events in meningioma surgery: a cohort study of 724 consecutive patients. PLoS ONE. 2013;8(11):e79170. https://doi.org/10.1371/journal.pone.0079170.
18. Hoefnagel D, Kwee LE, van Putten EHP, Kros JM, Dirven CMF, Dammers R. The incidence of postoperative thromboembolic complications following surgical resection of intracranial meningioma. A retrospective study of a large single center patient cohort. Clin Neurol Neurosurg. 2014;123:150–4. https://doi.org/10.1016/j.clineuro.2014.06.001.
19. Moussa WMM, Mohamed MAA. Prophylactic use of anticoagulation and hemodilution for the prevention of venous thromboembolic events following meningioma surgery. Clin Neurol Neurosurg. 2016;144:1–6. https://doi.org/10.1016/j.clineuro.2016.02.040.

Complications in Neuroendoscopy

Alberto Delitala and Benedetta Fazzolari

Abstract

Neuroendoscopy complications can be divided into three categories: vascular, neural, and technical failures. Moreover, cognitive sequelae can be considered as delayed complications of neuroendoscopic surgery. The purpose of this manuscript is to report the experiences published in the current literature in order to identify the causes of complications in neuroendoscopy and methods to manage and avoid them.

Keywords

Neurosurgery · Neuroendoscopy · Endoscopic ventricular surgery · Complications · Management · Avoidance

Abbreviations

ETV Endoscopic third ventriculostomy
MRI Magnetic resonance imaging

Introduction

Neuroendoscopy, understood as endoscopic intracranial surgery, has made progress in recent decades thanks to advances in optics, illumination, miniaturization, and computer technology, which allow surgeons to approach some pathologies with reduced parenchymal exposure, manipulation, and trauma. The intracranial endoscopy's field of interest includes disorders such as hydrocephalus, cysts, and neoplasms. Among these, ventricular endoscopy is a minimally invasive procedure that can be both diagnostic and therapeutic, but it is not risk-free, and the reported complications—intraventricular hemorrhage, parenchymal contusions, and technical failures—can be significant.

Materials and Methods

A bibliographic search of PubMed/Medline was performed using the following keywords: "endoscopic surgery complications," "neuro-endoscopy complications," and "ventricular surgery complications." Medline, Scopus, PubMed publishers, and DiscoverySapienza were searched as well. As inclusion criteria, we selected the original clinical studies that covered ventricular neuroendoscopy surgery. Papers referring to endoscopic endonasal transsphenoidal surgery were excluded, as were literature reviews. We identified one guideline document, published as "Complications in Neurosurgery" in 2018 in Elsevier. Relevant sections from works in the published literature and the guidance document were then assessed in full in two stages: the first aimed to determined key methodological steps, and the second aimed to reduce biases and eliminate irrelevant and low-quality studies.

Results

Rehder et al. [1] distinguished three orders of surgical complications: vascular injury, neural injury, and technical failure. Vascular injury is the most common complication presenting as intraventricular bleeding—often due to injuring small subependymal vessels. This can simply be managed via irrigation: choosing the endoscope (flexible or rigid) that is most suitable for the given type of procedure to be performed can largely avoid the occurrence of this type of complication. On the other hand, hemorrhage from a larger vessel can significantly impair operative visibility, and copious irrigation with Ringer's lactate solution will help treat the injury proper. However, leaving an external drainage and

A. Delitala
San Carlo di Nancy Hospital, Rome, Italy

B. Fazzolari (✉)
Neurosurgery Division, Lancisi Department, San Camillo Forlanini Hospital, Rome, Italy

K. Turel, E. M. Kasper (eds.), *Complications in Neurosurgery II*, Acta Neurochirurgica Supplement 133,
https://doi.org/10.1007/978-3-031-61601-3_6

ending the procedure may be necessary. During an intraventricular hemorrhage, irrigation must be carried out via the exit port of the endoscope, which must be open to allow the washout to occur without increasing the intracerebral pressure. The most feared bleeding is the one that occurs from injuring the basilar artery during endoscopic third ventriculostomy (ETV) while fenestrating the floor of the third ventricle. This catastrophic complication is reported in 1% of cases [2, 3]. How can this complication be avoided? Begin the fenestration of the floor of the third ventricle closer to the dorsum sellae, anteriorly in the third ventricle floor. Neural damage can occur along the endoscope trajectory, with an incidence ranging from 3% to 4% [4], and this can include damaging deep neural structures such as the fornices, mammillary bodies, hypothalamus, thalamus, brain stem, and cranial nerves, which could result in significant new neurological deficits. Lastly, technical failure occurs when procedural interruption is necessary to treat complications or life-threatening injuries (Figs. 1, 2, and 3).

Parenchymal tumors, as gliomas or oligodendrogliomas, are often associated with a higher than most metastatic tumors hemorrhage rate: copious warm lactate Ringer solution irrigation may allow for the visualization of the site of bleeding for the subsequent bipolar cautery of the site. Alternatively, a small cotton patty can be carried down the endoscope cannula and used for tamponade; in most cases, warm irrigation will cause the cessation of the bleeding. In cases of residual oozing, a ventricular drain is left in the endoscopy tract on completion.

Neurocognitive sequelae are likely underreported because of intraoperative damage caused to the fornix, mamillary bodies, anterior thalamus, hypothalamus, or hippocampal formation and fibers. The most common neurocognitive complication after ventricular neuroendoscopy is memory impairment, specifically anterograde amnesia, along with

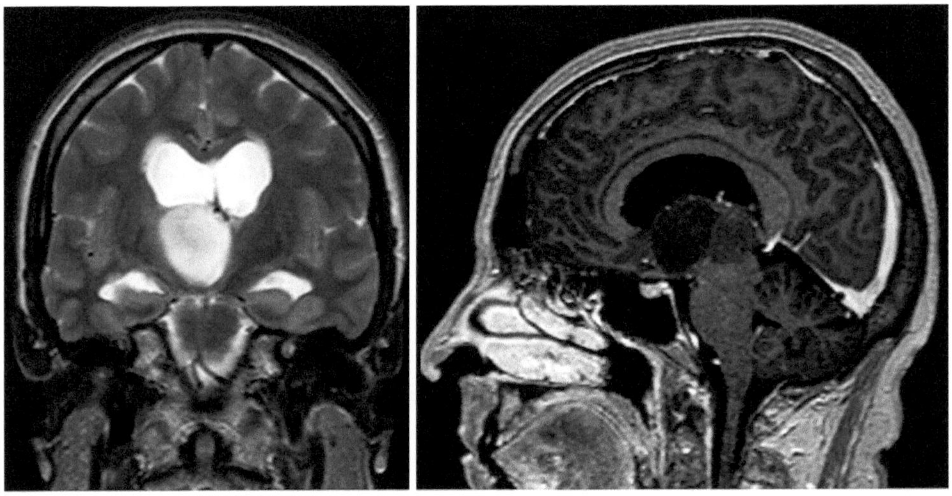

Fig. 1 (left, right) 55-year-old female patient. Anaplastic astrocytoma (III WHO) of the third ventricle: (left) T2-weighted MRI scan shows a hyperintense mass without a clear cleavage to the right diencephalon, which moves the lateral wall of third ventricle to the other side; (right) a sagittal T1-weighted gadolinium scan shows the continuity of the tumor with the hypothalami and the high vascularity around it

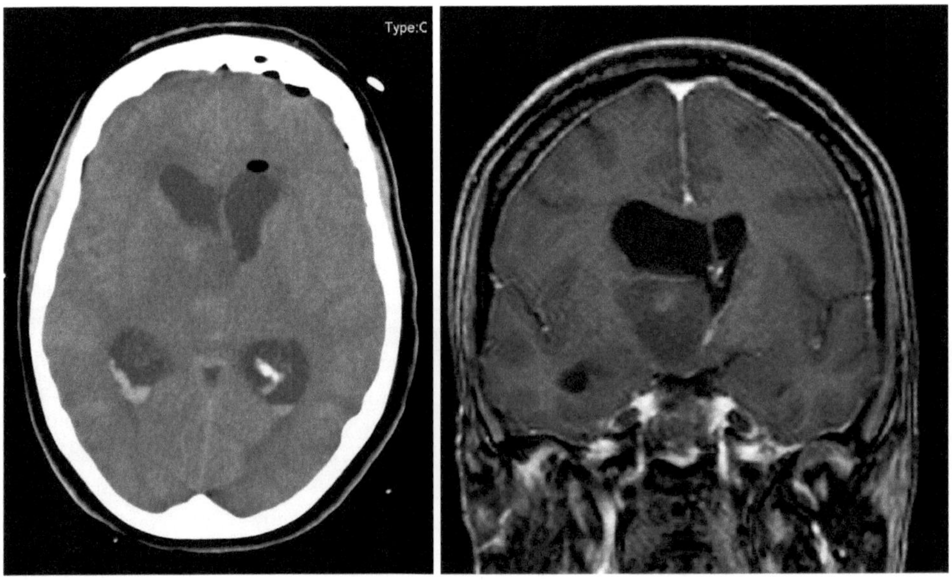

Fig. 2 (left, right) 55-year-old female patient. Anaplastic astrocytoma (III WHO) of the third ventricle: (left) during neuroendoscopic biopsy, severe bleeding was coming from the vascularity of the tumor, and the procedure needed to be interrupted and a ventricular drainage left; (right) MRI scan of T1-weighted gadolinium on the left and FLAIR-weighted on the right, during hospitalization, shows ependymitis and the residual tumor left

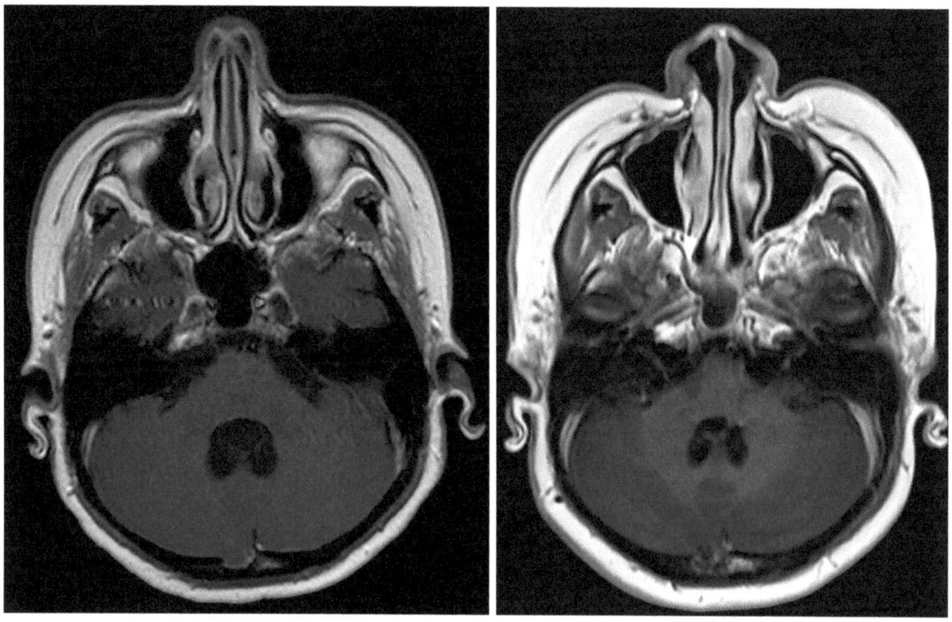

Fig. 3 (left, right) 36-year-old female patient. Fourth ventricle neurocysticercosis: (left) MRI T1-weighted scan of gadolinium in axial plane shows the rounded edge of the cyst. The patient has been submitted to endoscopic third ventriculostomy, but the ventricular walls were covered with a hard fibrous layer that did not allow for the correct recognition of the floor structures. An attempt was made to perforate the ependyma, but the peripontine cistern still could not be reached. A ventricular drainage was left. (right) MRI T1-weighted scan of gadolinium after six months, from ventricular peritoneal shunt positioning

psychiatric disorders and an associated decline in executive function. The fornix is the major tract connecting the hippocampal formation to the mamillary bodies, from which the projection goes to the hypothalamus, the thalamus, and the medial temporal regions—all these structures being involved in memory circuits and other important cognitive skills, such as executive functions [5]. Indeed, lesions in these structures are often associated with temporal lobe and diencephalic amnesia beyond executive function disorder. Furthermore, the fibers of the limbic system (fornix-hippocampus-mamillary bodies) are connected with the amygdala complex and the orbitofrontal cortex, both key areas involved in controlling emotions, decision-making, and social cognition.

Discussion

According to Rehder et al., "Unexpected events can be prevented by understanding the underlying causes of the pathologies. Overall, many complications can be avoided by selecting the right candidate for the procedure, having the most appropriate instrumentation, and having a thorough knowledge of the anatomy and pathology" [1]. The components of a distorted ventricular anatomy can thus be risk factors resulting in complications. Furthermore, patients with hydrocephalus or myelomeningocele can present with a number of anatomic variations: vertically oriented third ventricular floor, thickened massa intermedia, and hindbrain descent [6]. A careful preoperative analysis of magnetic resonance images (MRIs) should help to prevent a significant number of intraoperative complications. We strongly suggest using neuronavigation for intraoperative guidance by obtaining T1 gadolinium and T2 three-dimensional MRI sequencies, which are then loaded onto a surgical navigation system to guide the surgeon through the anatomy of the procedure. Chowdhry et al. [7] suggested "routinely" using neuronavigation for a more accurate selection of the entry point and trajectory; on the other hand, these authors stated that they did not use the pneumatic arm of the endoscope for every procedure but rather only in selected (usually lengthy) cases. Pneumatic device drift requires adjusting the position of the device at the beginning of each step during surgery to compensate for its downward drift.

Intraventricular neuroendoscopy permits the inspection of the ventricular system, tumor biopsy and resection, intraventricular cyst fenestration or resection, the irrigation and removal of hemorrhage, and the treatment of hydrocephalus. It is particularly useful for taking a biopsy of obstructive lesions within the posterior third ventricle because it allows for the concomitant treatment of the associated hydrocephalus with a third ventriculostomy. Employing endoscopic approaches in neurosurgery is optimal for tumors with an exophytic intraventricular component. Biopsy or tumor removal is suitable through cupped biopsy forceps, which can be rotated to free the tissue sample; tumor resection can be undertaken for small, low-vascularized lesions with a friable consistency. We suggest using neuronavigation strictly for the planning of a safe trajectory and for choosing the best entry site. For tumors extending below the ependymal surface, neuronavigation can be used to identify the location of the tumor through the ventricular ependyma.

A classic indication for endoscopic surgery is when patients present with third ventricle colloid cysts. These benign tumors are difficult to surgically remove because of their deep position, where they are surrounded by critical tributaries, veins, hypothalami, and fornices. Ventricular shunt placement alone has historically been used for the treatment of colloid cysts in patients who could not tolerate a craniotomy for many morbidities. Today, the endoscopic removal or aspiration of such a colloid cyst is considered the standard of treatment by many authors and can also be offered to patients with multiple comorbidities. A single intervention for only the aspiration of cysts has been found to be associated with a high rate of recurrence, and nowadays, the best option of treatment is total or subtotal endoscopic or microsurgical removal, which is curative. This leaves ventricular shunt placement as a temporary treatment for cases presenting with acute hydrocephalus. Alternatively, open microsurgical removal can be performed via a transcortical-transventricular route or via a classic transcallosal-transventricular approach with transforaminal/interforniceal or subchoroidal access to the third ventricle. However, neuroendoscopy has the advantage of being the fastest surgery by providing a small access corridor through the parenchyma and the ventricular cavities to reach the colloid cyst. This minimizes the dimension of the cortical and subcortical dissection and has been shown to reduce overall morbidity, reduce operative time, and decrease the duration of a patient's hospital stay. Many centers employ both endoscopic and microsurgical techniques, reserving microsurgery for the larger cysts or for complex cases. According to a literature review of large surgical series by Margetis and Souweidane [8], a comparison of microsurgery with the neuroendoscopy technique shows that endoscopic cases have a minor complication rate of 8.5%, whereas microsurgical cases have a rate of 10.5%—a difference that is not statistically significant. According to Gronding's system of classifying complications, resection is associated with a lower rate of major complications in endoscopic cases (ca 5%) than in microsurgical cases (ca 14%). However, the recurrence rate and subtotal resection rate were significantly higher in the endoscopically treated patient cohort.

During sharp dissection and electrocautery, the aspiration of cyst contents should be performed under the direct visualization of the cyst wall: During this step of the procedure, gauging the strength of the applied suction is very helpful in that it enables one to act swiftly if the choroid plexus is inadvertently aspirated. With a partial or complete evacuation, the cyst membrane can be carefully drawn into the foramen with grasping forceps. This maneuver positions the lesion into the line of sight for continued aspiration and further coagulation. Frequently, the cyst is entirely evacuated of contents, leaving only a cyst wall/adherent membrane. At this stage, sharp dissection may not always be safe, because of cyst membrane bleeding or dense adherences.

Moreover, some studies have analyzed the iatrogenic compromise of cognitive and emotional deficits following neuroendoscopy procedures. Despite the notion that neuroendoscopy has been considered as a minimally invasive surgery, some neurocognitive complications after ventricular neuroendoscopy are difficult to assess—e.g., hydrocephalus and lesions within the ventricles might be the cause for neurocognitive impairment. In a relevant study, Soleman et al. [5] reported a rate of 2% for transient cognitive impairment and 1% for permanent cognitive impairment after various ventricular neuroendoscopic surgeries. The most common complication during neuroendoscopic procedures with a rigid endoscope is a contusion of the fornix, which can be avoided by using a flexible endoscope. However, navigating within the ventricle by using a flexible endoscope requires some experience, and light intensity and optics are inferior in this setting. Endoscopic working channels are also more restricted than those available in a rigid endoscope.

Lastly, according to Agrawal et al. [9], the complication rates for any procedure decrease as the experience of the surgeon increases. The need to include formal training programs in neuroendoscopy is due to the longer learning curve for endoscopic surgery than the one for conventional microneurosurgery: Here, the use of the endoscope requires dexterity and hand-eye coordination, which some surgeons consider the main pitfalls of neuroendoscopy. Laboratory training should become an integral part of any super-specialty course.

Conflict of Interest Statement The authors have no conflict of interest to declare.

References

1. Rehder R, Cohen AR. Complications in ventricular surgery. In: Complication in neurosurgery, vol. 38. Amsterdam: Elsevier; 2018. p. 218–23.
2. Schroeder HWS, Oertel J, Gaab MR. Incidence of complications in neuroendoscopic surgery. Childs Nerv Syst. 2004;20:878–83.
3. Grand W, Leonardo J, Chamczuk AJ, Korus AJ. Endoscopic third ventriculostomy in 250 adults with hydrocephalus: patient selection, outcomes, and complications. Neurosurgery. 2016;78(1):109–19.
4. Beems T, Grotenhuis JA. Long-term complications and definition of failure of neuroendoscopic procedures. Childs Nerv Syst. 2004;20(11–12):868–77.
5. Soleman J, Guzman R. Neurocognitive complications after ventricular neuroendoscopy: a systematic review. Behav Neurol. 2020;2020:2536319.
6. Ganjoo P, Sethi S, Tandon MS, Singh D, Pandey BC. Perioperative complications of intraventricular neuroendoscopy: a 7-year experience. Turk Neurosurg. 2010;20(1):33–8.
7. Chowdhry SA, Cohen AR. Intraventricular neuroendoscopy: complication avoidance and management. World Neurosurg. 2013;79(2S):S15.
8. Margetis K, Souweidane MM. Endoscopic treatment of intraventricular cystic tumors. World Neurosurg. 2013;79(2S):S19.
9. Agrawal A, Kato Y, Sano H, Kanno T. The incorporation of neuroendoscopy in neurosurgical training programs. World Neurosurg. 2013;79(2S):S15.

Postoperative CSF Rhinorrhoea

Aniruddha Bhagwat, Chandrashekhar Deopujari, Nishit Shah, and Vikram Karmarkar

Abstract

Cerebrospinal fluid (CSF) rhinorrhoea is a well known complication following skull base surgery. Identifying the site of leak is the most important determinant for the appropriate approach in the further management of the case. Either transcranial or transnasal approaches may be used, alone or in combination, as deemed appropriate. The success of the repair depends on the site of the fistula, the timing of surgery, and patient factors. Discussion of two illustrative cases is presented here to describe the challenges faced by the neurosurgeon in the recognition and the immediate and definitive management of postoperative CSF rhinorrhoea and various strategies for a successful outcome in their repair.

Keywords

CSF rhinorrhoea · Endoscopic endonasal skull base repair · Clivectomy · Nasoseptal flap

Introduction

CSF leak remains a common complication of neurosurgical procedures with dural transgression, ranging from a simple burr hole for ventricular access to major craniospinal procedures. This has the potential to not only increase the morbidity but also to cause mortality, due to increased risk of infection. Some regions, in particular the skull base and the posterior fossa, appear more susceptible than others to developing a CSF leak [1–5].

Apart from the choice of a particular surgical procedure, patient factors such as accompanying hydrocephalus or persistent raised intracranial pressure (ICP) also influence the outcome. Like many postoperative complications, CSF leak is best anticipated and prevented rather than treated. This is especially true for skull base surgical procedures because any leak in direct communication with the paranasal sinuses translates into a greater chance of developing meningitis. Recently, increasing use of extended endoscopic skull base procedures involving the excision of large areas of dura and bone has amplified this issue, which has led to descriptions of several innovative reconstruction techniques.

In this report, we present two representative cases to illustrate the etiopathology of this complication for its timely recognition and management, and to emphasize adhering to the principles of preventive and prompt corrective measures.

Case 1

A 67-year-old male patient presented with generalized weakness, emotional lability, and short-term memory loss over the preceding few weeks. Examination revealed no sensorimotor or cranial nerve deficits. Contrast-enhanced MRI (CEMRI) revealed a large right frontal lesion across the midline, with solid and cystic areas and areas of patchy contrast enhancement. A high-grade glioma was suspected and, the patient was advised to undergo surgery for decompression and histopathological confirmation.

A bicoronal flap was raised and a right frontal craniotomy performed, with care taken to avoid opening the frontal sinus. Tumour decompression was carried out via the right middle frontal gyrus, and a maximal safe resection was performed. Large thrombosed vessels and necrotic areas were encountered, further confirming the diagnosis of glioblastoma (GBM). A radical decompression was carried out while avoiding opening of the ventricle. The dura was closed with monofilament absorbable sutures and augmented with a pericranial flap. The bone was replaced and fixed to the native bone. The wound was closed in layers. Histopathology confirmed the GBM.

The patient was mobilized the next day, and he developed clear nasal discharge after initial mobilization. A postopera-

A. Bhagwat · C. Deopujari (✉) · N. Shah · V. Karmarkar
Bombay Hospital and Institute of Medical Sciences, Mumbai, India

K. Turel, E. M. Kasper (eds.), *Complications in Neurosurgery II*, Acta Neurochirurgica Supplement 133,
https://doi.org/10.1007/978-3-031-61601-3_7

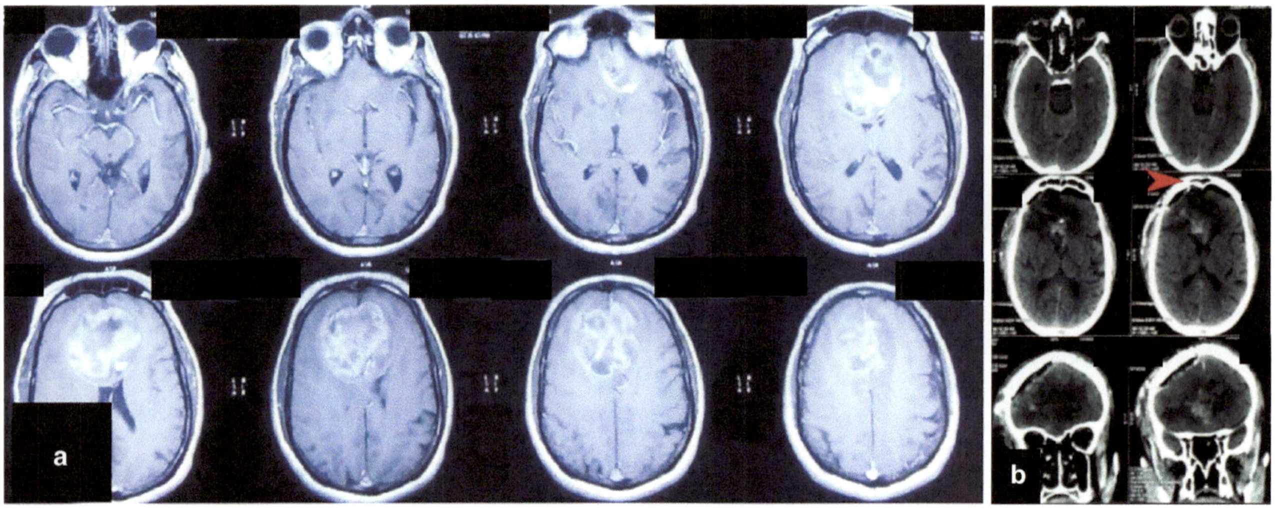

Fig. 1 (**a**) Preop CEMRI heterogeneously demonstrating an enhancing intra-axial lesion in the frontal midline that reaches the skull base. (**b**) Postop CT brain. No evidence of CSF collection in the frontal sinus, nasal cavity, or extradural space. The red arrowhead points to a possible injury to the superolateral recess of the right frontal sinus

tive computed tomography (CT) scan did not reveal any pneumocephalus, any bony defect either in the posterior wall of the frontal sinus or in the skull base, or any local CSF pooling (Fig. 1). The patient was advised conservative management consisting of bed rest with slow mobilization and antibiotics for a total of 7 days. No further episode of rhinorrhoea took place after his initial mobilisation in the following week, and he was discharged.

Radiotherapy was instituted two weeks after surgery. During the last week of fractionated radiotherapy, the patient developed another episode of CSF rhinorrhoea, which settled with conservative management, consisting of per oral (PO) acetazolamide to decrease CSF production and pressure. One month later, the patient presented with fever and signs of meningitis. A CT scan at this point in time revealed the possibility of a frontal abscess. Upon surgical exploration, a small opening in the frontal sinus was revealed, which was repaired after the abscess was drained. Postoperative antibiotic therapy was implemented, but unfortunately, the patient succumbed to the infection.

Case 2

A 28-year-old woman presented with complaints of tingling and numbness in all four limbs and imbalance while walking, for a duration of about 1 year. Examination revealed hyperreflexia in all limbs with bilateral extensor plantar responses. Hoffman's sign was present. Contrast-enhanced MRI revealed a lobulated lesion involving the clivus and anterior craniovertebral junction (CVJ) that reached the anterior arch of C1. There was considerable lateral extension as well as significant mass effect on the brain stem. The patient underwent a transoral surgery for biopsy at another centre and was subjected to fractionated radiotherapy. As the patient continued to worsen even 3 months after the completion of radiation, they were referred to us for further management.

The patient underwent, as a first step, an occipitocervical fusion up to the C3 lateral masses to treat the instability due to condylar and facetal erosion. This was followed by an endonasal endoscopic resection of the tumour, which required significant clivectomy and resection of the anterior arch of the C1 and dens. During surgery, considerable dural erosion and an intradural extension of the tumour were noted. Fragments of the tumour adherent to the vertebral arteries and in the extreme lateral recesses of the exposure were not aggressively removed. Because of considerable dural resection along with the tumour, a CSF fistula was created in the process. This defect was plugged with autologous fat, the dural defect was bridged with fascia lata. Lastly, a pedicled nasoseptal flap was placed and glued over the bony edges to create a three-layered reconstruction (Fig. 2). A nasal pack was placed to keep the graft in place.

The patient experienced CSF rhinorrhoea on postoperative day 5 after the removal of the nasal packs. She was taken back to the operating room (OR) the next day. The original repair was taken apart because a small leak from one of the graft corners was observed (at about the 1 o'clock position) with slight displacement off the flap. The arachnoid defect was further plugged with a larger blob of autologous fat, and sealed with fibrin glue. The dural defect was again covered with fascia lata, and then the entire construct was overlaid with readjustment of the same pedicled nasoseptal flap.

The patient recovered well, and oral feeding was resumed on postoperative day 5 of the second surgery. The patient was

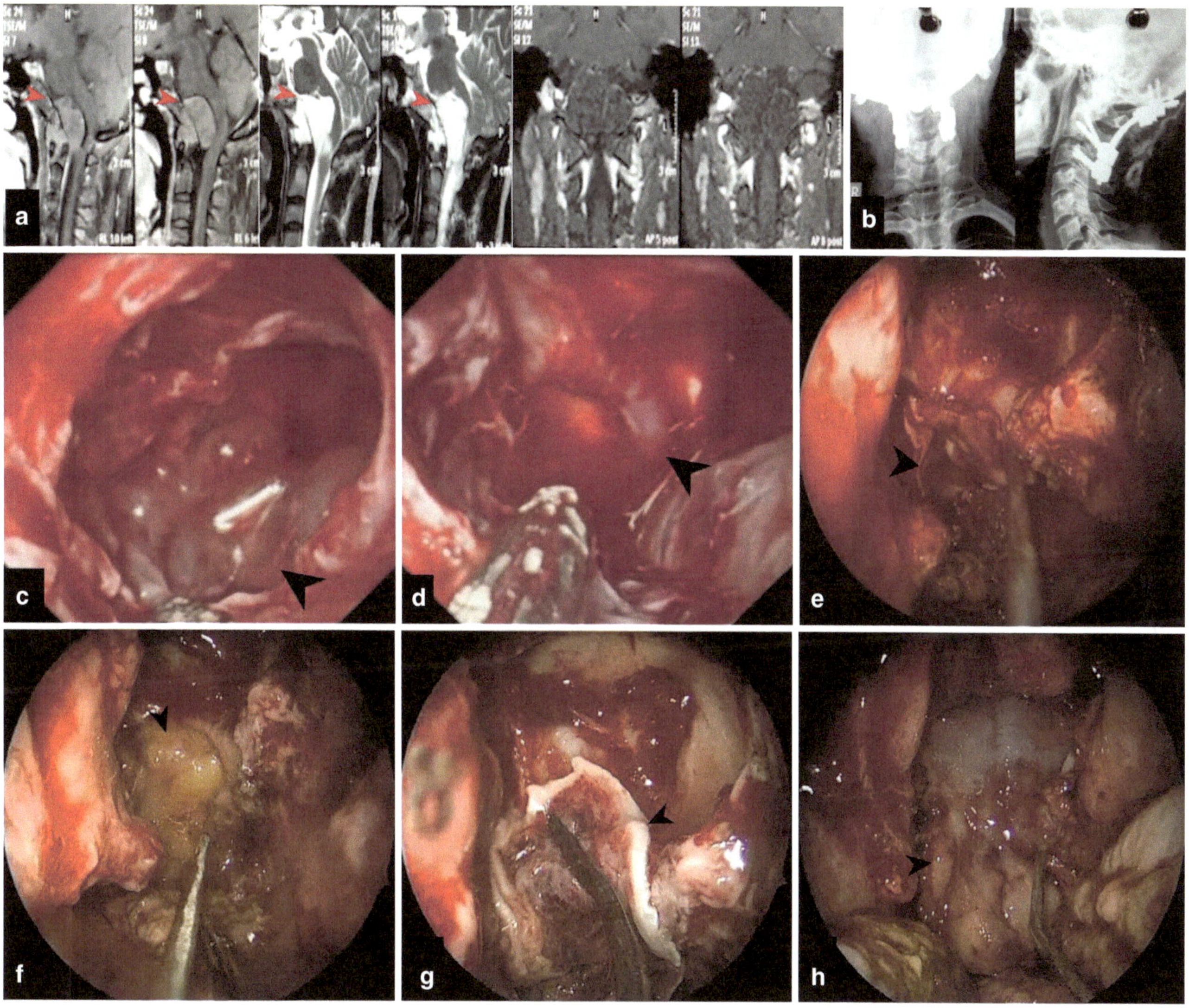

Fig. 2 (**a**) Preop CEMRI showing the lesion in the lower clivus extending to the CVJ. Its appearance is suggestive of a chordoma. (**b**) X-ray showing the instrumented fusion of CVJ performed before surgery. (**c**) Intraoperative view of the excision of the intradural component of the tumour. CSF fistula can be seen (black arrowhead). (**d**) Left vertebral artery seen cleared of tumour. (**e**) Dural opening repaired by using fascia lata graft and sealed with fibrin glue. (**f**) CSF leak repair using fat graft and sealed with fibrin glue. (**g**) Fascia lata graft laid over fat graft. (**h**) Pedicled nasoseptal flap placed over the fascia and sealed with fibrin glue

referred for proton beam therapy. She has responded well and has remained disease-free for over 6 years, at last follow-up.

Discussion

The phenomenon of CSF rhinorrhoea was first described by Greek physician Galen in the second century CE [6] in post-traumatic cases, and he postulated that fluid leaked into the nose through the pituitary and ethmoid regions. In 1826, Miller reported a case of CSF rhinorrhoea in a hydrocephalic child and described the communication between nasal and cranial cavities at autopsy. In 1926, Walter Dandy was the first surgeon to describe the intradural repair of a CSF fistula. The techniques were further developed and refined through the efforts of Dandy et al. [6].

In the context of surgical results, CSF neither forgives nor forgets, and a tardy or dural closure will frequently result in a CSF leak. This can become a frustrating, potentially recurrent problem for the surgeon, resulting in unanticipated morbidity and mortality and in the escalation of treatment costs [7]. The rates of postoperative meningitis may rise almost 15-fold because of a CSF leak [3].

More recently, a number of materials have been described for dural closure, including biological, semisynthetic, and synthetic dural substitutes as well as sealing glues. Such materials have been used individually and also in combination. The use of various techniques is frequently reported in the literature [8].

Postcraniotomy leaks can be classified according to their location: supratentorial, posterior fossa, or skull base. These differ in terms of incidence and difficulty in management [8]. The CRANIAL study sought to evaluate the incidence and determinants of postoperative CSF rhinorrhoea in endoscopic endonasal transsphenoidal and extended skull base surgeries, and the study also attempted to evaluate the techniques of CSF leak repair [9]. A preliminary analysis implicates the following factors: the size of the defect, the volume of the intraoperative CSF leak, the nature and size of the tumour/pathology, previous irradiation, systemic factors, a high body mass index (BMI), surgeon experience, and most importantly, the technique used for the reconstruction of the skull base defect. A survey conducted by the authors of the study revealed significant heterogeneity in the use of repair techniques by various neurosurgeons; however, most centres use a staged approach in constructing the repair, depending on the presumed probability of postoperative CSF fistula formation.

Planned or accidental frontal sinus opening during bifrontal craniotomy is rather common, especially when the lower edge of the craniotomy has to be flush with the floor of the anterior cranial fossa (ACF) [10]. The superior and lateral recesses of the frontal sinus are also susceptible to injury during unifrontal or pterional craniotomy [11]. The usual strategy to repair this type of opening is to exenterate the mucosal lining of the sinus, plug the frontonasal duct, perform the cranialization or obliteration of the frontal sinus proper, and carry out meticulous dural repair. To separate the intracranial compartment from the paranasal sinus environment, an autologous vascularised tissue layer is added, and the dura is usually overlaid with a pedicled galeopericranial flap as a buttress. When this is not available—because of a previous surgery, radiotherapy, or trauma—alternatives such as a pedicled temporalis fascia graft or a free tissue graft may be used. Adjuvant chemotherapy and radiotherapy have been known to impair healing and predispose patients to CSF leaks, at times even in place not close to the original site of the surgery [5, 12].

In cases (such as case 1 in this article) where the communication is not realized at surgery and only later discovered postoperatively when the leak occurs; he first task then is to localize the site—either the cribriform plate or the frontal sinus. This is most readily achieved by using a combination of high-resolution CT and MR cisternography. A cribriform leak is more amenable to conservative therapy, including diuretics, bed rest, and lumbar drainage, and its repair may be carried out through an extracranial approach, namely the endoscopic endonasal route, without having to reopen the craniotomy. A frontal sinus leak, on the other hand, is less likely to settle with conservative measures and therefore more likely to result in meningitis. It is also exceedingly difficult to approach endoscopically, especially in cases when the surgeon needs to reach the superior and lateral recesses [13]. Such a case would thus demand an immediate re-exploration of the craniotomy, with the formal opening and obliteration of the frontal sinus. In the case described above, the suspected leak stopped within a day, and a repair was not deemed necessary, especially because the surgery had been intraparenchymal without infringing the skull base dura, and the access site was repaired with adequate dural closure and galeopericranial flap augmentation. No frontal sinus opening was noted during surgery, and no pneumocephalus or paranasal sinus fluid collection was observed on the postoperative CT scan. Later, the repair was postponed at the local centre because the patient was nearing the end of his radiotherapy regimen for the GBM.

Clival region surgery is known to be prone to leaks owing to the high propensity of CSF to leak out of the posterior fossa [3, 7, 14] in surgeries involving dural opening or resection, as in case 2 in this report. The higher CSF pressure and direct communication with basal CSF cisterns exerts more pressure on any reconstruction and predisposes it to the formation of brain stem encephaloceles posterior to the pharynx [2]. The healing of midline mucoperiosteal incisions in the posterior nasopharyngeal wall is poorer than that of the rest of the nasal cavity [4]. Adding to this the contaminated nature of the corridor and constant pooling of secretions in transnasal/transoral approaches, such a setting makes postoperative CSF leak a potentially dangerous complication. Conservative management is therefore untenable in such circumstances, and an immediate revision of the surgical closure must be performed. The following steps may be taken during primary closure or secondary repair to minimize the possibility of a CSF leak:

- Use a fat graft to plug the arachnoid defect and obliterate dead space.
- Perform dural augmentation with a fascia lata graft.
- Seal the edges with fibrin glue.
- Close the pharynx in layers, where muscle and mucosa are closed separately.
- Use local pedicled flaps based on the sphenopalatine, ethmoidal, septal or pharyngeal arteries to close the defect.

We therefore recommend to create a nasoseptal flap for all skull base defects, and add a U-shaped pharyngeal flap for lower clival tumours, and overlap them [1].

Conclusion

CSF leak is a frustrating complication in neurosurgery, best managed by meticulous repair for prevention. This is especially important in patients who have undergone or who are likely to undergo radiation therapy for management of their disease. The contemporary neurosurgeon has many choices to augment the repair. Anterior skull base CSF leaks may be managed via endoscopic endonasal repair, except for frontal sinus leaks, which need urgent transcranial repair. Clival surgery is highly prone to CSF leaks. Any patient presenting with a postoperative leak must be managed with urgent definitive reconstruction, preferably using vascularized pedicled flaps to buttress the repair.

Conflict of Interest Statement The authors declare that they have no conflicts of interest.

References

1. Deopujari CE, Karmarkar VS, Shah NJ. Endoscopic approaches to the craniovertebral junction and odontoid process. World Neurosurg. 2014;82(6):S49–53.
2. Fraser S, Gardner PA, Koutourousiou M, Kubik M, Fernandez-Miranda JC, Snyderman CH, Wang EW. Risk factors associated with postoperative cerebrospinal fluid leak after endoscopic endonasal skull base surgery. J Neurosurg. 2018;128(4):1066–71.
3. Horowitz G, Fliss DM, Margalit N, Wasserzug O, Gil Z. Association between cerebrospinal fluid leak and meningitis after skull base surgery. Otolaryngol Head Neck Surg. 2011;145(4):689–93.
4. Jain VK, Behari S, Banerji D, Bhargava V, Chhabra DK. Transoral decompression for craniovertebral osseous anomalies: perioperative management dilemmas. Neurology. 1999;47(3):188–95.
5. Lee JJ, Kim HY, Dhong HJ, Chung SK, Kong DS, Nam DH, So YK, Hong SD. Delayed cerebrospinal fluid leakage after treatment of skull base tumors: case series of 9 patients. World Neurosurg. 2019;132:e591–8.
6. Tomasello F, Angileri FF, Cardali S. Prevention of cerebrospinal fluid leakage: an evergreen neurosurgical issue. World Neurosurg. 2014;81(2):261–2.
7. Grotenhuis JA. Costs of postoperative cerebrospinal fluid leakage: 1-year, retrospective analysis of 412 consecutive nontrauma cases. Surg Neurol. 2005;64(6):490–3.
8. Hutter G, Von Felten S, Sailer MH, Schulz M, Mariani L. Risk factors for postoperative CSF leakage after elective craniotomy and the efficacy of fleece-bound tissue sealing against dural suturing alone: a randomized controlled trial. J Neurosurg. 2014;121(3):735–44.
9. Khan DZ, Marcus HJ, Horsfall HL, et al. CSF Rhinorrhoea after endonasal intervention to the skull base (CRANIAL) - part 1: multicenter pilot study. World Neurosurg. 2021;149:e1077–89.
10. Wang G, Sun L, Li W, Yu J. Cerebrospinal fluid rhinorrhea in a bilateral frontal decompressive craniectomy patient caused by strenuous activity a case report. Medicine. 2018;97(47):e13189. https://doi.org/10.1097/MD.0000000000013189.
11. Woodworth BA, Schlosser RJ. Frontal sinus cerebrospinal fluid leaks. In: The frontal sinus. Heidelberg: Springer; 2005. p. 143–52.
12. Thornton BN, Sorenson JM, Shires CB. Post-radiation csf leak of skull base. Otolaryngol Neck Surg. 2014;151(1):P254.
13. Wang EW, Gardner PA, Zanation AM. International consensus statement on endoscopic skull-base surgery: executive summary. Int Forum Allergy Rhinol. 2019;9(S3):S127–44.
14. Hannan CJ, Kelleher E, Javadpour M. Methods of skull base repair following endoscopic endonasal tumor resection: a review. Front Oncol. 2020. https://doi.org/10.3389/fonc.2020.01614.

Blindness After Frontal Craniotomy

Andrey V. Dubovoy

Abstract

In our practice at our department, we have encountered two clinical cases involving the complete loss of vision and ophthalmoplegia after craniotomy on the vascular pathology of the brain. Both patients underwent microsurgery via bifrontal skin incision. In the first case, the subfrontal craniotomy on the right side was made, and then microsurgical resection of an arteriovenous malformation of the right frontal lobe was performed. In the second case, a fronto-basal interhemispheric craniotomy was made for aneurysm surgery. This surgery included an intracranial anastomosis in a side-to-side fashion between the A3 segments of both anterior cerebral arteries, and a clip was applied proximal to a fusiform aneurysm located in the A2 segment of the anterior cerebral artery. The intracranial part of the procedure was uneventful. However, upon awakening from anesthesia after surgical treatment, both patients developed bilateral amaurosis and ophthalmoplegia.

A thorough morbidity and mortality (M&M) analysis of these cases was performed, including a retrospective analysis of the clinical condition of patients and their ophthalmological status prior to surgery. Video recordings of the surgery and of anesthesia management and its records were carried out. Intraoperative iatrogenic direct damage to the cranial nerves and arteries was excluded.

From the data obtained, a putative intraoperative explanation of the decisive causative factor was highlighted: direct pressure on the eyeballs from the retracted skin flap during both surgeries.

A. V. Dubovoy (✉)
FSBI (Federal Neurosurgical Center), Ministry of Healthcare of Russia, Novosibirsk, Russia

Keywords

Postoperative loss of vision · Ischemic optic neuropathy · Frontal craniotomy complication · Postdecompressive optic neuropathy

Introduction

The loss of vision or the deterioration of vision after a craniotomy is rarely discussed in the literature, and many neurosurgeons are not even familiar with this potential complication. In neurosurgical practice, even doctors who performed an adequate surgical treatment of the indicated pathology without causing any intraoperative damage to the involved brain tissue and cranial nerves can encounter this complication in rare cases during the perioperative period. Comparable complications are known in spinal and cardiac surgery [1].

Materials and Methods

This chapter describes two cases featuring a complete loss of vision and ophthalmoplegia after surgical treatment for vascular pathologies of the brain.

Case I

A female patient, 27 years of age, was admitted to the Department of Vascular Neurosurgery of the Federal Center of Neurosurgery in Novosibirsk in February, 2016. She had been diagnosed with an arteriovenous malformation of the left frontal lobe (grade II according to Spetzler-Martin classification). As a concomitant medical condition, the patient was diagnosed with mild anemia. The patient had undergone repeated surgical treatments for high-grade myopia in 2009, 2012, and 2014. According to the data from an ophthalmological exami-

K. Turel, E. M. Kasper (eds.), *Complications in Neurosurgery II*, Acta Neurochirurgica Supplement 133,
https://doi.org/10.1007/978-3-031-61601-3_8

nation that took place prior to her neurosurgical intervention, no pathological changes of the eyeballs or pathways of vision were revealed. Visual acuity at the time of admission to the hospital was VIS = 0.7/0.7 Oculus Sinistra (OS) and Oculus Dextra (OD) (equivalent to 20/20 in other systems). The patient presented with a history of long-lasting headaches, for which she was examined and worked up with radiology (we performed MRI and DSA). This revealed a typical arteriovenous malformation (AVM) of the frontal lobe.

The patient was scheduled for admission, and a day later, standard surgical treatment was performed: A bifrontal (coronal) skin incision was made, the skin flap was retracted to the base of the skull, and a parasagittal frontal craniotomy on the left side was performed. After that, the arteriovenous malformation embedded in the left frontal lobe was resected uneventfully.

The intraoperative course was unremarkable: no intraoperative complications. The duration of the surgery was 5 h 30 min. In the early postoperative period, after emerging from anesthesia, the patient complained of a profound decrease in vision in both eyes to the level of mere light perception. Physical examination revealed reactive swelling of the upper eyelids, hyperemia of the eyelid skin in both eyes, an objective bilateral decrease in vision to the level of the light perception, and bilateral total ophthalmoplegia were noted (Fig. 1). Immediately after this physical compromise was identified, emergency CT and MRI scans of the brain and an angio-CT of the brain vessels were performed. The images revealed swelling in the retrobulbar and periorbital soft tissues on both sides, and significant enlargement of the veins in the upper half of the face.

After immediate conservative treatment measures (general and local hormone therapy with dexamethasone, antiplatelet agents, hemodilution, and anticholinesterase drugs), no clear sign of any recovery of visual functions was detected on clinical examination. In this setting, the patient underwent a formal assessment of the intracranial vasculature via DSA—which revealed that venous drainage through the orbital veins of both eyes into the cavernous sinus was reduced, whereas drainage through the facial veins was fully preserved. Unfortunately, the patient did not show any significant improvement in neurological function during her hospital stay. The patient was discharged from the hospital on the fifth day after surgery with persistent bilateral amaurosis, a progressive resolution of the swelling and hyperemia of the eyelid skin, and only an insignificant range of motion in both eyeballs (complete ophthalmoplegia).

Case II

A 39-year-old female patient was admitted to the Department of Vascular Neurosurgery of the Federal Center of Neurosurgery in Novosibirsk in July 2017 with a diagnosis of a fusiform aneurysm of the A2 segment of the right anterior cerebral artery. This patient also had mild anemia. According to an angio-CT scan, a fusiform aneurysm of the A2 segment of the right anterior cerebral artery was identified, and an incidental small en plaque meningioma in the anterior third of the falx, without compression on the brain, was also noted. Before surgery, imaging was reviewed, and the presence of a small intrinsic tumor in the intraorbital segment of the right optic nerve was diagnosed. Ophthalmologic examination demonstrated decreased vision in the right eye: VIS = 0.02 OD/1.0 OS, with some atrophy of the optic disc on the right side.

On the day after admission, the patient underwent surgical treatment, beginning with a standard bifrontal (coronal) skin incision, followed by retraction of the skin flap to the base of the skull. In this case, we took the fronto-basal interhemispheric approach. During surgery, the meningioma of the anterior third of the falx was removed. After adequately exposing the anterior circulation we created an intracranial side-to-side anastomosis between the matching A3 segments

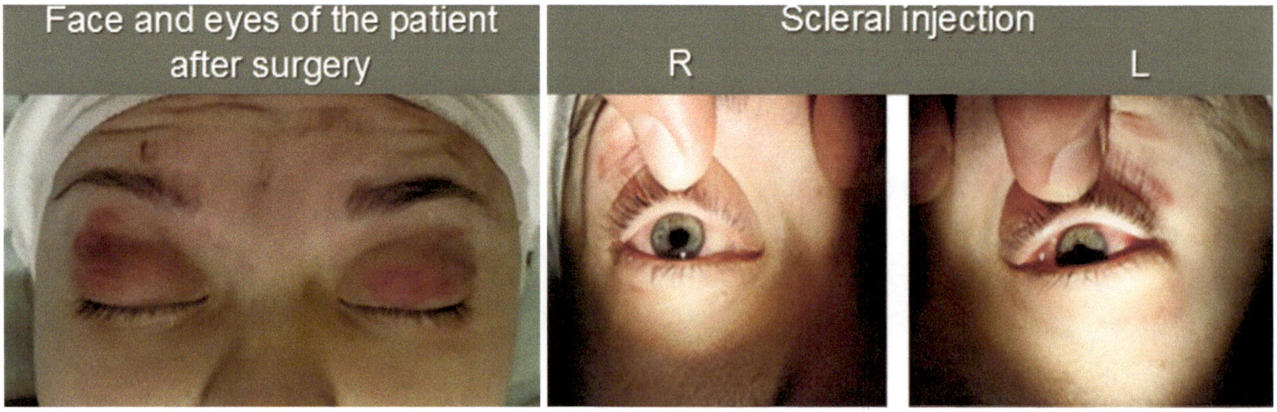

Fig. 1 Postsurgical upper eyelid swelling, scleral injection, bilateral ophthalmoplegia, and mydriasis

of the left and right anterior cerebral arteries. Afterward, a surgical clip was applied just proximal to the fusiform aneurysm of the right A2 segment.

The intraoperative course was without any intraoperative complications. The duration of the surgical case was 6 h 25 min. In the early postoperative period, after the patient recovered from anesthesia, the patient complained of a loss of vision in both eyes. On examination, she had hyperemia and swelling in the upper eyelids of both eyes, bilateral mydriasis, the bilateral absence of a pupillary light response, bilateral total ophthalmoplegia, and bilateral amaurosis.

After the examination revealed blindness, we immediately performed CT and MRI on the brain, as well as angio-CT on the brain vessels. Upon a review of the images, all cerebral arteries appeared patent, the intracranial anastomosis was functioning well, the aneurysm was no longer filling, and there were no foci of cerebral ischemia. However, there was swelling in the soft periorbital and retrobulbar tissues in both orbits. Accordingly, general and local pharmacological therapy with dexamethasone, antiplatelet agents, and hemodilution was started.

A study on the visual evoked potentials was urgently performed, which revealed signs of dysfunction in the optic tracts on both sides, with a complete loss of conduction on the right side. After conservative treatment, a slight change in neurological status was noted: the appearance of minimal movements of both eyeballs. Unfortunately, the visual function did not recover, and the patient was discharged from the hospital on the 11th day after surgery with bilateral amaurosis.

A thorough M&M analysis of these two cases was performed, and the general clinical condition of both patients before surgery was assessed. Attention was initially drawn to preoperatively pre-existing compromised vision in both cases: in the first case, repeated surgical treatment for high-grade myopia had been recorded, though the visual acuity was preserved; in the second case, a baseline impairment in vision on the right side was documented and due to the presence of a small tumor in a intraorbital segment of the right optic nerve. Also, mild anemia was identified as a comorbidity in both cases. To be thorough, the anatomical features of the skull shape of patients were studied. We paid particular attention to the prominence of the orbital ridges at the level of the eyebrow and the nasal bridge, as well as to the degree of physiological exophthalmos (Fig. 2). The intraoperative anesthesia management of both patients was studied from

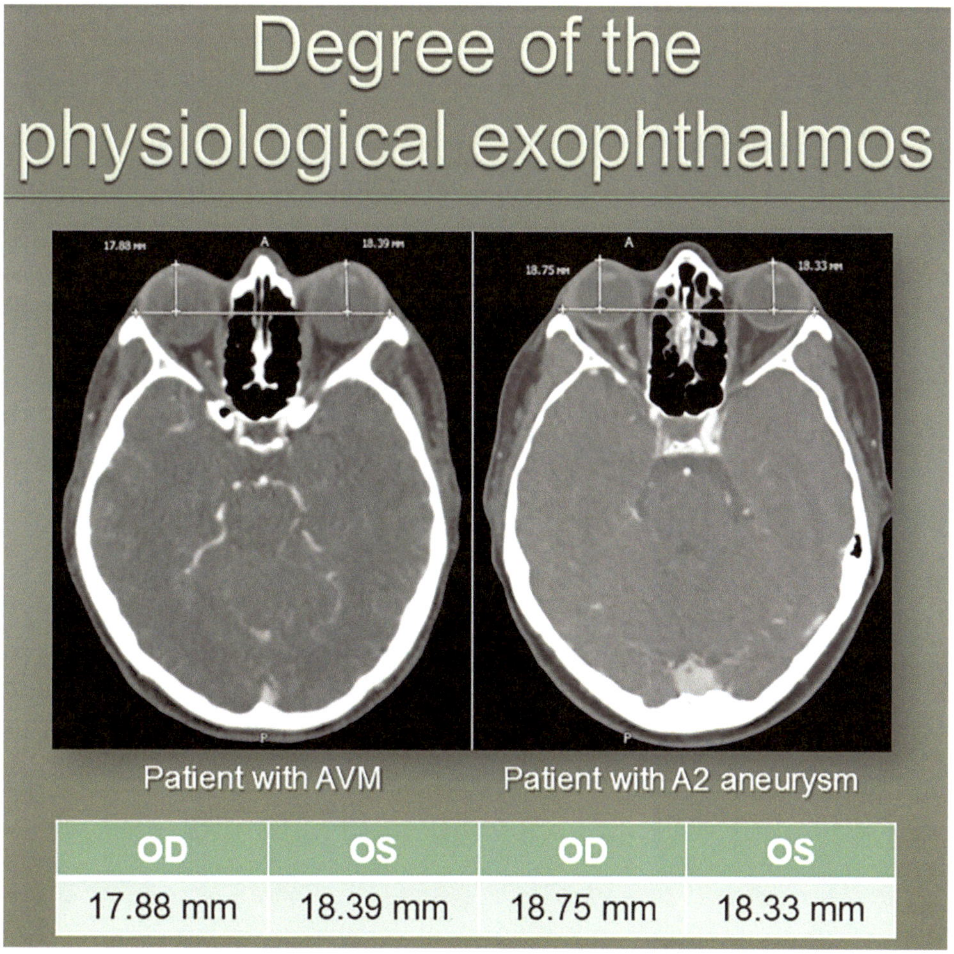

Fig. 2 Measurement of the physiological exophthalmos

the medical records. However, no hemodynamic disturbance (e.g., a drop in blood pressure), significant blood loss, or heart arrhythmia was revealed during surgery. Video recordings of the surgical steps in each case were studied, and intraoperative iatrogenic damage to the cranial nerves and arteries was excluded. Taken together, these observations pointed to a different pathomechanism for the sustained damages.

Results and Discussion

In 1937, Holmes described two cases of vision loss after the removal of brain tumors. One case showed blindness after the removal of a vestibular schwannoma. In the other, blindness occurred after the removal of a tumor in the frontal region. Unfortunately, the author did not give any specific explanation in the article for the occurrence of this complication [2].

In 1962, Rinaldi et al. described five clinical cases of postoperative vision loss that occurred after ventricular puncture in order to create internal decompression in patients with brain tumors [3]. The authors explained that the development of this complication was due to an intraoperative ischemia of the occipital region, which was a result of compression on the posterior cerebral arteries against the tentorial notch, due to a rapid drop in intraventricular pressure.

In 1985, Beck and Greenberg coined the term *postdecompressive optic neuropathy* [4]. These authors described five clinical cases of postoperative vision loss after craniotomy and the removal of brain tumors of various localizations. A sudden intraoperative decrease in the perfusion pressure of the eyeball supplying arteries, due to a tissue shift from a fast decrease in intracranial pressure, was assumed as the cause of this complication.

The literature also describes cases of postoperative vision loss as a result of direct external pressure on the eyeball with a skin flap during surgical treatment, leading to the occurrence of orbital infarction syndrome with subsequent blindness [5–8].

Takahashi, in his article, describes the development of such perioperative vision loss as being due to the development of an orbital compartment syndrome, which may be caused by excessive pressure on the eyeballs from a skin flap [8].

According to Payman, and as a result of prolonged mechanical compression on the eyeball, intraorbital pressure increases, whereas venous outflow from the eyeball decreases, resulting in a drop in perfusion pressure in the vascular system of the optic nerve at the level of the short posterior ciliary arteries, which leads to the development of posterior optic neuropathy and the atrophying of the optic nerve [9] (Fig. 3).

The reasons for the development of this complication can also be the result of complex effects—e.g., intraoperative hypotension, anemia with various origins, and embolism in the vessels feeding the eyeball, among others.

In our above-described clinical cases, the most probable factor that led to this complication was excessive external pressure exerted on the eyeballs by the retracted bicoronal skin flap during surgical treatment [10]. This could also be further influenced by certain anatomical features of the skull shape in patients, such as the prominence of the eyebrow ridges, the shape of the nasal bridge, and a high degree of physiological exophthalmos.

To prevent the development of this devastating complication, all the possible risk factors that can result in the loss of visual functions must be carefully assessed: the presence of concomitant diseases (anemia, atherosclerosis, or arterial hypertension); the anatomical features of the skull shape (the

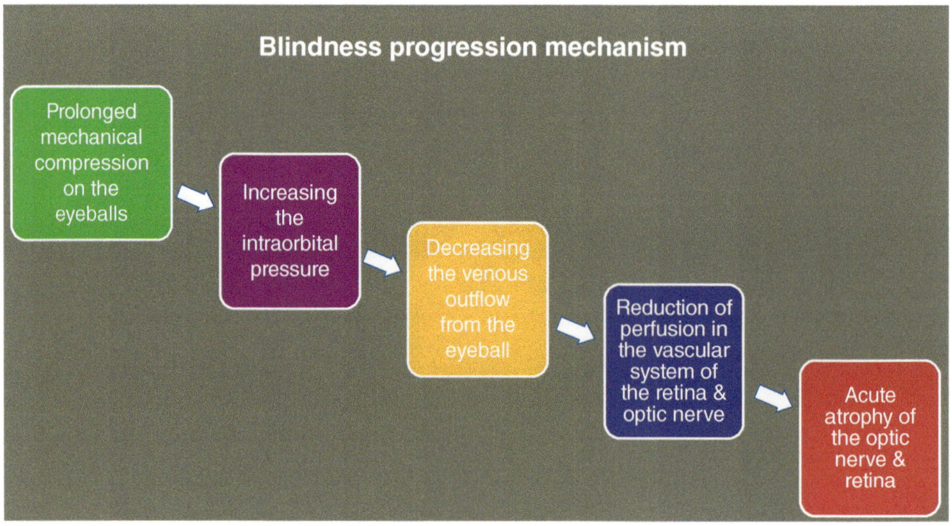

Fig. 3 Blindness progression mechanism

degree of physiological exophthalmos or the underdevelopment of the brow ridges and the nasal bridge); and the planned flap anatomy itself.

During surgery, carefully monitoring all the possible functions of the organ systems of the patient is important. Preventing a sudden drop in blood pressure and preventing massive blood loss are also important. Most relevant, though, is the opening step during craniotomy, when direct compression on the patient's eyeballs by a retracted skin flap must be avoided. These measures can prevent the development of postoperative vision loss in patients with neurosurgical pathologies.

Conflict of Interest The authors declare that they have no conflicts of interest.

References

1. Newman NJ. Perioperative visual loss after nonocular surgeries. Am J Ophtalmol. 2008;145(4):604–10. https://doi.org/10.1016/j.ajo.2007.09.016.
2. Holmes G. The prognosis in papilloedema. Br J Ophthalmol. 1937;21:337–42.
3. Rinaldi I, Botton JE, Troland CE. Cortical visual disturbances following ventriculography and/or ventricular decompression. J Neurosurg. 1962;19:568–76. https://doi.org/10.3171/jns.1962.19.7.0568.
4. Beck RW, Greenberg S. Post-decompression optic neuropathy. J Neurosurg. 1985;63:196–9. https://doi.org/10.3171/jns.1985.63.2.0196.
5. Choudhari KA, Pherwani AA. Sudden visual loss due to posterior ischemic optic neuropathy following craniotomy for a ruptured intracranial aneurysm. Neurology. 2007;55:163–5. https://doi.org/10.4103/0028-3886.32792.
6. Maier P, Feltgen N, Lagreze WA. Bilateral orbital infarction syndrome after bifrontal craniotomy. Arch Ophthalmol. 2007;125:422–3. https://doi.org/10.1001/archopht.125.3.422.
7. Mukherjee S, et al. Sudden-onset monocular blindness following orbito-zygomatic craniotomy for a ruptured intracranial aneurysm. BMJ Case Rep. 2016;2016:bcr2014208393. https://doi.org/10.1136/bcr-2014-208393.
8. Yamashita S, Takahashi H, Tanaka M. Bispectral index sensor as a possible cause of postoperative visual loss after frontal craniotomy. Br J Anaesth. 2009;103:134. https://doi.org/10.1093/bja/aep153.
9. Payman V, et al. Postcraniotomy blindness in the supine position: unlikely or ignored? Asian J Neurosurg. 2013;8(1):36–41. https://doi.org/10.4103/1793-5482.110278.
10. Takahashi Y, et al. Bilateral orbital compartment syndrome and blindness after cerebral aneurysm repair surgery. Ophthalmic Plast Reconstr Surg. 2010;26(4):299–301. https://doi.org/10.1097/IOP.0b013e3181c062ca.

The Nightmare of AVM Surgery: Early Rupture of the Venous Drainage—Lessons from Personal Experience and a Review of the Literature

Ioan Stefan Florian and Ioan Alexandru Florian

Abstract

We describe the case of a 72-year-old man who presented with signs of increased intracranial pressure, right-sided motor deficit, and repeated episodes of epilepsy due to a left frontal arteriovenous malformation (AVM) with a large superficial draining vein. Despite great efforts to protect the vein from the start, it ruptured shortly after we removed the bone flap. This required rigorous hemorrhage control, which in turn led to profuse bleeding from the nidus throughout the process of the dissection and coagulation of the arterial feeders. The postoperative course was initially uneventful; however, the patient declined neurologically and became unresponsive on the second day after surgery. Emergent CT revealed a significant hematoma occupying the space where the AVM nidus had been resected. The patient was taken back to the OR for emergency evacuation of the hematoma. Despite these efforts, the neurological status remained poor, and the patient was transferred to a territorial hospital after spending 3 weeks in the ICU.

An early rupture of the venous drainage represents a dreaded complication of AVM surgery, which can compromise the intervention before the start of the definite resection. We discuss our experience of and strategy for preventing and managing the intraoperative venous rupture of AVMs by describing our seven rules of "Don't." We also provide a brief overview of the relevant literature.

Ioan Stefan Florian and Ioan Alexandru Florian contributed equally with all other contributors.

I. S. Florian (✉) · I. A. Florian
Clinic of Neurosurgery, Cluj County Clinical Emergency Hospital, Cluj-Napoca, Romania

Department of Neurosciences, "Iuliu Hatieganu" University of Medicine and Pharmacy, Cluj-Napoca, Romania

Keywords

Arteriovenous malformation (AVM) · Surgical resection · Venous drainage rupture · Intraoperative hemorrhage

Introduction

Arteriovenous malformations (AVMs) are entanglements of abnormally developed brain vessels that shunt arterial blood directly into the venous system [1]. The surgical results of AVM resection are determined by a series of intrinsic characteristics of the lesions themselves: the larger and more-diffuse malformations, those with a deep-seated location or found in the posterior fossa, and the ones already presenting with hemorrhage are usually associated with poorer procedural outcomes [2]. Additionally, patient-related factors such as an age below 20 or above 40 years, significant comorbidities, and any compromise to the neurological status upon admission are also linked to less-favorable results [3]. An element that is less widely disputed is the influence of the experiences of surgeons themselves, which can be decisive even in the event that all other variables are favorable. Moreover, the rate of intraoperative AVM rupture, whether due to arterial bleeding or premature venous occlusion, appears to be influenced by the proficiency of the neurosurgeon [4].

The preservation of the draining vein until the very end of the dissection is critical to prevent intraoperative AVM rupture [5]. Yet this condition may prove more challenging than it would seem at first, in no small part due to the size of the draining vessels and their inherent brittleness. Herein, we present the illustrative case of a 72-year-old man with a left frontal AVM and its main draining vein, which had ruptured during surgery because of an accidental injury to the draining vein, leading to a severely compromised neurological outcome.

K. Turel, E. M. Kasper (eds.), *Complications in Neurosurgery II*, Acta Neurochirurgica Supplement 133,
https://doi.org/10.1007/978-3-031-61601-3_9

Case Report

A 72-year-old man, who had been previously diagnosed with an unruptured intracranial AVM and managed with surveillance imaging, was admitted in our department in an emergency setting for signs of increased intracranial pressure and unremitting seizures. Upon admission, he was uncooperative, deeply somnolent, and nauseous; had a GCS of 10 (M = 5, V = 2, O = 3) and severe speech difficulty; and showed signs of mild motor deficit and accentuated osteotendinous reflexes on the right side. The pupils were normal in diameter, and his sensory function could not be properly evaluated. The preoperative cerebral magnetic resonance angiogram (MRA), which had been performed about a week prior, revealed a Spetzler-Martin grade III AVM located in the left motor area, with a relatively focal nidus and a large superficial draining vein just underneath the dura mater (Fig. 1). He showed no signs of intracranial hemorrhage at this time. The emergency computed tomography (CT) scan demonstrated a panventricular hemorrhage and a calcified area within the AVM nidus (Fig. 2). After explaining to the family of the patient the

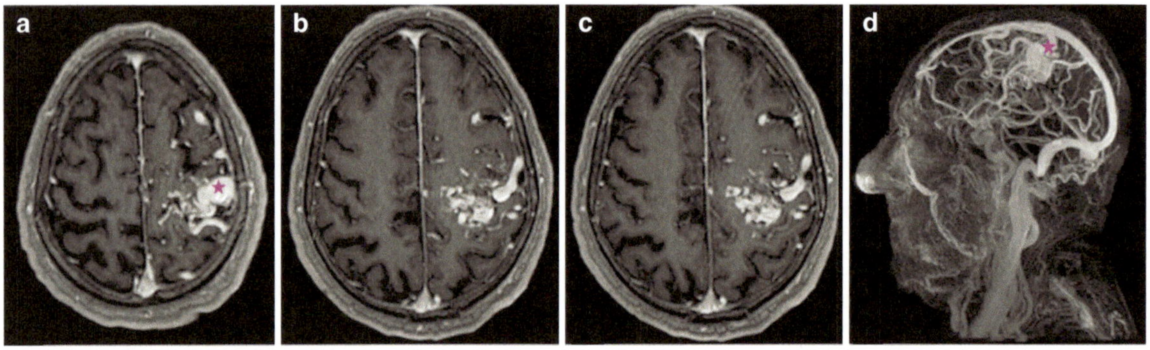

Fig. 1 Preoperative MRI angiography, approx. 1 week prior to rupture. (**a–c**) Gadolinium-enhanced T1 MRI angiography showing the left frontal arteriovenous malformation (AVM), with a prominent superficial vein (*magenta star*). (**d**) MRI angiography time-resolved imaging of contrast kinetics (TRICKS) displaying the AVM in relationship with neighboring vascular structures. The draining vein is also visible here (*magenta star*)

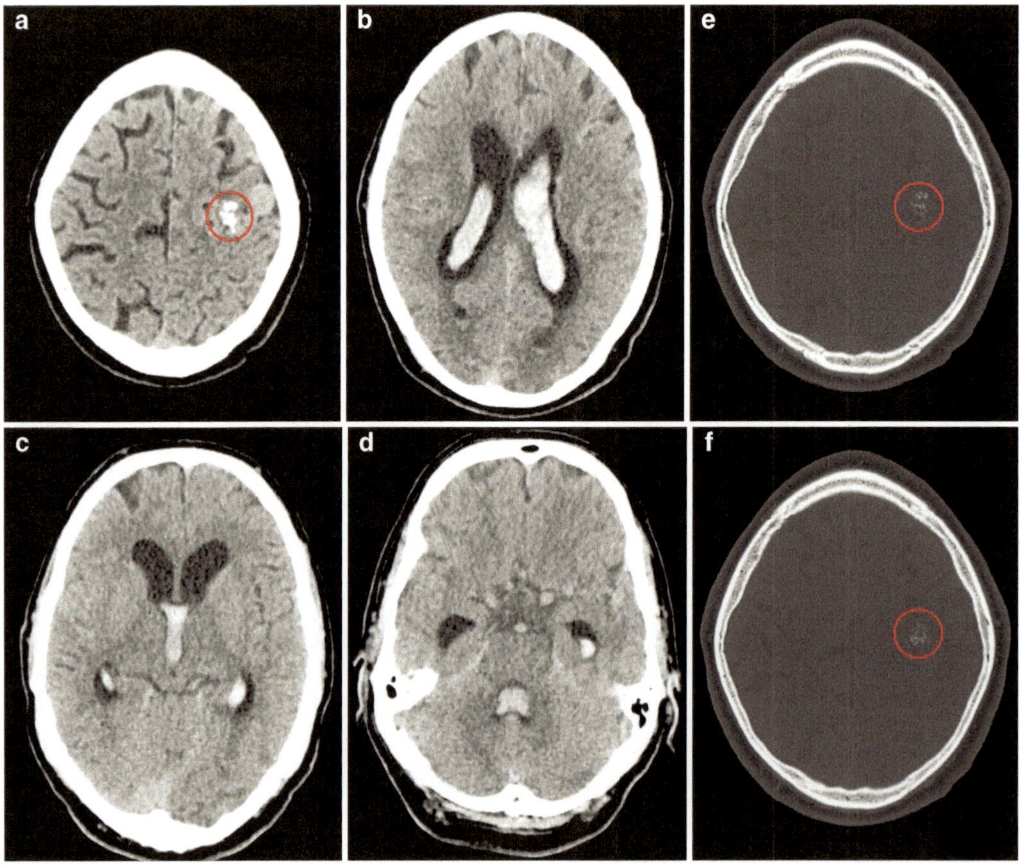

Fig. 2 Preoperative CT scan at the time of hemorrhagic stroke. (**a–d**) Axial nonenhanced sections displaying tetraventricular hemorrhage in the absence of parenchymal hematoma, as well as a spontaneously hyperdense area in the subcortical portion of the arteriovenous malformation (AVM) nidus (*red circle*). (**e, f**) The bone window demonstrates an osseous density of the previously described area, suggesting a calcified intranidal mass (*red circle*)

benefits and risks of surgery and after detailing the other treatment options available for such as endovascular embolization, they consented to surgery. He was taken into the operating room (OR) the day after admission.

Surgery

We performed a large frontoparietal craniotomy, and the superficial draining vein began to bleed profusely immediately after we lifted the bone flap off. The dura mater was immediately opened to allow us to pursue proper control of the bleeding. The hemorrhage was difficult to contain, barely manageable with suction and cottonoid patties, and it steadily continued before it was reduced via careful dissection and coagulation. After cutting off all arterial supply, the nidus was removed, and the draining vein was ligated and cut. Definitive hemostasis was performed with bipolar coagulation and Surgicel, and an external ventricular drainage (EVD) was placed in the left lateral ventricle. The dura mater was suspended and sutured, the bone flap was placed back and fastened with multiple sutures, and the skin was sutured in multiple layers above a subaponeurotic draining tube.

Postoperative Course

The postoperative course during the first 24 h in the intensive care unit (ICU) was unremarkable; however, the patient deteriorated later that day, becoming significantly more somnolent, experiencing increasing difficulty in moving the right side of the body, and ultimately becoming unresponsive. As the control cerebral CT scan demonstrated, he sustained a focal hemorrhage, most likely due to venous infarct (Fig. 3). This required a reintervention on the second postoperative day for the evacuation of the hematoma, when the EVD was also replaced. The final CT angiography revealed no traces of intraventricular or intraparenchymal hemorrhage and revealed the complete removal of the AVM nidus (Fig. 4). Afterward, the patient's clinical recovery stalled. He was maintained in the ICU, where the ventilator and EVD were removed 48 h after the second surgery. He was transferred to a territorial hospital 3 weeks later in a conscious state and able to speak, but he had a marked neurological deficit on his right side and a Glasgow Outcome Score (GOS) of 3. Unfortunately, the patient died while still hospitalized at the outside hospital, after having suffered from a deep venous thrombosis and a subsequent pulmonary embolism, despite being under daily treatment with subcutaneous prophylaxis.

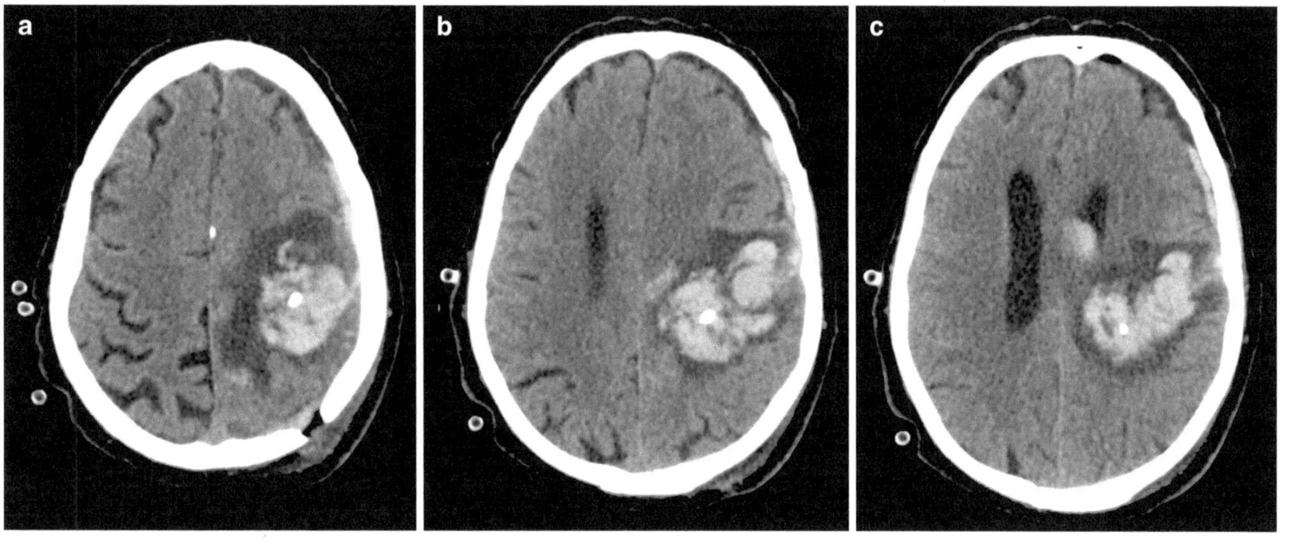

Fig. 3 Postoperative CT scan at 48 h after surgery. (**a**–**c**) A large intraparenchymal hematoma is clearly visible in the region where the arteriovenous malformation (AVM) resided. The external ventricular drainage (EVD) catheter can also be observed

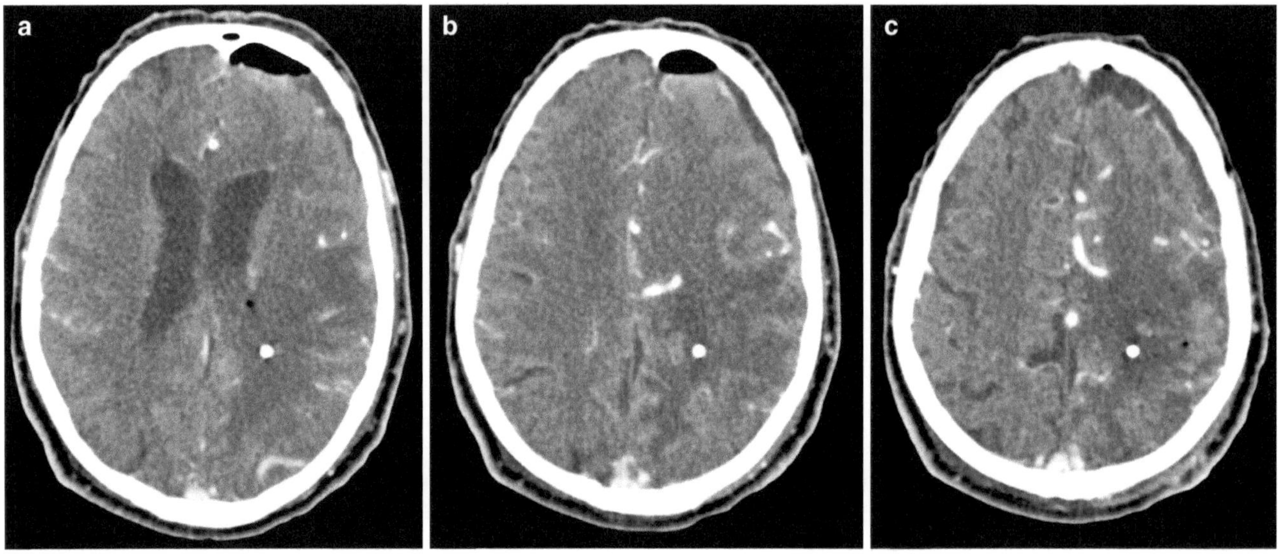

Fig. 4 Post-reinterventional CT angiography. (**a–c**) The arteriovenous malformation (AVM) has been completely removed. Furthermore, this shows no remaining trace of intraventricular or intraparencymal hematoma, and a minor amount of pneumocephalus can be noticed. A replacement external ventricular drainage (EVD) can also be seen

Discussion

Avoiding an accidental injury to the AVM draining veins seems simple enough in theory, yet it may sometimes be difficult to put into practice, especially when the vein itself has a caliber comparable to those of the feeding arteries. To this end, we recommend using the intraoperative microscope as soon as the bone flap has been lifted. Through it, the direction of the blood flow can be better recognized, and the surgeon can more easily differentiate between the vessel types. Remember that the blood inside the draining veins is arterialized; therefore, the difference in color between the two vessel types may be insignificant. If the draining vein also collects blood from functional areas of the brain, then a mixture between arterial and venous blood may be visible within its lumen. These subtle clues can be extremely helpful when considering which vessel to coagulate and which to preserve until the very end. While the feeders are progressively taken down, the mixed arterial and venous blood within a draining vein will steadily turn more toward a darker venous color. Once it is largely free of oxygenated blood, the draining vessel is hypothetically safe to coagulate, and any bleeding would at least be controllable. Alternatively, intraoperative fluorescein or indocyanine green (ICG) video microscopy/angiography, despite being invasive, can significantly simplify the identification process of feeders and drainers [6–8].

Intraoperative color Doppler ultrasonography can be utilized to accurately distinguish the vessels and differentiate between malformed arteries and veins [9–11]. Neuronavigation may also prove useful in identifying the components of the AVM in real time [10, 12]. With these two methods, by themselves or in combination, identifying the vein from the very start could be easier and much less frustrating.

Even when employing neuronavigation, one must also take into account possible brain shift, which might displace vessels by a few millimeters in whichever direction. Once the draining vein has been correctly identified, it needs to be protected and preserved until the very end of the dissection, when it is safe to ligate. As these AVM veins are fragile, preventing venous stretching is imperative. Do not use brain retractors excessively, as these might strain the veins and cause catastrophic bleeding. If the veins are in the way of proper dissection, the strategy is to always perform a dissection around them first and with great care. Using constant irrigation with saline or Ringer's lactate solution, or cottonoid patties imbued with either, will lessen the risk of venous stretching. Nevertheless, the most important aspect in preventing draining vein rupture is to utilize a fine and gentle microsurgical technique.

As Lawton pointed out in one of his seminal works, and our own experience can also attest to this, every surgery has a few specific moments when the rupture of the AVM draining veins might occur [13]. In case the veins are superficial and prominent and corrode the inner table of the skull vault, they can be notched or sheared when performing the craniotomy. This is possibly the worst-case scenario because it might compromise the entire surgery before it has even properly started. If a cortical vein is closely adherent to the dura mater, it may also be damaged during durotomy. Another possible moment when these veins may break is during the dissection of the AVM when the brain is being retracted too forcefully. Therefore, avoid applying too much strength while using the aspirator or spatula. In short, a surgeon should anticipate that the draining veins may rupture at any given point during the intervention and take precautions.

The first sign of an accidental or premature coagulation of the vein is the rapid enlargement of the nidus, which becomes firm and starts to pulsate intensely. Immediately afterward, profuse bleeding may ensue from any part of the AVM. If, despite the best efforts to preserve it, the vein breaks or leaks, one might be tempted to coagulate or clip it. This should never be done, because reducing venous outflow will only worsen the hemorrhage. The bleeding may be controlled via direct gentle pressure or by using patties and mild suction with the aspirator. The bipolar can also be used in remodeling the vein around the point of rupture to reduce the diameter of the leak, but not so much as to completely occlude the vessel. More importantly, the arterial inflow of the AVM needs to be reduced urgently. This can be achieved by identifying and temporarily clipping the major feeders, inducing arterial hypotension, or by asking the anesthesiologist to perform an ipsilateral carotid artery compression. Once the bleeding has been reduced, both the amplitude and force pulsations within the nidus steadily decrease and the AVM becomes soft and easy to mobilize. The neurosurgeon must then quickly ensure the coagulation of all feeders, the complete circumferential dissection of the nidus, and proper hemostasis.

When faced with this dreaded intraoperative complication, we propose following our seven rules of "Don't" so that control can be swiftly regained:

1. Don't worry: It will bleed regardless. The risk of supratentorial AVMs to rupture during surgery is slightly higher than that of posterior fossa lesions [4]. Regardless, intraoperative bleeding is lower for AVMs than it is for intracranial aneurysms. The experience of the surgeon is valuable not only in precluding intraoperative bleeding but also in managing it. Having a second suction on hand is always helpful in ensuring that the excessive amount of blood does not compromise surgical field visibility.
2. Don't rush it: You will waste more time. Indiscriminately coagulating every visible blood vessel in an attempt to control the bleeding as soon as possible will only lead to more neurological damage because the arteries surrounding the AVM usually supply functioning parenchyma. Nor is mildly or quickly cauterizing the feeding arteries of the AVM a solution, because the high blood flow will reopen them. Take your time when identifying the feeders, and thoroughly coagulate them one by one.
3. Don't panic: Surgery on living patients means that sometimes intraoperative hemorrhage is inevitable. One should use this both as a gentle reminder that the patient is still alive and an incentive to keep them that way. For precluding heavy losses of blood, intraoperative perfusions and transfusions are invaluable. In AVM surgery, intraoperative blood-saving devices and procoagulants such as recombinant factor VIIa are both potential game changers that can reduce the necessity of transfusion [14, 15]. Consider preoperative embolization with N-butyl cyanoacrylate (NBCA) or Onyx, which can also prevent a catastrophic intraoperative bleed, particularly for higher grade lesions [16–19]. Single-stage embolization and resection has also shown promising results, being associated with a lower intraoperative bleeding and favorable outcomes in both the short term and the long term [20].
4. Don't allow the AVM to take the lead: You are and should always be in charge. With each feeder coagulated, the goal of hemostasis comes closer. Continue trying to control the hemorrhage, and if possible, do not attempt to immediately remove the nidus (the so-called commando resection). Otherwise, the bleeding will become even more severe, possibly recurring after the surgery is over. For the deeper feeders, the Thulium laser has been proven effective in controlling hemorrhages [21]. "Dirty coagulation," or the practice of coagulating the small vessels and the thin layers of surrounding brain tissue, may help [22] because it safe as long as the surgeon does not delve too deeply into the parenchyma. Nevertheless, we advise against overusing this technique so as not to induce a permanent focal deficit if the lesion is located in an eloquent area.
5. Don't lose your patience: Otherwise, you will lose your patient. Seeing that the hemorrhage is unremitting despite the numerous feeders already cauterized may seem daunting, yet this is merely a result of simple physics: The same amount of blood is rushing out of fewer and fewer abnormal vessels. Do not worry that this is a sure sign of normal perfusion pressure breakthrough (NPPB); this only rarely occurs after AVM resection, and its reported offshoots are inconstant or debatable [23–25]. After a while, the last remaining feeders will not be able to carry as much blood, and the hemorrhage will slow down. All it takes is patience and perseverance.
6. Don't abuse your power (coagulator) or force (aspirator): You will only worsen the damage if you do. Again, cauterizing every visible vessel with increased bipolar intensity will only lead to cortical damage and potential neurological deficit. Nor do we recommend using excessive pinching force at the tip of the coagulating bipolar forceps, because it has been demonstrated to injure the more fragile vessels [26]. At times, coagulation can prove even more difficult to achieve, especially in AVMs with intensely calcified vessels [27]. On the other hand, using the aspirator too vigorously may result in drawing in some of the fragile vessels or, in a worst-case scenario, the functioning brain parenchyma. The aspirator should be kept neatly in place, as close as possible to the source of bleeding without being actually in contact with it.
7. Don't hesitate to ask for help: You always have a team behind you. The anesthesiologist is arguably the most vital player in the operating room, and you can ask them to provide temporary hypotension or ipsilateral carotid compression, which might limit the intensity of the hemorrhage. In turn, this would grant the surgeon the opportunity to identify what is acting on the AVM feeders. Additionally, the anesthesiologist can compensate for the patient's blood loss, including transfusions with whole blood or red blood cells in case the arterial pressure drops too much. Although not widely studied, transient pharmacological asystole induced via adenosine administration could be a safe and efficient method of expediting the

surgical resection of complex AVMs [28]. Moreover, intraoperative adenosine practically decreases the need to place temporary clips on crucial parent arteries, markedly diminishing their associated complications. When feasible, rapid ventricular pacing (RVP) during cerebrovascular surgery can also assist in achieving flow arrest and facilitating the dissection and resection of AVMs [29], although this has to be planned beforehand and should not be attempted once surgery has begun (Table 1).

Table 1 The seven rules of "Don't"

	Rule	What to avoid	What to do
1	Don't worry	Overconfidence or the expectation that the AVM will surely not bleed	Always be prepared for the AVM to bleed and then act accordingly; look through the operative microscope and assess the direction of the blood flow—where inwards means feeder and outwards means draining vein
2	Don't rush it	Coagulating indiscriminately	Take your time to ensure the proper coagulation of arterial feeders
3	Don't panic	Losing your nerve at the sight of blood	Preoperative embolization may help; use blood savers, recombinant factor VIIa, and/or a secondary aspirator
4	Don't allow the AVM to take the lead	Forgetting the first two crucial steps of the surgical resection of AVMs	Continue with the circumferential dissection and progressive coagulation: In time, the feeders will lessen in number, and the hemorrhage will diminish
5	Don't lose your patience	Losing the precision and caution of microsurgical gestures	Keep using finesse and minute manipulations while dissecting the AVM, especially in its innermost aspect—here you may find another draining vein that should be preserved at all costs until all feeders have closed
6	Don't abuse your power (coagulator) or force (aspirator)	Relying too much on your coagulator and/or aspirator	Keep the bipolar coagulator at the same intensity as before, and coagulate only once you have correctly identified the feeders; maintain the aspirator in a single spot, as close to the source of hemorrhage without coming into contact with the leaking vessels
7	Don't hesitate to ask for help	Disregarding the rest of the surgical team	The anesthesiologist is your friend: Ask them to temporarily decrease systemic blood pressure or compress the ipsilateral carotid artery, and allow them to provide the patient with perfusion or administer procoagulants

AVM arteriovenous malformation

Conclusions

An intraoperative venous rupture of a brain AVM is a dreaded complication that can be avoided with sufficient experience. It may happen at any given moment during or after craniotomy. In the event that it does occur, surgery must resume with the standard steps, albeit at a more alert pace. We recommend following the seven rules of 'Don't' to ease the procedure and ensure optimal surgical results.

Acknowledgments None.

Conflicts of Interest The authors have no conflicts of interest to disclose.

Ethical Statement The consent to present and publish this case was given by the family of the patient.

Funding No funding was received for the writing of this manuscript.

References

1. Kalb S, Gross BA, Nakaji P. Vascular malformations (arteriovenous malformations and dural arteriovenous fistulas). In: Ellenbogen RG, Sekhar LN, Kitchen ND, editors. Principles of neurological surgery, vol. 20. 4th ed. Amsterdam: Elsevier; 2018. p. 313–24.
2. Kim H, Abla AA, Nelson J, McCulloch CE, Bervini D, Morgan MK, Stapleton C, Walcott BP, Ogilvy CS, Spetzler RF, Lawton MT. Validation of the supplemented Spetzler-Martin grading system for brain arteriovenous malformations in a multicenter cohort of 1009 surgical patients. Neurosurgery. 2015;76(1):25–31. https://doi.org/10.1227/NEU.0000000000000556. PMID: 25251197; PMCID: PMC4270816.
3. Florian IA, Stan HM, Florian IS, Cheptea M, Berindan-Neagoe I. Prognostic factors in the neurosurgical treatment of cerebral arteriovenous malformations. In: Kandasamy R, editor. World federation of neurosurgical societies symposia 2018 proceeding book. Bologna: Editografica; 2019. p. 232–41.
4. Torné R, Rodríguez-Hernández A, Lawton MT. Intraoperative arteriovenous malformation rupture: causes, management techniques, outcomes, and the effect of neurosurgeon experience. Neurosurg Focus. 2014;37(3):E12. https://doi.org/10.3171/2014.6.FOCUS14218.
5. Rutledge WC, Lawton MT. Brain AVM: current treatments and challenges. In: Su H, Lawton MT, editors. Molecular, genetic, and cellular advances in cerebrovascular diseases. Singapore: World Scientific; 2018. p. 69–81.
6. Zhao X, Belykh E, Cavallo C, Valli D, Gandhi S, Preul MC, Vajkoczy P, Lawton MT, Nakaji P. Application of fluorescein fluorescence in vascular neurosurgery. Front Surg. 2019;6:52. https://doi.org/10.3389/fsurg.2019.00052. PMID: 31620443; PMCID: PMC6759993.
7. Shimada K, Yamaguchi T, Miyamoto T, Sogabe S, Korai M, Okazaki T, Kanematsu Y, Satomi J, Nagahiro S, Takagi Y. Efficacy of intraarterial superselective indocyanine green videoangiography in cerebral arteriovenous malformation surgery in a hybrid operating room. J Neurosurg. 2020. https://doi.org/10.3171/2020.3.JNS20319.
8. Takagi Y, Sawamura K, Hashimoto N, Miyamoto S. Evaluation of serial intraoperative surgical microscope-integrated intraoperative near-infrared indocyanine green videoangiography in patients with cerebral arteriovenous malfor-

mations. Neurosurgery. 2012;70(1):34–42. https://doi.org/10.1227/NEU.0b013e31822d9749.

9. Xu H, Qin Z, Xu M, Chen C, Zhang J, Chen X. Clinical experience with intraoperative ultrasonographic image in microsurgical resection of cerebral arteriovenous malformations. World Neurosurg. 2017;97:93–7. https://doi.org/10.1016/j.wneu.2016.09.089.
10. Akdemir H, Oktem S, Menkü A, Tucer B, Tuğcu B, Günaldi O. Image-guided microneurosurgical management of small arteriovenous malformation: role of neuronavigation and intraoperative Doppler sonography. Minim Invasive Neurosurg. 2007;50(3):163–9. https://doi.org/10.1055/s-2007-985376.
11. Walkden JS, Zador Z, Herwadkar A, Kamaly-Asl ID. Use of intraoperative Doppler ultrasound with neuronavigation to guide arteriovenous malformation resection: a pediatric case series. J Neurosurg Pediatr. 2015;15(3):291–300. https://doi.org/10.3171/2014.10.PEDS14249.
12. Zeeshan Q, Carrasco Hernandez JP, Sekhar LN. Localization and microsurgical resection of left postcentral gyrus spetzler-martin grade 3 arteriovenous malformation by intraoperative neuronavigation and tracing of subcortical draining vein: 3-dimensional operative video. Oper Neurosurg. 2020;19(2):E185–6. https://doi.org/10.1093/ons/opz383.
13. Lawton MT. Seven AVMs: tenets and techniques for resection. New York: Thieme; 2014. p. 352.
14. Novak V, Petrović B, Calija B, Mitov L, Rancić Z. Recombinant factor VII (NovoSeven) in intraoperative blood saving during neurosurgical treatment of the brain arteriovenous malformation. Vojnosanit Pregl. 2007;64(2):151–4. https://doi.org/10.2298/vsp0702151n.
15. Penington A. Surgical resection of an arteriovenous malformation. J Vasc Anomalies. 2021;2(2):e009. https://doi.org/10.1097/JOVA.0000000000000009.
16. Catapano JS, Frisoli FA, Nguyen CL, Wilkinson DA, Majmundar N, Cole TS, Baranoski JF, Whiting AC, Kim H, Ducruet AF, Albuquerque FC, Cooke DL, Spetzler RF, Lawton MT. Spetzler-martin grade III arteriovenous malformations: a multicenter propensity-adjusted analysis of the effects of preoperative embolization. Neurosurgery. 2021;88(5):996–1002. https://doi.org/10.1093/neuros/nyaa551.
17. Luzzi S, Del Maestro M, Bongetta D, Zoia C, Giordano AV, Trovarelli D, Raysi Dehcordi S, Galzio RJ. Onyx embolization before the surgical treatment of grade III Spetzler-Martin brain arteriovenous malformations: single-center experience and technical nuances. World Neurosurg. 2018;116:e340–53. https://doi.org/10.1016/j.wneu.2018.04.203.
18. Thakur R, Haider AS, Thomas A, Vayalumkal S, Khan U, Osumah T, Doughty K, Finn S, Layton KF. Preoperative embolization in tandem with surgical resection for cerebral arteriovenous malformations. Cureus. 2018;10(1):e2042. https://doi.org/10.7759/cureus.2042. PMID: 29541563; PMCID: PMC5843387.
19. Pasqualin A, Zampieri P, Nicolato A, Meneghelli P, Cozzi F, Beltramello A. Surgery after embolization of cerebral arteriovenous malformation: experience of 123 cases. In: Tsukahara T, Esposito G, Steiger HJ, Rinkel G, Regli L, editors. Trends in neurovascular interventions, vol. 119. Cham: Springer; 2014. p. 105–11. https://doi.org/10.1007/978-3-319-02411-0_18.
20. Santin MDN, Todeschi J, Pop R, Baloglu S, Ollivier I, Beaujeux R, Proust F, Cebula H. A combined single-stage procedure to treat brain AVM. Neurochirurgie. 2020;66(5):349–58. https://doi.org/10.1016/j.neuchi.2020.03.004.
21. Cenzato M, Dones F, Marcati E, Debernardi A, Scerrati A, Piparo M. Use of laser in arteriovenous malformation surgery. World Neurosurg. 2017;106:746–9. https://doi.org/10.1016/j.wneu.2017.07.101.
22. Kozyrev DA, Thiarawat P, Jahromi BR, Intarakhao P, Choque-Velasquez J, Hijazy F, Teo MK, Hernesniemi J. "Dirty coagulation" technique as an alternative to microclips for control of bleeding from deep feeders during brain arteriovenous malformation surgery. Acta Neurochir. 2017;159(5):855–9. https://doi.org/10.1007/s00701-017-3138-8.
23. Chyatte D. Normal pressure perfusion breakthrough after resection of arteriovenous malformation. J Stroke Cerebrovasc Dis. 1997;6(3):130–6. https://doi.org/10.1016/s1052-3057(97)80229-7.
24. Nagasawa S, Kawanishi M, Kondoh S, Yamaguchi K, Kajimoto S, Tada Y, Ohta T. Normal perfusion pressure hyperperfusion in cerebral arteriovenous malformation surgery: model study on the hemodynamics and mechanisms. J Clin Neurosci. 1998;5(Suppl):30–2. https://doi.org/10.1016/s0967-5868(98)90007-8.
25. Rangel-Castilla L, Spetzler RF, Nakaji P. Normal perfusion pressure breakthrough theory: a reappraisal after 35 years. Neurosurg Rev. 2015;38(3):399–404. https://doi.org/10.1007/s10143-014-0600-4.
26. Sugiyama T, Gan LS, Zareinia K, Lama S, Sutherland GR. Tool-tissue interaction forces in brain arteriovenous malformation surgery. World Neurosurg. 2017;102:221–8. https://doi.org/10.1016/j.wneu.2017.03.006.
27. Florian IA, Popovici L, Timis TL, Florian IS, Berindan-Neagoe I. Intracranial gorgon: surgical case report of a large calcified brain arteriovenous malformation. Am J Case Rep. 2020;21:e922872. https://doi.org/10.12659/AJCR.922872.
28. Al-Mousa A, Bose G, Hunt K, Toma AK. Adenosine-assisted neurovascular surgery: initial case series and review of literature. Neurosurg Rev. 2019;42(1):15–22. https://doi.org/10.1007/s10143-017-0883-3.
29. Saldien V, Menovsky T, Rommens M, Van der Steen G, Van Loock K, Vermeersch G, Mott C, Bosmans J, De Ridder D, Maas AI. Rapid ventricular pacing for flow arrest during cerebrovascular surgery: revival of an old concept. Neurosurgery. 2012;70(2):270–5. https://doi.org/10.1227/NEU.0b013e318236d84a.

Sudden Loss of Motor-Evoked Potentials (MEPs) During the Resection of A Nondominant Insular Glioma: Case Report and Management Review

Cristina Gómez-Revuelta, Carlos Martorell Llobregat, Javier Abarca-Olivas, Maria Dolores Coves Piqueres, and Pablo González-López

Abstract

A 43-year-old man was admitted into the emergency room at our hospital after presenting with a tonic-clonic seizure. MRI showed a right-side operculo-insular tumor. This was treated by performing a craniotomy under general anesthesia with intraoperative monitoring. Tumor resection was started by exploring the temporal and frontal opercula without problems. However, during the resection of the insular compartment, a sudden loss of MEPs was observed. Surgery was stopped immediately, and all the relevant anesthetic parameters, vital signs, anesthetic drugs were reviewed. No retractors had been used at that time, so vasospasm was suspected as the underlying cause of the signal change. An ICG bolus injection confirmed vasospasm in one of the M2 branches running over the insula. A direct vessel massage was performed yet resulted in no apparent improvement in the appearance of the vessel when ICG was injected. Therefore, repeated massage with nimodipine was performed, which resulted in the resolution of the vasospasm. MEPs progressively recovered to base line levels, and surgery could then be finished without further incident. During the postoperative recovery period, no focal deficit was identified, and the postoperative MRI showed a planned subtotal resection without apparent ischemia. The goal of this report is to review the potential causes of such a loss of intraoperative MEPs and its best management in order to prevent postoperative motor deficit and to manage the situation should it occur.

Keywords

MEP drop · Complication · Asleep surgery · Insular glioma · Vasospasm

C. Gómez-Revuelta · C. M. Llobregat · J. Abarca-Olivas · M. D. C. Piqueres · P. González-López (✉)
University General Hospital of Alicante, Alicante, Spain
e-mail: gonzalez_pab@gva.es

Introduction

The insular cortex is a common location for gliomas and is involved in 25% of all low-grade gliomas and 10% of all high-grade gliomas [1]. Insular gliomas were traditionally considered inoperable because of their deep location, surrounded by highly eloquent cortical and subcortical areas and vascular structures [1, 2]. These include the speech-related cortex (e.g., frontal and temporal opercula), the motor cortex and corticospinal tract, and key cerebral vessels (lenticulostriate arteries and M2 branches) [3] (Fig. 1a–c). However, ever since Yasargil published his surgical results after dealing with lesions in this area [4], insular glioma surgery has become popular, with good neurological and oncological results. We cannot ignore that the extent of resection is the most important prognostic factor of recurrence-free survival. However, the preservation of function is of equal importance, so in the modern era, a risk–benefit analysis must occur before any attempt to resect such tumors [2].

One should always include intraoperative neurophysiological monitoring in the surgeon's armamentarium to diminish the risk of postoperative neurological deficits, and the options are either awake surgery (especially in the dominant hemisphere) or continuous motor monitoring via motor-evoked potentials (MEPs) in asleep surgery. This strategy allows the surgeon to detect changes in the motor pathways' response, before a permanent deficit is caused when working around relevant motor-related structures, such as the precentral region and the M2 branches, or working close to the corticospinal tract [5, 6]. Most cases of postoperative paresis are caused by vascular complications. Therefore, when a problem is detected intraoperatively, one needs to check the preservation and integrity of all the vessels in the field and also rule out any potential vasospasm [7, 8].

In this report, we present the case of a 43-year-old man who displayed a sudden intraoperative loss of MEPs from a vasospasm of a distal segment of the M2 superior division, which

K. Turel, E. M. Kasper (eds.), *Complications in Neurosurgery II*, Acta Neurochirurgica Supplement 133,
https://doi.org/10.1007/978-3-031-61601-3_10

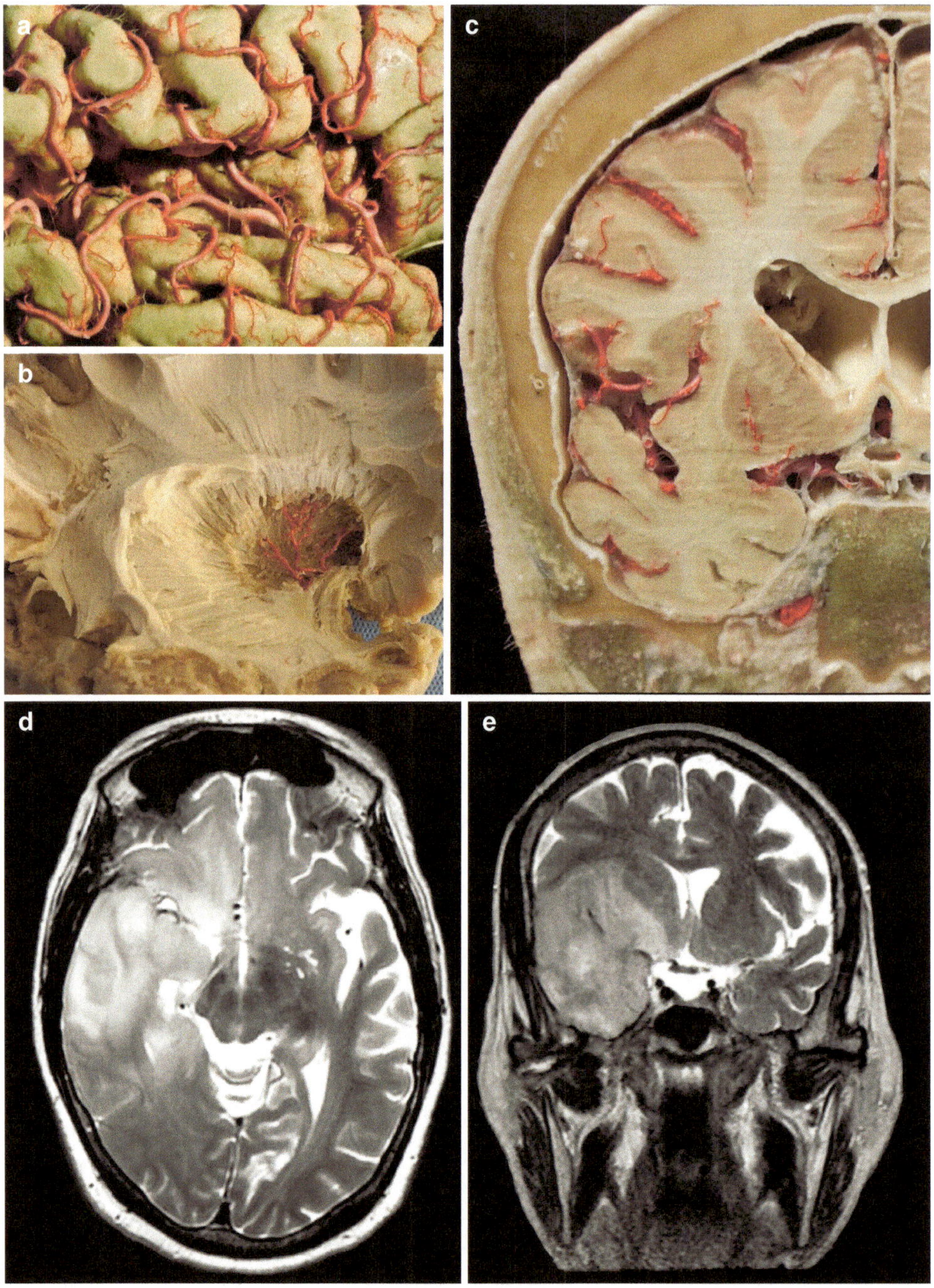

Fig. 1 Anatomical images of insular vascular relationships: (**a**, **b**) M2 branches running over the insular surface (**a**) and lenticulostriate arteries crossing the anterior perforated substance and entering the basal ganglia that have been removed from this image to improve understanding (**b**). (**c**) Coronal cut of a right hemisphere that shows the lenticulostriate arteries entering through the anterior perforated substance to the basal ganglia and the middle cerebral artery branches: M2 over the insula with its perforating branches, M3 over the opercula, and M4 corresponding with the cortical vessels. (**d**, **e**). Axial (**d**) and coronal (**e**) T2-weighted preoperative MRIs: hyperintense T2 lesion involving the insula, frontal opercula, and temporal opercula and extending to the temporal pole and temporo-mesial structures (Yasargil type 5B)

was successfully resolved after direct nimodipine massage. We aim to use this case to further analyze the differential diagnosis of MEP loss during glioma surgery, especially in reversible scenarios, to aid surgeons in increasing the chances of recovery from this severe intraoperative complication.

Case Report

An otherwise-healthy 43-year-old man was referred to our department after a brain tumor had been discovered during the work-up for tonic-clonic seizures. He had experienced no episodes of headache or vomiting and had no other symptoms of intracranial hypertension. No focal deficits were found during his physical examination, and neither sensory-motor affection nor verbal alterations (aphasia or dysarthria) were identified. Brain MRI showed a T2-hyperintense lesion centered in the right insula, also involving the frontal operculum and the temporal lobe, including temporo-mesial structures and the parahippocampal gyrus (Yasargil type 5B). Imaging showed well-defined planes with normal parenchyma medial to the lesion at the level of the basal ganglia. The lesion showed no contrast enhancement after a standard application of intravenous (IV) gadolinium. Therefore, a low-grade glioma was suspected, and surgery was considered (Fig. 1d, e).

Surgery

Because the location of the tumor was on the right side (nondominant hemisphere) and because extensive frontotemporal involvement reached the lateral aspect of the basal ganglia, the whole insular lobe, and the temporo-mesial structures, we decided to carry out the surgery as an asleep craniotomy with intraoperative monitoring. Intraoperative monitoring included somatosensory evoked potentials (SSEPs) and motor-evoked potentials (MEPs). Direct monopolar subcortical white matter stimulation was also part of the surgical plan to be employed when getting close to the deepest and posteromedial part of the insular component of the tumor (Fig. 2a).

The patient was positioned supine, with the head rotated 20 degrees to the left. A right pterional craniotomy was performed, and the primary motor area was identified by using the N20 wave-inversion technique. A flat grid was placed over the motor area to register the motor response (Fig. 2b). Tumor resection started at the level of the temporal lobe, performing a 2/3 anterior temporal lobectomy, followed by the resection of the amygdala and hippocampal. The upper surface of the temporal lobe (in the depth of the Sylvian fissure) was subpially resected, trying to maintain the integrity of the arachnoid layers to protect the middle *cerebral* artery (MCA) branches. Once the temporal aspect of the lesion had been anatomically resected, the frontal component was removed without any issues. Lastly, the insular part was approached subpially from both the frontal and temporal windows through the anterior and inferior periinsular sulci where MCA branches were running (Fig. 2c). The insular resection was carried out satisfactorily when a progressive loss of the contralateral superior limb motor responses was noticed. This signal loss lasted for 3 min (Fig. 3a, b), and resection was immediately stopped. The position of the subdural grid that had been placed over the motor area was checked first, and no displacement had been noted since the beginning of the resection. No changes in the blood pressure parameters or any unwanted alterations in anesthesia drugs were noted. No retractors were used in this case, so no direct damage to the motor area during dissection was suspected. Another possible explanation that was considered was any potential direct damage to the internal capsule with its corticospinal tract component; however, subcortical white matter stimulation showed that there was no concern of proximity, as demonstrated by 15 mA subcortical stimulation in the closest area.

After some of the most common causes of an intraoperative loss of MEPs were thus analyzed and ruled out, a vascular problem was suspected. To assess this further, an indocyanine green (ICG) injection was performed, which revealed a clear stop to intraluminal blood flow in a distal segment of the superior division of M2 at the level of the insula, which was most likely caused by vasospasm (Fig. 3c). A direct microscopic massage of the vessel segment was performed to increase the blood flow, but it did not work (Fig. 3d). The maneuver was repeated with a cottonoid embedded in nimodipine (Fig. 3e), finally resulting in the resolution of the vasospasm, being confirmed after a new ICG injection (Fig. 3f). After this had been accomplished, MEPs progressively improved over the next few minutes until their base line level had been reached. The surgical resection continued without further troubles.

Postoperative Course

The patient was extubated in the operating room without incident. Initially, a mild left hemiparesis was found, which showed complete recovery after 3–4 h. The postoperative MRI performed on the next day showed a near total resection without signs of ischemia (Fig. 3g, h). The patient was discharged on the eighth postoperative day without motor deficits.

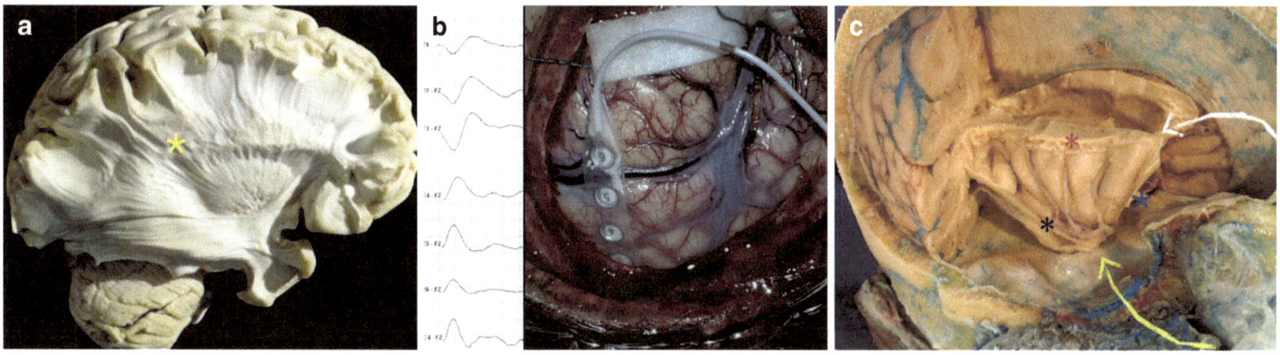

Fig. 2 Surgical planning: (**a**) White matter dissection specimen showing direct subcortical stimulation that was used when getting close to the deepest part—the posteromedial part—of the insular compartment of the tumor (*yellow asterisk*). (**b**) The primary motor area was identified by using the N20 wave-inversion technique. (**c**) Anatomical dissection showing how the insular approach is limited by the limitans sulcus of the insula (*red asterisk* for the superior sulcus; blue for the anterior; and black for the inferior): subpially from both the frontal window (white arrow) and the temporal window (*yellow arrow*)

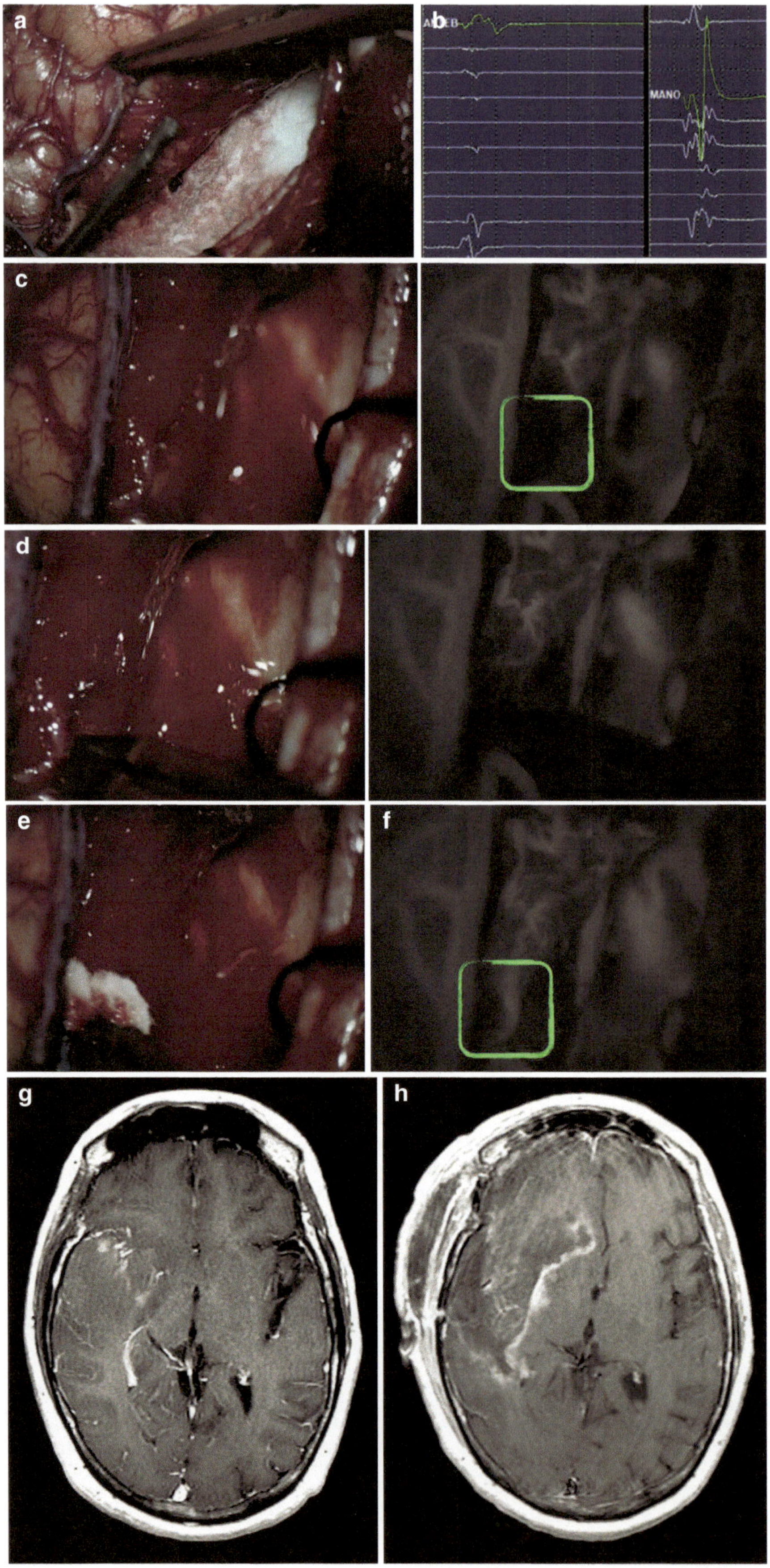
a
b
MANO
c
d
e
f
g
h

Discussion

When facing tumors in the insular region, three important questions must be answered: (1) Is surgery feasible with only minor risks of postoperative deficits? (2) How must the procedure be carried out in terms of anesthesia and intraoperative monitoring (awake vs. asleep and which modality of intraoperative monitoring is to be used)? (3) Last but not least, how will the surgeon address any case of an intraoperative neurological deficit if one is detected?

Although the resectability and determination of extent of resection (EOR) is the shortest and clearest question, it is also probably the most difficult one to answer. To know whether a complete excision is possible in cases of insular gliomas, one must check its medial radiographic extent and limit, as most authors have recommended, with the intention to stop the resection at the level of the white matter layer just lateral to the putamen (external capsule). This avoids potentially compromising the lenticulostriate arteries (LSAs) and therefore avoids causing ischemic damage to the internal capsule [6]. Moreover, a poorly delineated medial limit was correlated with partial resections and an increased risk of vascular complication due to a lesion of the LSAs, especially on its basal aspect, near the anterior perforated substance [9] (Fig. 1a–c). In our case, the tumor had a distinct border lateral to the basal ganglia, and no involvement of the anterior perforated substance was noted. Given the age of our patient, his good neurological status, and the fact that he presented with seizures only in the setting of a well-demarcated tumor in his nondominant hemisphere, microsurgical resection was offered. In cases where these factors are not favorable and a safe resection cannot be achieved (especially in high-grade gliomas), some authors have proposed pursuing only a biopsy, followed by chemotherapy and radiotherapy, which appears to offer a good alternative [10].

When deciding on the type of surgery, one should seriously consider the available intraoperative tools such as the use of intraoperative monitoring in cases of insular gliomas. Some authors have considered performing awake surgery for lesions in both hemispheres regardless of dominance as appropriate [1]. Our policy is to undertake awake procedures for lesions that are involving or near eloquent brain regions and that cannot be tested while the patient asleep. That is why diligent preoperative neuropsychological assessment is crucial. Our case turned out to be an extensive glioma of the nondominant hemisphere, in which the motor and sensory fibers were those at the highest risk of damage. On the other hand, the size and extension of the tumor influenced our decision to perform the procedure asleep, aiming to avoid the tiredness of the patient from a prolonged case under awake conditions. In these cases, monitoring is performed via MEPs to continuously check the integrity of the corticospinal tract, and surgery is further aided by subcortical stimulation as the resection gets closer to the posteromedial limit of the insula, where corticospinal motor fibers are located.

The use of direct subcortical stimulation, provides the advantage of allowing the surgeon to realize how close the resection is getting to the relevant fibers. However, this technique is not sufficient for a complete monitoring, as it cannot provide direct information about a potential vascular compromise [11]. However, the use of MEPs allows the surgeon to detect complications that might happen ''far away'' from the operative field, which is specially relevant when dealing with operculo-insular gliomas as most of the complications are caused by vascular injuries to the white matter tracts that may be far away from th working area.

Although different criteria have been suggested, the most widely accepted "alarm criterion" consists of a decrease in MEP amplitude of 50% from the base line levels (the potential acquired before opening the dura) [12, 13]. This situation usually represents a reversible problem affecting the corticospinal tract, while a complete loss of MEPs is usually irreversible in most cases because it correlates mostly to an ischemic lesion that will be visualized on postoperative MRI [9, 11, 14].

To answer our last question, what the surgeon needs to consider in cases of intraoperative signal loss, we have to keep in mind a clear scheme to check all the possibilities that may apply in this situation to especially not forget any of the reversible causes. That requires drawing a clear diagram of checks and decisions in our mind. First of all, we have to make sure that all the intraoperative monitoring equipment is working properly. From the surgical point of view, the correct position of the electrodes should be checked. Afterward, other causes outside the direct surgical field should be ruled out. Changes in anesthesia can interfere with the correct reading of MEPs [13]. Also, changes in blood pressure (especially hypotension) can decrease the MEP amplitudes. Therefore, when a decrease in the MEPs is observed, the anesthesiologist should increase the blood pressure and check whether this improves the affected responses [14].

Fig. 3 Intraoperative findings: (**a–f**) Insular resection was started without problems (**a**) until a loss of the contralateral superior limb MEPs was found (**b**). A vascular lesion was suspected, so an ICG injection was performed, showing a vasospasm in one M2 branch over the insula (**c**; *green square*). A direct massage was performed to increase the vessel flow, but it had no effect (**d**), so it was repeated with nimodipine (**e**), finally resolving the vasospasm (**f**; *green square*). (**g**, **h**). Axial cuts of postoperative MRI showing near total resection without ischemic lesions

Some authors have even considered performing bilateral stimulation or checking specific parameters to differentiate this general alteration from real problems in the surgical field [15]. Finally—or, even better, while these checks are taking place—the surgeon must think about the latest surgical steps that have been performed and reassess the area in which the resection is actually being carried out. Most importantly, this will require considering which structures were and are at risk in this surgery and what could have occurred: damage to the lenticulostriate arteries, a direct lesion of the precentral region, a disruption in the internal capsule, or an alteration of the MCA branches.

As said at the beginning of the discussion, an extended resection at the inferomedial limit of the tumor might disrupt the lenticulostriate arteries. For this reason, the resection must be stopped at the level of the white matter external to the basal ganglia (external capsule) and especially medial to the limen insulae, which lies just lateral to the anterior perforating substance, assuming that a subtotal resection in a neurologically intact patient is much better than a total resection in a hemiparetic patient or an aphasic patient [6, 7].

In certain circumstances, the precentral region can be altered by an intense retraction of the frontal opercula, especially when facing a purely insular glioma (Yasargil type 3A) when approached via a transylvian route [16]. Therefore, releasing all the retractors is one of the first maneuvers to be performed by the surgeon [7, 16]. In this sense, in our minds, dynamic retraction (using large cottonoids and surgical instruments) appears more suitable. Also, because of the excessive manipulation, some edema may be found, so an extra bolus of corticosteroids has been recommended by some authors [8].

A direct lesion of the corticospinal tract is rare and difficult to assume owing to its medial position, which is protected by the basal ganglia. However, at the most postero-superior part, down to the posterior insular point, where the corona radiata converges and forms the corticospinal tract, it runs over the basal ganglia, and this is a risky point for damaging this tract [5]. Moreover, we can have a vascular lesion of the corona radiata, which is supplied by three types of arteries: lateral striated arteries, long insular arteries, and medullary arteries (branches of M3 and M4) [5, 10].

Finally, a vasospasm of the M2 branches can also lead to an ischemic event of the corticospinal tract. This might be due to a compromise of the long insular arteries (LIA) that are perforating the M2 branches that supply the corticospinal tract [3, 6]. These arteries constitute approximately 3–5% of all insular branches and are in the posterior region of the insula. For this reason, special care should be taken when working near the postero-superior limiting sulcus [5, 7, 10, 17]. Although rare in subpial dissection, close manipulation near the distal MCA branches, as happened in the case that we are presenting, increases the risk of this phenomenon.

Our case proved that this kind of vasospasm can be confirmed via ICG injection and that—when this complication is suspected—irrigation with nimodipine can help to diminish the degree of vascular spasm. To reduce the possibility of this complication, a subpial dissection is widely recommended, although it does not entirely protect the sylvian vessels against blood products and direct manipulation [7, 14], as seen in our case.

Conclusion

In the modern era, surgery on the insular gliomas should not be carried out without intraoperative neurophysiological monitoring to detect compromise to the distal corticospinal tract early. When any alteration in MEPs is found during the case, the surgeon should have a clear scheme in mind on how to rapidly assess all the potential causes. This should especially include a mental review of all the anatomical structures that can be at risk in this approach: lenticulostriate arteries, the corticospinal tract, the prefrontal cortex, and the M2 branches.

Conflict of Interest The authors have no conflicts of interest concerning the reported materials or methods.

References

1. Gravesteijn BY, Keizer ME, Vincent AJPE, Schouten JW, Stolker RJ, Klimek M. Awake craniotomy versus craniotomy under general anesthesia for the surgical treatment of insular glioma: choices and outcomes. Neurol Res. 2018;40(2):87–96.
2. Di Carlo DT, Cagnazzo F, Anania Y, Duffau H, Benedetto N, Morganti R, Perrini P. Post-operative morbidity ensuing surgery for insular gliomas: a systematic review and meta-analysis. Neurosurg Rev. 2019;43(3):987–97.
3. Hirono S, Ozaki K, Ito D, Matsutani T, Iwadate Y. Hammock middle cerebral artery and delayed infarction in the lenticulostriate artery after a staged resection of giant insular glioma: a case report. World Neurosurg. 2018;117:80–3.
4. Yasargil MG, von Ammon K, Cavazos E, Doczi T, Reeves JD, Roth P. Tumours of the limbic and paralimbic systems. Acta Neurochir. 1992;118:40–52.
5. Neuloh G, Pechstein U, Schramm J. Motor tract monitoring during insular glioma surgery. J Neurosurg. 2007;106:582–92.
6. Saito R, Kumabe T, Inoue T, Takada S, Yamashita Y, Kanamori M, Sonoda Y, Tominaga T. Magnetic resonance imaging for preoperative identification of the lenticulostriate arteries in insular glioma surgery: technical note. J Neurosurg. 2009;111:278–81.
7. Lang F, Olansen NE, De Monte F, Gokaslan ZL, Holland EC, Kalhorn C, Sawaya R. Surgical resection of intrinsic insular tumors: complication avoidance. J Neurosurg. 2001;95:638–50.

8. Mammadkhanli O, Bozkurt M, Caglar YS. Assesment of functional results for the lesions located in eloquent areas with using intraoperative cortical-subcortical stimulation and cortical mapping. Turk Neurosurg. 2020;30(6):854–63.
9. Moshel YA, Marcus JDS, Parker EC, Kelly PJ. Resection of insular gliomas: the importance of lenticulostriate artery position. J Neurosurg. 2008;109:825–34.
10. Kumabe T, Higano S, Takahashi ST, Tominaga T. Ischemic complications associated with resection of opercular glioma. J Neurosurg. 2007;106:263–9.
11. Plans G, Fernández-Conejero I, Rifà-Ros X, Fernández-Coello A, Rosselló A, Gabarrós A. Evaluation of the high-frequency monopolar stimulation technique for mapping and monitoring the corticospinal tract in patients with Supratentorial gliomas. A proposal for intraoperative management based on neurophysiological data analysis in a series of 92 patients. Neurosurgery. 2017;81:585–94.
12. Boex C, Haemmerli J, Momjian S, Schaller K. Prognostic values of motor evoked potentials in insular, Precental, or postcentral resections. J Clin Neurophysiol. 2016;33(1):51–9.
13. Jasiukaitis P, Lyon R. A motor evoked potential trending system may discriminate outcome: retrospective application with three cases. J Clin Monit Comput. 2019;33(3):481–91.
14. Gempt J, Krieg SM, Hüttinger S, Buchmann N, Ryan YM, Shiban E, Meyer B, Zimmer C, Forscher A, Ringel F. Postoperative ischemic changes after glioma resection identified by diffusion-weighted magnetic resonance imaging and their association with intraoperative motor evoked potentials. J Neurosurg. 2013;119:829–36.
15. Jasiukaitis P, Lyon R. Trending algorithm discriminates hemodynamic from injury related TcMEP amplitude loss. J Clin Monit Comput. 2020;34(1):131–7.
16. Lu VM, Goyal A, Quiñones-Hinojosa A, Chaichana KL. Updated incidence of neurological deficits following insular glioma resection: a systematic review and meta-analysis. Clin Neurol Neurosurg. 2019;177:20–6.
17. Iwasaki M, Kumabe T, Saito R, Kanamori M, Yamashita Y, Sonoda Y, Tominaga T. Neurol Med Chir (Tokyo). 2014;54:321–6.

The Safe and Appropriate Use of a High-Speed Drill

Kazuhiro Hongo, Tetsuyoshi Horiuchi, and Tetsuya Goto

Abstract

A high-speed drill is an essential tool for any skull base surgery. However, if not appropriately used, it may cause serious inadvertent complications. Here, the authors present one case of surgery for a paraclinoid aneurysm of the internal carotid artery, in which tissue grabbing occurred during the drilling of the anterior clinoid process. This resulted in venous injury to the vessels of the nearby Sylvian fissure. Fortunately, the injury was manageable and caused no significant problems. The authors discuss the basic and other important points for the safe use of a high-speed drill. Discussion includes basic ways of drill handling, the appropriate selection of burrs, and so on. Bone curettage is also mentioned as a safe alternative tool.

Keywords

Burr · Complication · Grabbing · High-speed drill · Surgery

Introduction

When taking a skull base approach under an operating microscope, bone removal near the critical neural structure is an important part of the procedure. Currently, nonrotating tools, such as bone curettes, are available for bone removal. However, high-speed drills are also still widely used. Employing a high-speed drill is efficient, but knowing its appropriate use is mandatory to ensure safety during the procedures. If not, the drill may cause tissue damage through a direct injury, soft tissue grabbing, a heat injury, and so on. Several recommendations have been on how to safely use a high-speed drill. In this manuscript, the authors present a case in which intraoperative complications were caused by the inappropriate handling of the drill. We review the pertinent steps and discuss how to safely use a high-speed drill to avoid such complications.

Case Presentation

A 43-year-old woman was incidentally found to have a paraclinoid aneurysm arising from her left internal carotid artery (Fig. 1). Open microsurgical repair was planned, as requested by the patient. After the proximal internal carotid artery was exposed and secured to be prepared for any premature rupture of the aneurysm at the neck, a standard left pterional approach was carried out. The anterior clinoid process was intradurally drilled away under the operating microscope to expose the proximal neck of the aneurysm, which included unroofing the optic canal. All the cottonoid patties were removed from the operating field, and the adjacent cerebral cortex was covered with rubber sheets. When the lateral edge of the anterior clinoid process was being drilled away (Fig. 2a), the burr slightly slipped off the bone and instantaneously grabbed the rubber sheet (Fig. 2b), causing a slash injury to nearby vessels. Venous bleeding occurred from a nearby Sylvian vein; however, venous injury was rather limited, and normograde venous flow was confirmed with a Doppler flowmeter after controlling the field. Hemostasis was obtained in this instance with cottonoid patty placement, and aneurysm clipping was carried out as usual without any problems.

K. Hongo (✉)
Department of Neurosurgery, Ina Central Hospital, Ina, Japan
e-mail: khongo@shinshu-u.ac.jp

T. Horiuchi
Department of Neurosurgery, Shinshu University School of Medicine, Matsumoto, Japan

T. Goto
Suwa Red Cross Hospital, Suwa, Japan

K. Turel, E. M. Kasper (eds.), *Complications in Neurosurgery II*, Acta Neurochirurgica Supplement 133,
https://doi.org/10.1007/978-3-031-61601-3_11

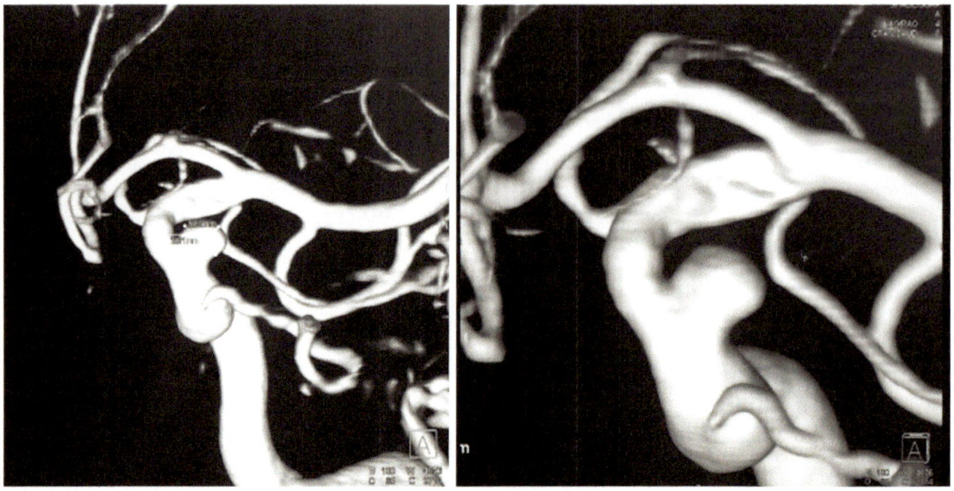

Fig. 1 MR angiograms of the case. Left: Anterior posterior view of the left internal carotid artery. An aneurysm is confirmed in the paraclinoid portion. Right: Magnified and oblique view showing the aneurysm

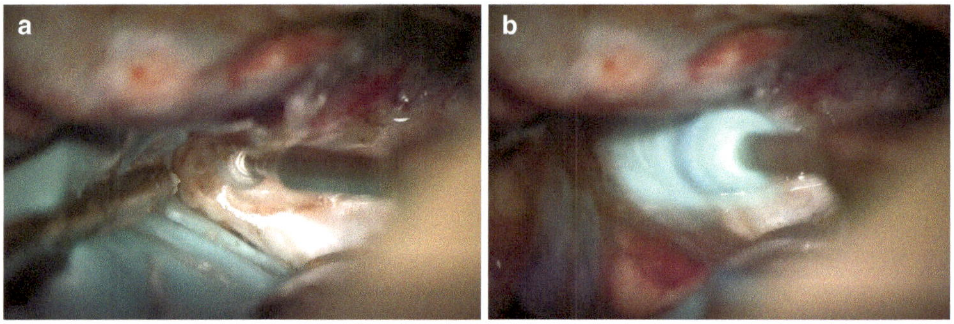

Fig. 2 Intraoperative photos at the time of drilling the left anterior clinoid process. (**a**) The drilling of the lateral edge of the anterior clinoid process. (**b**) Immediately after tissue grabbing

Discussion

Neurosurgeons should know the basic characteristics of high-speed drilling in order to use the device safely and without causing inadvertent complications. This requires their having detailed knowledge of the tool because various shapes of burr tips are available, and one therefore needs to select the most suitable burr. Basically, two types of burr tips can be employed: diamond burrs and cutting burrs (Fig. 3). The efficiency of bone removal is superior when using a cutting burr; however, it has a higher risk of grabbing tissue. Heat generation and heat dissipation are higher when using a diamond burr, which can cause adjacent tissue injury too. When a cutting burr is used, the spinning direction of the burr rotation (usually clockwise = right-side rotation) should be kept in mind. The most efficient site of burr action during bone removal is at the level of the equator of the burr (the maximal diameter), whereas the very tip (pole) of the burr has the least efficiency (Fig. 4a, b). When the lateral edge (equator site) of the burr is in use, bone working can be efficiently carried out just with "soft holding" and by applying minimal pressure; however, when the other sites are being used (including the pole), one needs to employ some additional power to the drill, and these are the moments that have a higher chance of damaging the surrounding critical structures (Fig. 5). The direction of burr handling is also important. Burr handling should be carried out in a direction that points away from the critical tissue and toward the safer side of the surgical field in order to avoid tissue grabbing (Fig. 6).

Given the aforementioned characteristics of a high-speed drill, mainly those relevant to the burr and its proper use, drill operators must abide by the following list of the important points of safely handling a high-speed drill:

1. Remove all the cottonoid patties from the operative field. This is to avoid grabbing the cottonoid patties, which easily damages the brain, vessels, and/or nerves.
2. Protect the cerebral surface with rubber sheets. Rubber sheets are safe in that they protect against grabbing and are also helpful to protect the brain surface from a direct injury to a critical structure.
3. Hold the drill shaft gently and steadily with minimal pressure. Gently holding the shaft is recommended. When the shaft is held firmly, the maneuverability of the burr handling is reduced.
4. Switch the drill on or off only at the operating field. The burr should be on/off at the site of the bone work in the operative field. When drilling is to be finished, after confirming that a burr has stopped its rotation, the shaft should be moved out of the operative field.

Fig. 3 Comparison of characteristics: diamond burr and cutting burr

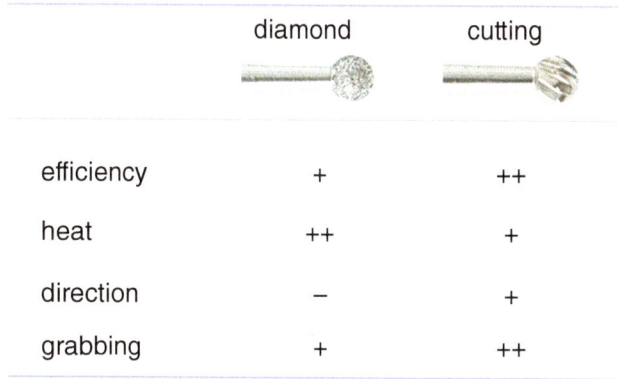

	diamond	cutting
efficiency	+	++
heat	++	+
direction	–	+
grabbing	+	++

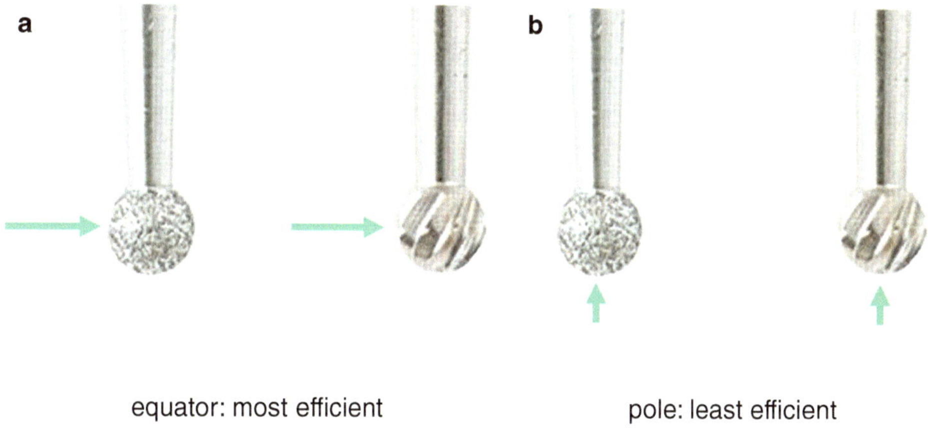

Fig. 4 Schemas showing that the drilling efficiency of burrs depends on the site of the work. (**a**) Schema showing the equator works the most efficiently. (**b**) Schema showing the tip and pole work the least efficiently

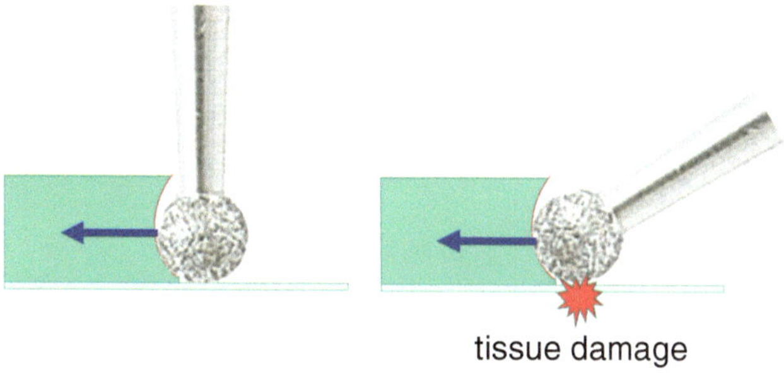

Fig. 5 Schemas showing the appropriate angle of burr handling. Left: The correct way to handle a burr. Right: The incorrect way to handle a burr, which may damage the surrounding structures

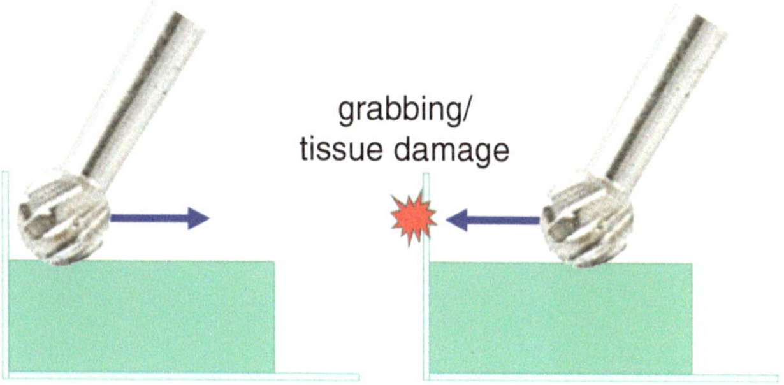

Fig. 6 Schemas showing the appropriate direction of burr handling. Left: The correct and safe way. Right: The incorrect way, which may grab and damage the tissue ahead

5. Adequately irrigate the drill burr with saline to prevent causing a heat injury. A heat injury to nearby structures, such as the optic nerve or other cranial nerves, depending on the site of the bone work, may occur when the field has not been irrigated well. One may see that the drilled bone dust changes to yellow, which indicates that the temperature is too high. This situation should be avoided.
6. Select the appropriate burr size (in mm), tip design (round vs. matchstick), and material (sharp steel vs. diamond splits). To efficiently and safely conduct bone work, the selection of a suitable burr is important. When no critical structures are in proximity or when the work happens far enough away from critical structures, a cutting burr can be selected, which is more efficient. On the other hand, when critical structures are nearby, a diamond burr should usually be selected. As mentioned above, the efficiency of bone removal is reduced when using a diamond drill, so it needs more time to complete this task. One should not hold the shaft firmly or work in haste, because this may cause inadvertent complications.

7. Apply a protective dural flap method. Another safe and useful method for a high-speed drill is to use the so-called protective dural flap method, as has been proposed elsewhere. [1] This is a safe procedure for drilling the anterior clinoid process and porus acusticus internus that avoids injury. Briefly, the semicircular dural flap is pulled out with a thread over the anterior clinoid process. The flap is extended over the underlying structures with a tapered spatula to create adequate space for bone drilling.

In the case presented here, at the time of drilling the anterior clinoid process, the aforementioned points were all kept in mind, and drilling was performed cautiously. However, an inadvertent move by the surgeon caused a slip of the burr tip, and soft tissue from the Sylvian vessels was grabbed. In hindsight, we suspect that the direction of burr handling might not have been appropriate, and the edge of the rubber sheet might not have fit well—it apparently was too near to the working site at the bone's edge. One alternative method for bone removal could have been to use a bone curette [2]. Its tip works via high frequent vibration and torsion without any rotation. Although limited in its application by the bone's consistency, no grabbing occurs with this tool, which also needs adequate irrigation. This needs to be explored further.

Conclusions

A case of paraclinoid aneurysm surgery is presented, in which the grabbing of a protective rubber sheet occurred when drilling the anterior clinoid process. To safely use a high-speed drill, neurosurgeons need to know the basic characteristics of the drill in use. When a bone curette is available, it is an alternative tool for safer bone drilling.

References

1. Tanaka Y, Hongo K, Tada T, Kakizawa Y, Kobayashi S. Protective dural flap for bone drilling at the paraclinoid region and Porus acusticus—technical note. Neurol Med Chir (Tokyo). 2003;43:416–8.
2. Chang HS, Joko M, Song JS, Ito K, Inoue T, Nakagawa H. Ultrasonic bone curettage for optic canal unroofing and anterior clinoidectomy. Technical note. J Neurosurg. 2006;104:621–4.

Dura Opening in Cases with Acute Traumatic Subdural Hemorrhage

Ekkehard M. Kasper and Serdar Kaya

Abstract

The most common pathophysiological etiology of traumatic subdural hematoma is the rupture of bridging veins that drain the venous blood from the brain parenchyma into the superior sagittal sinus. Treatment of choice for such a hematoma would be craniotomy and evacuation. Opening dura in a stellate fashion during in acute traumatic subdural hematoma surgery might decrease the risk of added injury to bridging veins and decrease possible morbidity due to brain edema.

Keywords

Subdural hematoma · Complication · Dura

Acute Traumatic Subdural Hematoma (ASDH)

The most common pathophysiological etiology of traumatic subdural hematoma is the rupture of bridging veins [1]. Bridging veins normally drain the venous blood from the brain parenchyma via the surface veins of the cerebral cortex into the superior sagittal sinus (SSS), and in doing so, they traverse (bridge) the subdural space when they come close to the SSS in the parasagittal space. Here, the cranial end of the bridging veins is firmly anchored and fixed to the dura mater, whereas the cerebral end of the emerging vein is fixed to the surface of the movable hemispheres. The subdural space proper provides no additional structural support to the bridging veins. Lateral movements of the brain are minimized by the presence of the falx. However, it has no protection against antero-posterior movement. Therefore, any severe impact to the head causing such an antero-posterior translocation or significant rotation can lead to the rupture of the bridging veins [2]. Once the bridging vein has broken, the blood extravasates and fills the surrounding cerebrospinal fluid (CSF) space with hemorrhage, forming an acute subdural hematoma. This bleeding must stop spontaneously (via clotting and obliteration of the bleeding site). However, once a surface vein is lost from the index trauma or surgical treatment (see below), significant brain swelling can occur. Lastly, the hematoma that now resides over the hemisphere can cause significant mechanical/chemical irritation and the compression of the underlying brain and cause profound symptoms, which often depend on the location of the clot. In such cases, surgical decompression and clot evacuation are indicated.

Brain Swelling

Although the terms *brain swelling* and *cerebral edema* are frequently used interchangeably, they do have different meanings. *Brain swelling* refers to an increase in brain volume, whereas *cerebral edema* refers to an abnormal accumulation of water within the brain tissue. Thus, brain swelling can be a result of hemorrhage, tumor, or cerebral edema [3]. Cerebral edema, on the other hand, is a more gradual process, due to some form of injury, that can lead to the formation of cytotoxic, ionic, or vasogenic edema.

The first, cytotoxic edema, is defined by the disrupted transmembranous transport of osmolytes due to the depletion of cellular adenosine triphosphate (ATP), which occurs in the setting of stroke. Cell death therefore results in an

E. M. Kasper (✉)
Boston University, Chobanian and Avedisian School of Medicine, Boston, MA, USA

Department of Neurosurgery, Boston University, Chobanian and Avedisian School of Medicine, Boston, MA, USA
e-mail: kaspere@mcmaster.ca

S. Kaya
Department of Neurosurgery, St Elizabeth's Medical Center and Brigham and Women's Hospital, Boston, MA, USA

K. Turel, E. M. Kasper (eds.), *Complications in Neurosurgery II*, Acta Neurochirurgica Supplement 133,
https://doi.org/10.1007/978-3-031-61601-3_12

increase in intracellular Na^+ and water thanks to osmosis, which results in cell swelling [4]. Cytotoxic edema occurs because of the disruption of the actively maintained (and energy-dependent) transendothelial Na^+ gradient. Loss of oxygen supply leads to the breakdown of the energy supply, preventing the accumulation of electrolytes and water in the extracellular compartment of brain parenchyma, which now follows the movement of water from the intravascular to the extracellular spaces. This process is termed *ionic edema* and represents the state of extracellular edema with an intact blood–brain barrier (BBB) [5].

Second, any brain injury caused by inflammatory mediators and oxidative stress damages the blood–brain barrier, causes an increase in the permeability of the astrocytic BBB, and will permit the extravasation of water and plasma proteins, ultimately resulting in extracellular edema, commonly also known as vasogenic edema [6].

Lasty, direct brain tissue trauma causes damage in two stages. In the first stage, primary mechanical deformation leads to altered membrane permeability and disturbances in ion fluxes, which, if sustained, lead to edema and brain swelling. The edema specific to traumatic brain injury (TBI) has generally been considered to be of vasogenic origin, secondary to a traumatic opening of the BBB. However, as the brain injury evolves, these three forms of cerebral edema are likely to overlap significantly, instead of evolving in a sequential manner, and contribute to brain swelling [7].

Once the hematoma resides over the hemisphere, its mass effect exerts compression on the underlying brain, and the venous outflow obstruction may exacerbate an already-swollen brain. This supports the indication for surgical decompression and clot evacuation in these cases.

Surgery for the Decompression and Evacuation of Hematoma

Commonly used surgical techniques for the evacuation of acute traumatic subdural hematoma (ASDH) include osteoplastic craniotomy, large decompressive hemicraniectomy, focal trephination/craniostomy, or a combination of these procedures. The choice of surgical procedures may depend on the surgeon's expertise and training, the neurological status of the patients, the duration of deterioration, the preoperative radiological findings, and the degree of intraoperative brain swelling.

In principle, the purpose of surgery is to alleviate brain compression and intracranial hypertension, and both aspects help to avoid secondary injury [8]. As postulated by the Monro–Kellie doctrine, the sum of all intracranial components is defined by the compartments for brain tissue, brain blood volume, and the CSF space. Once the physiological reserve to compensate for any increase in any of the three components in these compartments has been exhausted, any further intracranial components or brain swelling will cause an increase in intracranial pressure (ICP) because of the predetermined and fixed total volume of the enclosed cranial cavity. Given the inherent limitation of brain tissue (it has no "compressibility"), the pressure will increase steeply once the compressible (shiftable) compartments have been used up and can no longer act as available spaces for the accommodation of further volume. The resulting raised ICP in turn forces a reduction in capillary perfusion and leads to tissue hypoxemia [9]. Thus, a large craniotomy with hematoma evacuation may be the principal procedure of need. When intra- and/or postoperative brain swelling is strongly expected, decompressive craniectomy may be suitable [8]. However, taking the bone off alone will not suffice. The constriction that is caused by the meninges also needs to be addressed, and the dura must be rapidly opened to release the pressure of the intradural compartment.

Dura

The dura can be opened in several ways, and we often do not think much about this step of the surgery. The most common one is cutting the dura parallel to the craniotomy edges. Other common alternatives are cruciate, four flap, fish mouth, slit, and stellate openings [10, 11]. Although opening the dura parallel to the craniotomy line seems to provide the fastest and largest opening, and the one that least obstructs the reach of the surgeon in any other required step, it has significant drawbacks: As mentioned above, brain swelling is very common in traumatic brain injury cases. In addition, some "chemical" irritation is caused by the blood products in the subdural space as well as some blocking of the Virchow–Robin spaces, which provide extracellular clearance pathways to the brain parenchyma, and intraoperative brain swelling will thus be expected intra- and/or postoperatively. Even if the dura is left open to accommodate brain swelling, the veins over the swollen brain will often end up compressed against the free dural margin. This may lead to venous stasis or thrombosis, venous blockage, and subsequently the further worsening of cerebral edema or hemorrhagic infarct [12], thus aggravating a vicious cycle of increased ICP and decreased cerebral perfusion.

Another key aspect of this seemingly very simple step of rapid durotomy is the profound problem that can be inflicted with this opening via an iatrogenic injury to the bridging veins. Since the flow of these veins is mainly toward the SSS, the use of surgical scissors as an opening move carried out perpendicular to their course may cause iatrogenic injury.

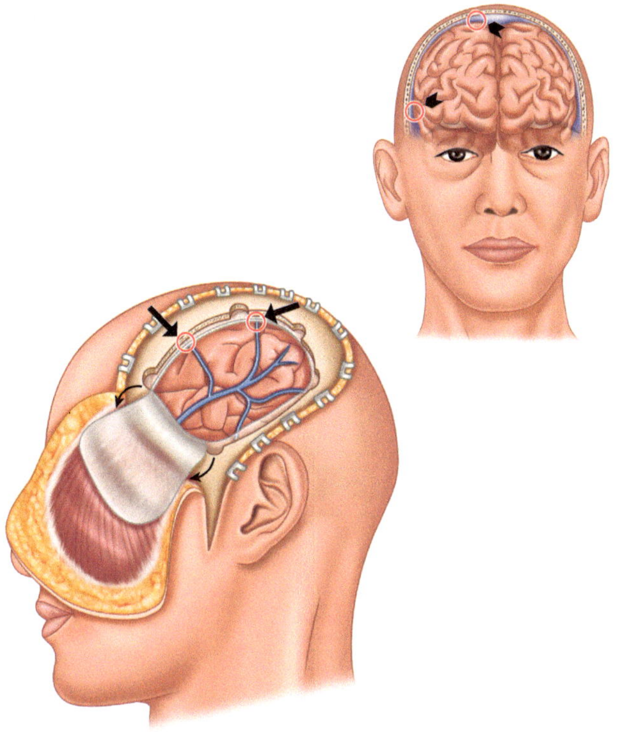

Fig. 1 Bridging veins at risk from trauma (arrows) are at further risk from iatrogenic injury during dural opening via trauma flap (arrow heads)

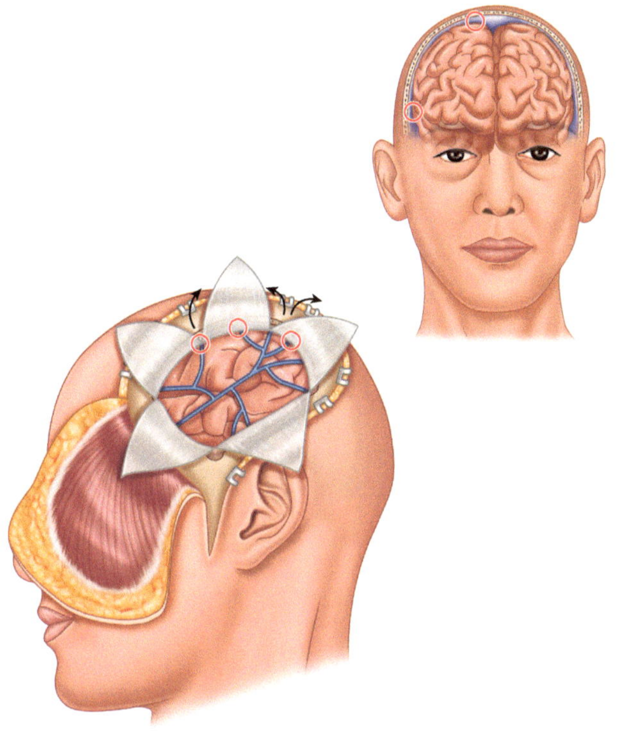

Fig. 2 Complication avoidance: By switching from a classic C-shaped durotomy to a stellate durotomy in trauma cases, the iatrogenic risk to the bridging veins can be avoided

This occurs especially when a large hemicraniectomy is planned and carried out and when the superior margin of the craniotomy is close to the SSS. Here, any further injury/loss of bridging veins has highly detrimental effects on the already-compromised venous flow: When a large bridging vein is cut (or cauterized), then a significant part of the cortical drainage pathway is disrupted or completely taken away, and—in the absence of suitable collateral flow—the venous outflow backs up like a traffic jam, where high venous pressure affects the parenchyma, which can lead to significant venous hemorrhage (Fig. 1).

To avoid this often-devastating complication, which can occur from a rushed and somewhat careless durotomy under often-stressful conditions, we prefer to open the dura in a way that does *not* run parallel to the superior craniotomy edges. Instead, we aim for a much smaller central durotomy or a cruciate durotomy with "relaxing" incisions that widely extend high up toward the midline and SSS at a right angle to the bone margins. Variants of this pattern look like an opening in a stellate fashion (Fig. 2). This will not only avoid the loss of larger dural bridging veins from an iatrogenic injury but also mitigate any venous compression—which is caused by conventional dural margins seen in cuts running parallel to the craniotomy border.

For dural closure, some authors prefer to perform an expansile duraplasty by adding some form of dural onlay graft or by inserting and watertight suturing autografts or allografts [13].

Lastly, vascularized pedicled pericranial flaps can be utilized to form a suitable layer of closure and protection. This step is more important in case with the large anterior craniotomy flaps, which open into the frontal sinus; in cases where the surgeon violates air cells rather low in the access corridors to the middle fossa; and in cases contaminated by a penetrating injury because these cases have increased risks of delayed meningitis and subdural empyema. However, in most cases, dura leaves can be left folded back on the brain and can be supported with artificial or biological dura substitutes without any increase in the rate of postoperative complications [14]. This idea is supported by emerging evidence that watertight duraplasty may not be necessary in standard supratentorial craniotomies [15] (Figs. 3 and 4).

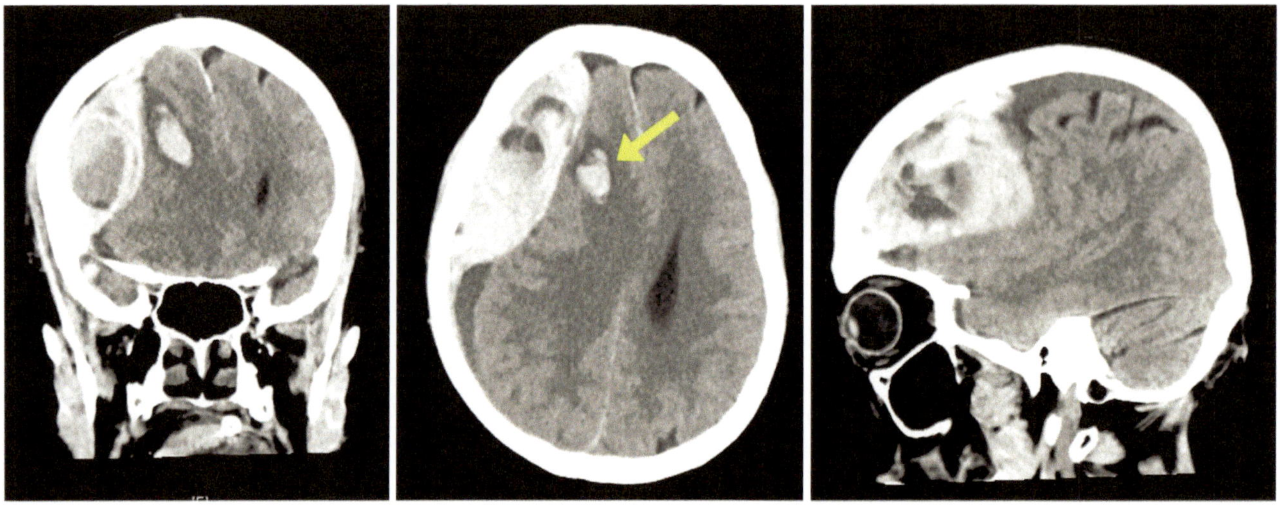

Fig. 3 Pre-OP computed tomography (CT) scan of a 69-year-old female patient who had sustained head trauma in a motor vehicle accident, causing a large hyperacute right frontal subdural hematoma with a 1.3 cm midline shift; note the second focus of the right-side deep-seated parenchymal hemorrhagic contusion (*arrow*)

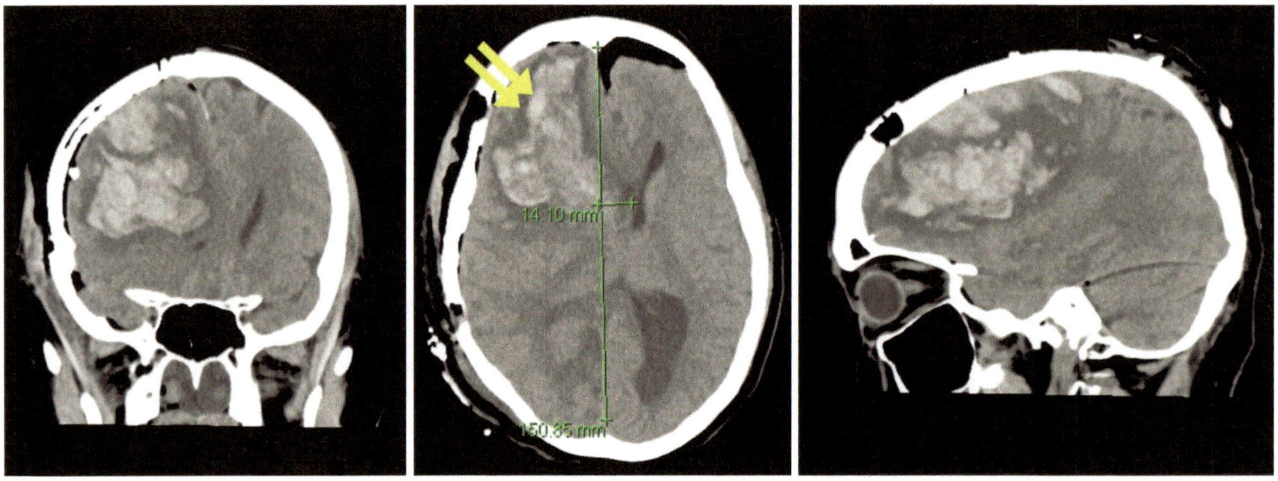

Fig. 4 Post-OP CT scan of the same patient with matching cuts: Despite the excellent evacuation of the extra-axial acute subdural hematoma, a new significant right-side intraparenchymal hematoma developed (*double arrow*); although the contusion might blossom, it is more consistent with venous outflow obstruction and back bleeding from a bridging vein that was taken during surgery

Conclusion

The development of brain swelling following a traumatic brain injury is the most significant predictor of outcomes and accounts for up to 50% of mortalities [16]. Hence, any modification in surgical technique that can alleviate brain swelling should be pursued.

Opening dura in a stellate fashion in acute traumatic subdural hematoma cases appears a simple yet very effective way of gaining access to the site of clot evacuation without introducing any procedural delay. More importantly, though, it is a very safe move that will help decrease the chances of iatrogenic cerebral venous injury, and it does not pose any additional risk that might compromise the already-precarious scenario of brain swelling. We think that this simple maneuver deserves further consideration within the neurosurgical community.

References

1. Miller JD, Nader R. Acute subdural hematoma from bridging vein rupture: a potential mechanism for growth. J Neurosurg. 2014;120(6):1378–84. https://doi.org/10.3171/2013.10.JNS13272.
2. Famaey N, Ying Cui Z, Umuhire Musigazi G, Ivens J, Depreitere B, Verbeken E, Vander Sloten J. Structural and mechanical characterisation of bridging veins: a review. J Mech Behav Biomed Mater. 2015;41:222–40. https://doi.org/10.1016/j.jmbbm.2014.06.009.
3. Shah S, Kimberly WT. Today's approach to treating brain swelling in the neuro intensive care unit. Semin Neurol. 2016;36(6):502–7. https://doi.org/10.1055/s-0036-1592109.
4. Stokum JA, Kurland DB, Gerzanich V, Simard JM. Mechanisms of astrocyte-mediated cerebral edema. Neurochem Res. 2015;40(2):317–28. https://doi.org/10.1007/s11064-014-1374-3.
5. Simard JM, Kent TA, Chen M, Tarasov KV, Gerzanich V. Brain oedema in focal ischaemia: molecular pathophysiology and theoretical implications. Lancet Neurol. 2007;6(3):258–68. https://doi.org/10.1016/S1474-4422(07)70055-8.
6. Klatzo I. Presidental address. Neuropathological aspects of brain edema. J Neuropathol Exp Neurol. 1967;26(1):1–14. https://doi.org/10.1097/00005072-196701000-00001.
7. Marmarou A. A review of progress in understanding the pathophysiology and treatment of brain edema. Neurosurg Focus. 2007;22(5):E1. https://doi.org/10.3171/foc.2007.22.5.2.
8. Karibe H, Hayashi T, Hirano T, Kameyama M, Nakagawa A, Tominaga T. Surgical management of traumatic acute subdural hematoma in adults: a review. Neurol Med Chir. 2014;54(11):887–94. https://doi.org/10.2176/nmc.cr.2014-0204.
9. Stokum JA, Gerzanich V, Simard JM. Molecular pathophysiology of cerebral edema. J Cereb Blood Flow Metab. 2016;36(3):513–38. https://doi.org/10.1177/0271678X15617172.
10. Ghosh AK. Different methods and technical considerations of decompressive Craniectomy in the treatment of traumatic brain injury: a review. Indian J Neurosurg. 2017;2017(6):36–40.
11. Yao Y, Mao Y, Zhou L. Decompressive craniectomy for massive cerebral infarction with enlarged cruciate duraplasty. Acta Neurochir. 2007;149(12):1219–21. https://doi.org/10.1007/s00701-007-1415-7.
12. Gopalakrishnan MS, Shanbhag NC, Shukla DP, Konar SK, Bhat DI, Devi BI. Complications of decompressive Craniectomy. Front Neurol. 2018;9:977. https://doi.org/10.3389/fneur.2018.00977.
13. Malliti M, Page P, Gury C, Chomette E, Nataf F, Roux FX. Comparison of deep wound infection rates using a synthetic dural substitute (neuro-patch) or pericranium graft for dural closure: a clinical review of 1 year. Neurosurgery. 2004;54(3):599–604. https://doi.org/10.1227/01.neu.0000108640.45371.1a.
14. Horaczek JA, Zierski J, Graewe A. Collagen matrix in decompressive hemicraniectomy. Neurosurgery. 2008;63(1 Suppl 1):ONS176–ONS181. https://doi.org/10.1227/01.neu.0000335033.08274.1c.
15. Barth M, Tuettenberg J, Thomé C, Weiss C, Vajkoczy P, Schmiedek P. Watertight dural closure: is it necessary? A prospective randomized trial in patients with supratentorial craniotomies. Neurosurgery. 2008;63(4 Suppl 2):352–8. https://doi.org/10.1227/01.NEU.0000310696.52302.99.
16. Donkin JJ, Vink R. Mechanisms of cerebral edema in traumatic brain injury: therapeutic developments. Curr Opin Neurol. 2010;23(3):293–9. https://doi.org/10.1097/WCO.0b013e328337f451.

Dysgraphia Following the Resection of a Left Parietal Glioma

Eduardo Robatto Plessim de Almeida,
Lucival Silva Santos, and Igor Lima Maldonado

Abstract

We report herein the case of a 41-year-old man operated on for a small inferior parietal lobule ganglioglioma with a sleep-awake-sleep protocol and language mapping to avoid major speech disorders. Postoperatively, however, writing disturbance was characterized by persistent graphemic errors that lasted for about 8 months. The topic is discussed in light of recent literature, exploring the possible relationship between writing difficulties and disconnections produced by a combination of resecting supramarginal gyrus components and interrupting arcuate fasciculus fibers. Awake mapping of eloquent structures is typically done using direct brain stimulation to maximize the extent of the resection while minimizing permanent neurological deficits. However, most intraoperative language tests focus on language skills such as oral and reading skills. Therefore, the detection of dysgraphia requires a high degree of attention from the surgical team and direct examination intra-and perioperatively. To this end, employing an intraoperative writing test during awake surgery may be considered. Advances in this field may aid in increasing the accuracy during parenchymal dissections, influencing the extent of the resection, improving the patient's functional prognosis and long-term quality of life.

Keywords

Parietal lobe · Brain mapping · Brain tumor · Dysgraphia · Language · Aphasia · Ganglioglioma

Introduction

Surgery on the temporoparietal junction in the dominant hemisphere is a neurosurgical challenge because of the proximity to eloquent brain areas, which requires that surgeons have an accurate knowledge of functional neuroanatomy at both the cortical and subcortical levels. Mapping these eloquent structures can be performed via direct brain stimulation with the patient awake, which maximizes the extent of the resection while minimizing permanent neurological deficits.

At the cortical level, Wernicke's area is located in the posterosuperior portion of the temporal lobe, which often corresponds to the lower portion of the exposed cortex if a temporoparietal or frontotemporoparietal craniotomy is undertaken. As the definition of Wernicke's area is functional, its precise delineation has considerable individual variability. In the anterior portion of the surgical field, the surgeon deals with the sensory and motor cortices in the postcentral gyrus and the precentral gyrus separately.

At the subcortical level, the white matter of the inferior parietal lobule (IPL) is traversed by important fasciculi. This is the case for the ventral (opercular) component of the superior longitudinal fasciculus (SLF-III) and, more deeply, the posterosuperior portion of the arcuate fasciculus (AF) [1, 2]. Numerous studies on subcortical mapping have pointed out the importance of the SLF-III and the AF for articulatory and phonological functions, respectively [3–6]. Both fasciculi have been considered important anatomical correlates of the dorsal stream of the language network. In this context, the use of speech and naming tests has been deemed important for "safe" surgical resections, though not only during cortical mapping but also as the surgeon progresses into the depth

E. R. P. de Almeida
Escola Bahiana de Medicina e Saúde Pública, Fundação para o Desenvolvimento das Ciências, Salvador, Brazil

L. S. Santos
Hospital Santa Izabel, Santa Casa de Misericórdia da Bahia, Salvador, Brazil

I. L. Maldonado (✉)
Instituto de Ciências da Saúde & Hospital Universitário Professor Edgard Santos, Universidade Federal da Bahia, Salvador, Brazil

INSERM, Imaging Brain & Neuropsychiatry iBraiN U1253, Université de Tours, Tours, France
e-mail: limamaldonado@univ-tours.fr

K. Turel, E. M. Kasper (eds.), *Complications in Neurosurgery II*, Acta Neurochirurgica Supplement 133,
https://doi.org/10.1007/978-3-031-61601-3_13

of the parenchyma. Transient speech disorders are relatively common after the surgical manipulation of these structures, but when the structural integrity of these functional areas is properly preserved, medium-term recovery is usually excellent [7].

In this manuscript, we report the case of a 41-year-old man who underwent surgery for a small inferior parietal lobule ganglioglioma, where we employed a sleep-awake-sleep protocol and intraoperative language mapping to avoid major speech impairment. Postoperatively, however, the patient was surprised by the presence of writing disturbances characterized by persistent graphemic errors lasting for about 8 months. This case draws attention to the fact that common examination protocols during awake surgery are less sensitive to this kind of problem because they focus mostly on language skills such as oral and reading skills. The topic is discussed in the context of recent literature, as is the possible relationship between such writing difficulties and the surgical manipulation of the AF in the depth of the supramarginal gyrus.

Case Report

History, Clinical Examination, and Imaging

A 41-year-old male accountant who was also a law school student presented himself for consultation, referred from another service. The man played guitar, spoke two languages (Portuguese and English), and was studying a third one (Mandarin). The patient did not present with any cognitive, sensory, or motor neurological deficits. Two secondarily generalized seizures had prompted magnetic resonance imaging (MRI). The MRI showed an intraparenchymal tumor of small volume intrinsic to the supramarginal gyrus and invading the white matter at its depth (Fig. 1). Radiographic appearance was compatible with a tumor of glial origin. Surgical removal including awake brain mapping was proposed.

The patient was evaluated by three examiners trained in the surgical protocol: a neurosurgeon, an anesthesiologist, and a speech therapist. No signs or symptoms other than the preceding seizure were identified. At the time of the initial assessment, he was instructed on the procedure and trained to perform the language tests in the awake phase. He was also asked to report abnormal sensations such as paresthesia or dysesthesia along with their specific locations. The neurological examination was normal, as were the mini-mental status, counting, verbal fluency, spontaneous speech, picture-naming, and line bisection tests.

Surgical Procedure

The patient was placed in the right lateral decubitus position and underwent general anesthesia, which used a laryngeal mask and an anesthetic scalp block. The head was placed in a Mayfield holder. A frontotemporoparietal craniotomy was performed, which was centered on the left parietal prominence, allowing the exposure of the IPL, part of the temporal lobe, and the postcentral gyrus. An intraoperative ultrasound helped to delineate tumor boundaries as well as sulci and gyri. After the craniotomy, the patient was awoken, and electrical stimulation was used to map eloquent areas and to guide neurosurgical resection. A Ojemann-style bipolar electrode (Micromar, Diadema, Brazil) with 5 mm spacing between tips was used to apply electrostimulation with a current intensity between 1.0 and 6 mA (60 Hz pulse frequency,

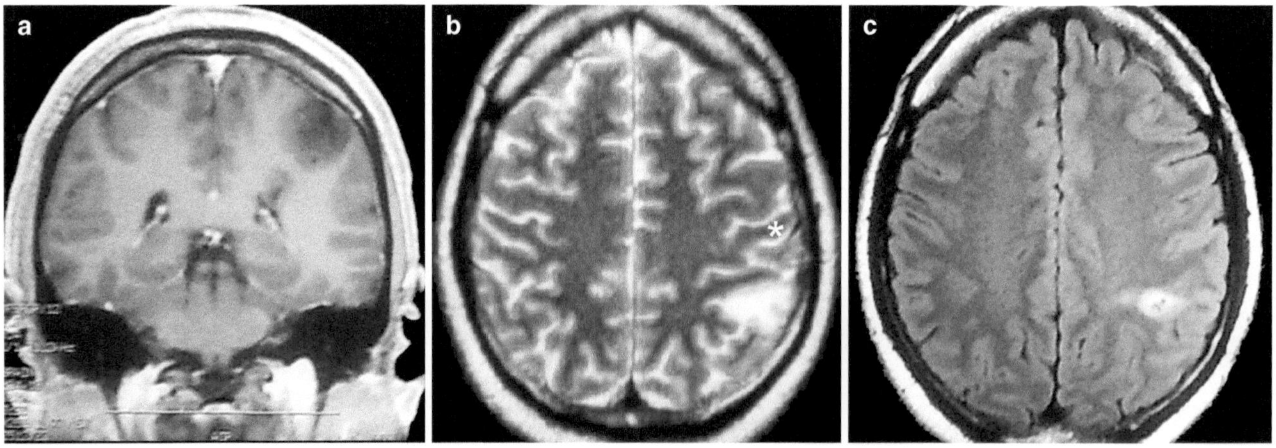

Fig. 1 Preoperative MRI examination showing a left parietal tumor suggestive of low-grade glioma. (**a**) Coronal T1-weighted image after an intravenous injection of gadolinium. No contrast enhancement was observed. (**b**) Axial T2-weighed image allowing the study of the sulcal and gyral anatomy. The tumor infiltrated the supramarginal gyrus, in the inferior parietal lobule. (**c**) Axial fluid attenuated inversion-recovery image showing a zone of hypersignals corresponding to the infiltration of the adjacent white matter. *postcentral gyrus

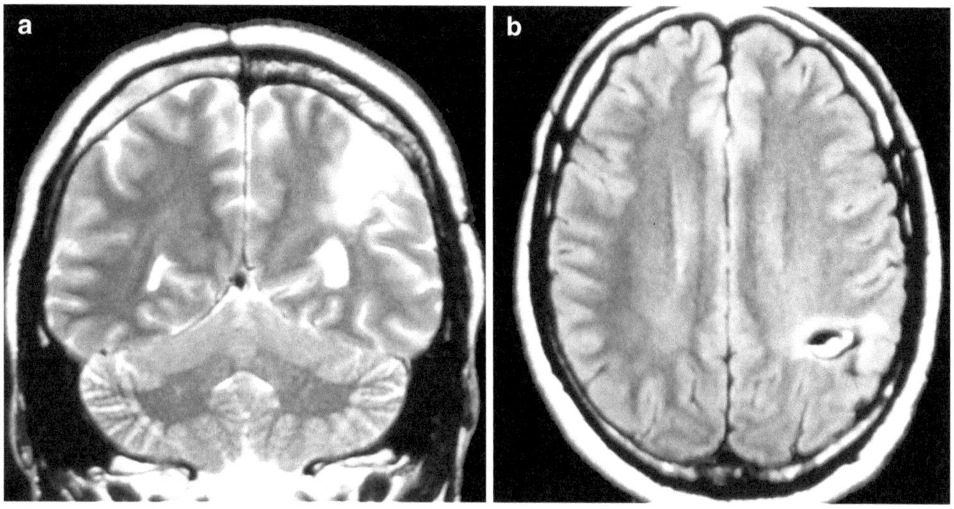

Fig. 2 Postoperative MRI after tumor resection that was assisted by awake brain mapping and used the asleep-awake-asleep technique. (**a**) Coronal T2-weighted image. (**b**) Axial fluid attenuated inversion-recovery image

1 ms pulse width). The intraoperative examination included repetitive counting, motor function, sensory examination, spontaneous speech, a DO-80 picture-naming test, line bisection, and a dual task composed of simultaneous upper limb movements and picture naming. Stimulation was systematically alternated with tumor resection, which was progressively carried further until the limits of resection were reached, at the depth of the IPL. Reproducible phonological paraphasias were triggered by stimulating the white matter in the depth of the operative cavity in topographical proximity to the arcuate fasciculus. The occurrence of these paraphasias delineated the functional limit that surgical resection should not exceed. Dysarthria and anomia were not observed during white matter stimulation. The patient underwent general anesthesia again, for closure.

Follow-Up

The awakening from anesthesia was uneventful. A postoperative MRI examination was performed shortly after the procedure and repeated after 3 months (Fig. 2). It showed complete tumor removal and confirmed that the floor of the operative cavity was in proximity to the AF topography (Fig. 3). From the first day after the surgical procedure, the patient displayed numerous phonological paraphasias that became progressively less frequent and less impactful on speech. The evolution of these paraphasias was typical of the transient language disturbances often seen after awake surgery, most likely related to transient postoperative edema. The patient was then discharged on corticosteroid therapy and was reassessed at 15 days after the surgery. At this time, he began to show his recovery from his impairment.

At the next follow-up visit, carried out 1 month after the procedure, speech was very much improved. Although less frequent, his phonological paraphasias were still present, but the patient presented with fluid and very understandable speech. Because he was also a musician, the neurological examination was completed by testing his instrumental interpretation and singing. No difficulty in playing guitar was reported or perceived. Interestingly, the phonological paraphasias were completely absent during singing. The patient's main complaint, however, was not related to oral language but rather to writing. He reported that he noted (retrospectively) that texts that he had written after the surgery contained numerous spelling mistakes. This description by the patient encouraged us to undertake a written picture-naming test to better characterize the impairment. No motor difficulty was observed; the handwriting was legible and corresponded to his usual handwriting. However, the words were often wrong in that they featured either substituted or omitted letters (Fig. 4). These mistakes made in written language were much more impactful than the phonological paraphasias in oral language (Table 1). The patient was meanwhile followed by a speech therapist. While his speech has become practically normal at about 3 months, the dysgraphia lasted for a total of about 8 months, with significant effects on his daily and professional life during that period.

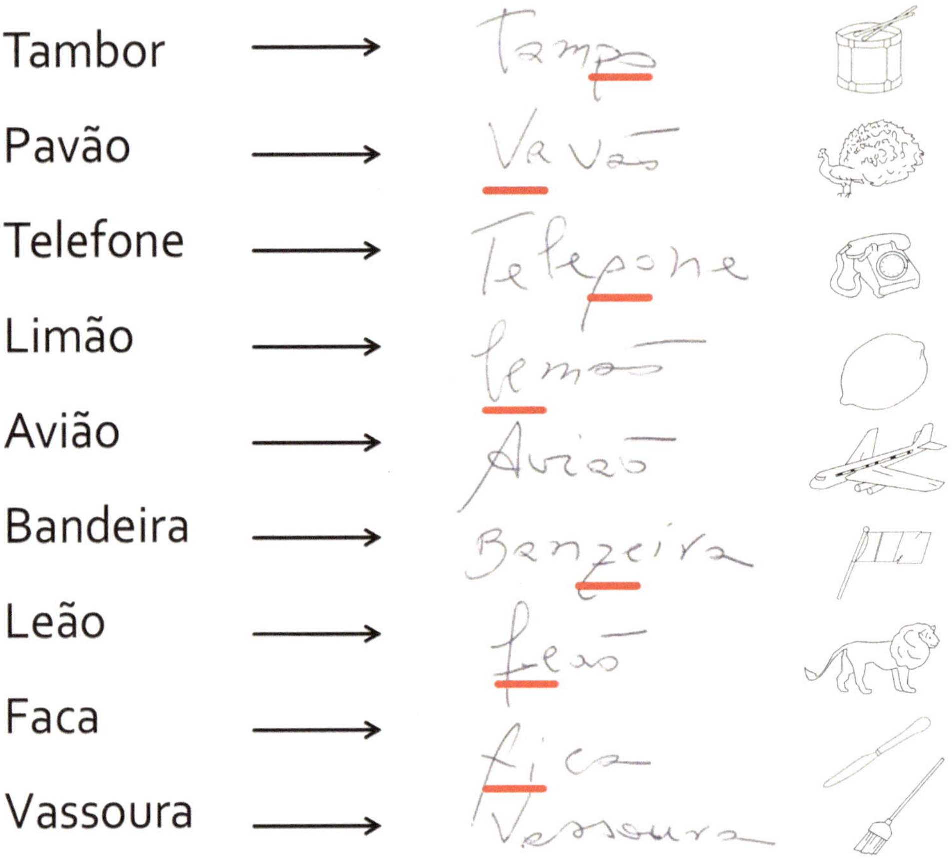

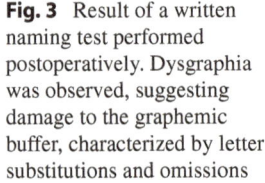

Fig. 3 Result of a written naming test performed postoperatively. Dysgraphia was observed, suggesting damage to the graphemic buffer, characterized by letter substitutions and omissions

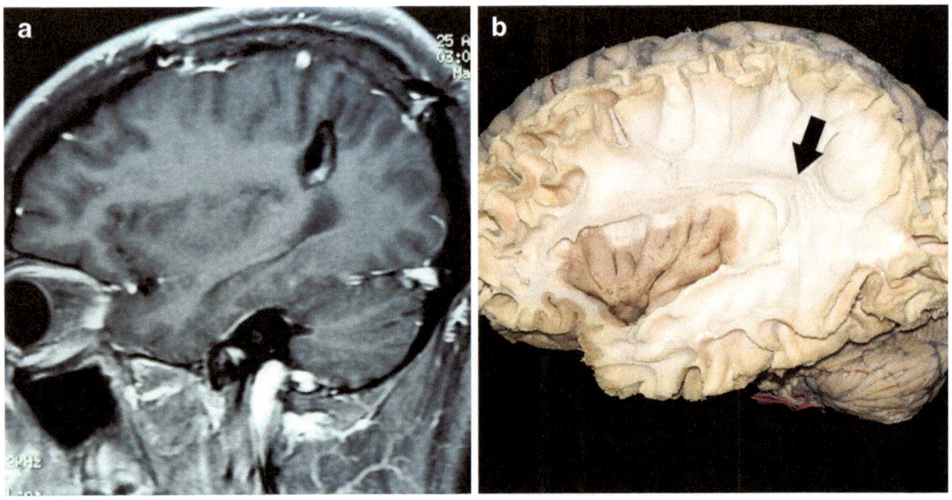

Fig. 4 Relevant white matter anatomy in the depth of the operative cavity. (**a**) Sagittal T1-weighted image after an injection of gadolinium-based contrast medium. The depth of the operative cavity is located on the white matter, in contact with the postero-superior portion of the arcuate fasciculus. At this point, direct cerebral stimulation triggered reproducible pholonogical paraphasias. (**b**) Anatomical specimen showing relevant anatomy for the case. Fiber dissection of arcuate fasciculus (*arrow*), around the limitant sulcus of the insula

Table 1 Summary of results of picture-naming test (DO-80) 1 month after the surgical resection, showing graphemic errors and less-frequent phonological paraphasias

Errors	Nb
Written	
Spelling errors	26
Ommission	1
Substitution	19
Insertion	2
Mixed	4
Visual paraphasia	1
Oral	
Phonological paraphasias	10
Perseveration	7
Anomia	2

Discussion

We report herein the case of a young right-handed male adult who presented with long-lasting dysgraphia after surgery that involved superficial and deep portions of the dominant IPL.

Written language impairment has previously been reported in the context of acute brain damage, especially stroke [8]. These disabilities occur more frequently after damage to the left cerebral hemisphere. In the context of a cerebral intraparenchymal tumor, the slowly infiltrating character of the disease, which leaves room for adaptations and brain plasticity, seems to be the main explanation for the rarity of this phenomenon in treatment-naïve patients [9]. It may, however, manifest prominently after surgical treatment. Frontal, parietal, and temporal structures have been related to the occurrence of spelling mistakes after glioma surgery, although properly documented evidence of postoperative deficits is remarkably scarce [10].

Theories on the topographical distribution of linguistic functions were strengthened by the studies of Broca and Wernicke. In addition to describing one more language-related brain area, Wernicke reinforced the concept of the further existence of connections between the two areas, for which the AF is the main anatomical correlate [11]. Other routes, shorter but highly robust, indirectly connect these regions. The inferior parietal lobe, more specifically the supramarginal gyrus, is an area of convergence for fiber pathways originating from these two language areas and serves as an intermediate relay station [12]. This peculiarity is why this zone is referred to as the Geschwind territory in studies on structural connectivity, in honor of Norman Geschwind and his studies on disconnection syndromes. Modeling language brain circuits, Hickok and Poeppel (2004) proposed that language would be organized in at least two parallel integration pathways [13]. According to this model, the dorsal pathway is preferentially articulatory-phonological, while the ventral pathway is semantic. The dorsal pathway appears to correspond to the elements of the connective system comprising the superior longitudinal fasciculus and the AF [2, 6].

Different forms of dysgraphia have been recognized, but cognitive models propose two basic mechanisms for writing words: writing with phonological mediation (the conversion of phonemes into graphemes) and the lexical route with access to words as a whole [14, 15]. The latter is faster and used for writing familiar words. This mechanism allows the correct spelling of irregular words. After damage to the graphemic buffer has been sustained, difficulties in lexical access and phoneme–grapheme conversion are observed. The patient usually writes well-formed graphemes, but the replacement, omission, or addition of words happens, as in the present case [8, 10]. In another scenario, so-called peripheral dysgraphia involves errors in converting orthographic information into movement. In this situation, the patient usually has spatial, perceptual, or apraxic difficulties with writing tasks.

In the specific case of our patient, the absence of motor disturbances (in writing and fine gestures of the upper extremities) makes apraxia or a disturbance in motor function an unlikely underlying mechanism. The absence of articulatory disturbances during speech and the presence of concomitant phonological paraphasias makes us hypothesize that a relationship may exist between the observed disturbances and the partial disconnection of the AF (Fig. 4). Added to the resection that was carried out in the supramarginal gyrus, this dual impact probably functionally disconnected the frontal and temporal language areas. Letter-level errors after glioma resection with damage to the AF has been reported by classic and contemporary studies [16, 17]. Nevertheless, a clear relationship with this topography is difficult to establish given that this clinical impairment has also been observed in patients with cerebral lesions in other locations and given that it has not been reported as a constant finding after AF damage. A more extensive discussion on the clinical observation is further complicated by the fact that data on the phenomenon remain scarce.

The occurrence of dysgraphia after surgery on the temporoparietal junction leads us to rethink the sensitivity of the current clinical examination protocols during awake surgery to detecting this phenomenon. Most tests focus on language skills such as oral and reading skills. Therefore, to detect dysgraphia in this setting, a high degree of attention is required on the part of the team involved in surgery, and an intra-and perioperatively conducted examination is needed. To this end, the use of a writing test during the awake phase of the surgical mapping and resection may be considered. Advances in this field, particularly concerning white matter procedures, may contribute to increasing the precision of parenchymal surgeries, thus positively affecting the extent of resection, the prognosis for functional status after surgery, and, lastly, patients' long-term quality of life.

Acknowledgments None.

Conflict of Interest Statement The authors have no conflicts of interest to declare.

References

1. Vavassori L, Sarubbo S, Petit L. Hodology of the superior longitudinal system of the human brain: a historical perspective, the current controversies, and a proposal. Brain Struct Funct. 2021;226:1363. https://doi.org/10.1007/s00429-021-02265-0.
2. Yagmurlu K, Middlebrooks EH, Tanriover N, Rhoton AL. Fiber tracts of the dorsal language stream in the human brain. JNS. 2016;124(5):1396–405.
3. Duffau H, Gatignol P, Denvil D, Lopes M, Capelle L. The articulatory loop: study of the subcortical connectivity by electrostimulation. Neuroreport. 2003;14(15):2005–8.
4. Duffau H, Moritz-Gasser S, Mandonnet E. A re-examination of neural basis of language processing: proposal of a dynamic hodotopical model from data provided by brain stimulation mapping during picture naming. Brain Lang. 2014;131:1–10.
5. Maldonado IL, Moritz-Gasser S, de Champfleur NM, Bertram L, Moulinié G, Duffau H. Surgery for gliomas involving the left inferior parietal lobule: new insights into the functional anatomy provided by stimulation mapping in awake patients. J Neurosurg. 2011;115(4):770–9.
6. Maldonado IL, Moritz-Gasser S, Duffau H. Does the left superior longitudinal fascicle subserve language semantics? A brain electrostimulation study. Brain Struct Funct. 2011;216:263–74.
7. Zetterling M, Elf K, Semnic R, Latini F, Engström ER. Time course of neurological deficits after surgery for primary brain tumours. Acta Neurochir. 2020;162(12):3005–18.
8. de Rodrigues JC, da Fontoura DR, de Salles JF. Acquired dysgraphia in adults following right or left-hemisphere stroke. Dement Neuropsychol. 2014;8(3):236–42.
9. Desmurget M, Bonnetblanc F, Duffau H. Contrasting acute and slow-growing lesions: a new door to brain plasticity. Brain. 2006;130(4):898–914.
10. van Ierschot F, Bastiaanse R, Miceli G. Evaluating spelling in glioma patients undergoing awake surgery: a systematic review. Neuropsychol Rev. 2018;28(4):470–95.
11. Catani M. The connectional anatomy of language: recent contributions from diffusion tensor tractography. In: Johansen-Berg H, Behrens TEJ, editors. Diffusion MRI. From quantitative measurement to in-vivo neuroanatomy. Amsterdam: Academic Press; 2009. p. 403–13.
12. Catani M, Jones DK, Ffytche DH. Perisylvian language networks of the human brain. Ann Neurol. 2005;57(1):8–16.
13. Hickok G, Poeppel D. Dorsal and ventral streams: a framework for understanding aspects of the functional anatomy of language. Cognition. 2004;92(1–2):67–99.
14. Miceli G, Capasso R. Spelling and dysgraphia. Cogn Neuropsychol. 2006;23(1):110–34.
15. Rodrigues J, Pawlowski J, Müller J, Bandeira D, Salles J. Comparison of errors in the writing of words between adults post-stroke in the cerebral hemispheres. Neuropsicol Latinoamericana. 2013;5(4):1–14.
16. Köhler K, Bartels C, Herrmann M, Dittmann J, Wallesch C-W. Conduction aphasia-11 classic cases. Aphasiology. 1998;12(10):865–84.
17. Tomasino B, Marin D, Maieron M, D'Agostini S, Medeossi I, Fabbro F, Skrap M, Luzzatti C. A multimodal mapping study of conduction aphasia with impaired repetition and spared reading aloud. Neuropsychologia. 2015;70:214–26.

Ethical Considerations in Complications of Surgical Procedures

H. Maximilian Mehdorn and Anne-Sophie Mehdorn

Abstract

Surgical procedures carry certain risks of complications, which need to be considered and discussed when any procedure is suggested to a patient. In this article, some ethical problems will be discussed concerning the communication of problems after they have occurred. Some clinical case studies will serve to clarify the need for having standards of ethical behavior, even in difficult situations. Further information will be given from experience gained from a medicolegal commission for malpractice complaints.

Keywords
Ethical behavior · Complication · Surgical error · Medicolegal issue · Arbitration

Introduction

Behavior as a doctor caring for patients should follow the ethical principle of primum nil nocere—which translates into English as "first do no harm." Under this rule and the rule of the self-determination of the patient, medical treatment and surgical procedures are allowed only if they have been clearly indicated, the patient has been well informed about the risks and benefits, and the patient has consented to the intervention. As can be seen across centuries and various cultural backgrounds, modifications have been made to these rules. Still, the most important rules certainly mean taking a patient-centered approach in which the patient is considered the partner of the doctor in fighting the disease. This approach should aim to benefit neither the doctor nor the patient's relatives in specific and must include a vigorous consideration of how the physician would feel about undergoing whatever diagnostics and treatment they recommend to the patient if they were in that patient's place. With this in mind, good doctor–patient relationships could develop over centuries, both overall in society and among individuals. This should be kept in mind despite the changing sociocultural environments and financial rules governing neurosurgical practice [1]. The increasing number of court rulings, litigation proceedings, and even aggressive behaviors by relatives against doctors in various countries may contradict the old saying "trust me; I'm a doctor," which might have turned into "the doctor—while needed—is rather the enemy." Is the doctor today rather conceived as a moneymaking individual or still as a well-educated and well-trained person? Are they honest with their patients, and do they teach their patients and their staff such that progression along a learning curve and good clinical judgment are evident?

A PubMed search was carried out to help answer the preceding question, yet it showed only an increasing number of publications in recent years when the two search phrases "ethics and complications" (5983 in 2019 vs. 22.284 in June 2021) and "ethics and complications and neurosurgery" (181 vs. 799) were used, while a query for "the ethical implications of complications and neurosurgery" yielded only 22 hits, which did not help to further define this problem. The increasing number of retrieved studies is influenced partly by referring to "ethics committee involvement" in those studies. However, the way that healthcare is delivered to an individual patient within a given framework obviously influences the doctor–patient relationship [1].

Therefore, in this chapter, this problem is extensively discussed on the basis of the personal neurosurgical experience of nearly 50 years, covering a neurosurgical career that has been burdened by a number of complications from which the senior author has tried to learn throughout his life, as well as

H. M. Mehdorn (✉)
Departments of Neurosurgery, University Hospitals of Schleswig-Holstein Kiel, Kiel, Germany
e-mail: mehdorn@nch.uni-kiel.de

A.-S. Mehdorn
General, Visceral, Transplantation, Thoracic and Pediatric Surgery, University Hospitals of Schleswig-Holstein Kiel, Kiel, Germany

K. Turel, E. M. Kasper (eds.), *Complications in Neurosurgery II*, Acta Neurochirurgica Supplement 133,
https://doi.org/10.1007/978-3-031-61601-3_14

the lessons learned from the problems of other surgeons, which he as a member of the medicolegal college for arbitration learned about over many years.

Ethical issues may be derived from the financial implications of increasingly expensive modern medicine, the further development of modern (neuro-)surgery, and the application of evidence-based medicine. Especially the latter has contributed to, for example, the routine use of prophylactic antibiotics, the postoperative adjudication of intensive care unit (ICU) beds for otherwise-healthy patients (the need of which has been discussed recently on the basis of single center studies), the length and quality of survival under conservative therapy for indications for surgery in world health organization (WHO) grade II glioma patients, and the further reductions in the length of hospital stay and in costs thanks to performing awake craniotomy for most intrinsic brain tumors [2], to name only a few. However, the topic extends into organizational problems—e.g., when or whether to send patients only to high-volume centers, which might make sense for specific diseases like movement disorders or cerebrovascular problems requiring an interdisciplinary approach to achieve the best possible results. Further suitable examples are the application of intraoperative indocyanogreen (ICG) fluorescence for intracranial vascular surgery and the modern extended use of neuronavigation and/or intraoperative computed tomography (CT) or magnetic resonance (MR) imaging. Do these technologies need to be used, or are they just gadgets? Would continuing to perform surgeries without these adjuncts (which are often not scientifically evaluated in multicenter randomized double-blind studies, given that this may not even be possible) be ethical?

Such organizational problems might also be touched on when a patient or their relative is confronted with a complication that occurred in an individual case recently treated by a responsive (neuro-)surgeon.

Yet the focus of this article should be more on individual patient care than on discussing problems of hospital organization.

Defining the Problem

A patient usually seeks help from a specific individual doctor and therefore usually considers a doctor a partner whom the patient can trust—because they (unfortunately) had no other choice depending on an emergency or referral situation. From a legal point of view, obtaining a correct indication of treatment according to the present standard of care and obtaining informed consent for elective interventions are the two primary prerequisites for a good discussion with the patient and their relatives. However, when something goes wrong—that is, when the patient is not satisfied with the result—it has one of three major explanations:

1. The optimal results of a procedure could not be achieved, because of the preoperative situation.
2. Inherent complications have occurred.
3. A mistake has been made.

With the personal experience of the senior author as a member of a large medicolegal board of arbitration covering northern Germany (dealing with approx. 2000 arbitrations every year), we reviewed 205 consecutive complaints brought forward in the years 2014 and 2015 against spine surgeons. These complaints were filed mostly because of persistent or worsened pain or the postoperative deterioration of the patient's neurological/functional status. After a careful review of the materials, we found that in 26.3% of cases, some damage indeed occurred that could have been prevented if treatment (including postoperative care) would have been performed properly (according to the rules), while most cases with alleged damages (65.7%) were not due to malpractice induced by treatment but rather remaining consequences from the original disease. Lastly, noncompensable iatrogenic damage occurred in 7% of cases. This means that slightly more than a quarter of all malpractice complaints in spine care brought forward to the arbitration board were considered justified—after a written case-testimony by an independent peer expert was evaluated by a group of lawyers and surgeons—and resulted in reasons for patients to be financially compensated. This is a relevant number given the high number of spine surgeries performed by neurosurgeons, orthopedic surgeons, and trauma surgeons in the area covered by this committee. Fortunately, in our experience, the total number of cases brought forward for review seems to have decreased over recent years. Yet this number does not include the patients who immediately went to court or who failed to complain and instead accepted their fate.

After these arbitration institutions had been created by the regional Medical Chambers in Germany in the mid 1970s, we evaluated all cases from a large region in Germany (industrial North Rhine–Palatine, centered on Duesseldorf) for the years 1976–1988 [3]. Neurosurgical cases were considered by the arbitration panel as due to wrongdoing in 15.6% of all claims brought forward against neurosurgeons (1.65% out of all claims brought to the arbitration panel), and this number could be divided into spinal cases (18.4%) vs. cranial cases (10.2%), which compared favorably to the 22.9% seen in the entire study group (Mehdorn et al., 1990). Most neurosurgical mistakes were due to a delay in the diagnostic or therapeutic intervention once a postoperative worsening of the neurological status had occurred, and this is true for spinal surgery, the treatment of peripheral nerves, and trigeminal neuralgia cases.

Over the course of the assessment, we also contacted the 11 hospitals in the area under review to possibly find local variations in error frequencies among the approx. 4500 spinal and 2400 brain tumor operations every year. This would correspond to a requested independent evaluation of 0.13% of the total volume of spinal cases, and only 0.024% of the total number of rendered treatments were considered as indicative of wrongdoing. The respective figures for brain tumor surgery were 0.035% (alleged wrongdoing) and 0.0032% (actual treatment mistakes made). In conclusion, brain tumor surgeries had remarkably small numbers of alleged wrongdoings and factual wrongdoings.

Individual Cases and Personal Experience

These percentages may suggest a very low relevance of the problem. However, each case of alleged wrongdoing has a profound psychological impact on the doctor and should encourage the surgeon to prevent the next one by optimizing their treatment algorithms and their communication with patients. Some personal experiences should help to clarify this need:

1. When still a resident in the early 1980s, the senior author (MM) had to operate—assisted by a staff member—on a frontal meningioma diagnosed by CT scan. At this time, marking the laterality on CT scans was not yet standardized which was implemented only shortly after, and positioning of the patient for surgery was performed by an experienced nurse assistant. In those days, the surgeons would come in to start the skin incision—after a booking denoted as "simple, for frontal meningioma." After the craniotomy, the dura was incised but no meningioma found. Looking carefully at the CT scans it became evident that the wrong side had been operated on. Consequently, the dura was closed and the bone flap fixated before craniotomy was performed on the correct side and the meningioma was completely removed. When finishing the case, the assisting staff member discussed with me that I should have to compensate the patient for my wrongdoing. I went to see the patient the afternoon after surgery and on the following days, and I explained to him, "we had also looked on the other side and had not found another tumor." No issue was raised even when he developed a meningioma a few years later that was contralateral to the primary surgery, its origin obviously being at the level of the falx.

   Was the excuse/explanation that I gave to the patient a lie? At least it did calm him, and we did not do any harm. After this occurrence, we changed the hospital policy, and from then on, the surgeon had to be in the operating room (OR) starting from the introduction of anesthesia—which is very rapid these days—and the surgeon was responsible for positioning the patient's head as the first step of the procedure.
2. As the head of the Neurosurgery Department at the University in Kiel/Germany, I had to operate, in the early 1990s, on a recurrent lumbar vertebral body tumor via a retroperitoneal approach, and access to the spine was provided by the head of the general surgery department. After having removed the tumor and performed stabilization as required, we jointly closed the access wound. Later that afternoon, the X-ray control panel showed that we had left an abdominal swab inside that required our redoing the surgery. The patient, a locally well-known pharmacist, accepted my immediate explanation and apology, but he wondered in an angry fashion why the abdominal surgeon—whom I had asked/urged to do the same—had not shown up to apologize himself.

   Who was to be blamed, and who would have been held legally responsible for leaving the swab inside?
3. When performing an implantable pulse generator (IPG) exchange in a Parkinson's patient who had undergone a successful deep brain stimulation (DBS) operation a few years earlier, which is considered a minor surgery and which I did alone with a nurse, hemostasis was usually achieved by inserting sponges soaked with H_2O_2. A few days post-OP, one small swab was discovered to have been left behind, and I had to take the patient back to surgery, which I had to explain to the patient, a high-ranking business executive. I apologized and explained everything carefully. The patient fully understood my mistake and accepted my reason because he had not suffered any harm; he even volunteered to discuss his excellent surgical results from DBS on a TV show a few days later. Formal discussion at our departmental morbidity and mortality (M&M) conference and the implementation of a rule to repeat swap counting were the procedural consequences aiming to prevent this from happening again.
4. The misplacement of pedicle screws—which itself is an inherent possiblity of surgery and not itself to be considered a mistake—may lead to neural damage or long-lasting pain. In such a setting hardware misplacement should be revised when safely possible and when openly discussed with the patient. The discussion is not always easy, particularly after a difficult surgery has exhausted the surgeon, but it can help to prevent arbitration or a court proceeding. Instead of informing the patient, would it be better for the patient to suffer from radicular pain or an unstable spine, potentially causing further harm—in which case the patient would learn about the mistakes later on from another surgeon?
5. In a 77-year-old female patient, the posterior third of her superior sagittal sinus was injured by a younger staff member during craniotomy when the staff member gained access to a tentorial notch meningioma. Hemorrhage from the site of injury could not be stopped, and she died

on the table. As I was the head of the department and was the one who had finalized the indication for surgery, I felt responsible for this case, so I called her husband immediately and explained everything to him by phone. In addition, I immediately wrote a letter to the hospital chair the very same day explaining the details, and I had the young staff member present his case in detail at the next M&M conference for all neurosurgeons and OR personnel, to prevent gossiping. No lawsuit was filed by the patient's family, and official persecution by the coroner's office was not pursued, because none of details of the events had been hidden in this case. Being transparent—yet not accusatory—in the department's M&M conference and drawing conclusions on the handling such cases in the future relieved much of the psychological pressure that had affected the young staff member and should help to prevent such events in the future.

Conclusions from these Cases

Because a patient suffering from complications will usually—sooner or later—realize what occurred or learn about the problems that were encountered during surgery or the delivery of care, their surgeon needs to explain what precisely happened and why. A patient would never consider a doctor to be without fault but would expect that they would deliver all care to the best level possible, and this is what we should strive to do every day.

The best way of dealing with a complication in surgery is for the performing surgeon to frankly inform the patient about the complication without blame. Doing so is a much-needed learning process for young surgeons, which they also have to be taught—nowadays possibly through recorded sessions with informed actors.

Problems that occur during surgery should be discussed in the presence of a witness or a few witnesses, with at least one on the side of the doctor, and such disclosure conversations must be documented afterward. If major problems (such as in the last case presented above) have occurred, involving the head of the department in the explanation of the unfortunate situation may be helpful.

Above all, when the patient or their relative requests an appointment with the chairperson of a unit in which a complication occurred, I believe that this should be freely arranged because many of the allegations brought to the arbitration counsel have come from the patient's or their relative's understandable perception of not being heard by senior personnel.

The timing of when to provide the information to a patient experiencing significant pain or a patient who may be overwhelmed by a newly diagnosed deficit is also crucial: This should be done very early on so that the patient understands the need for additional surgical or conservative therapy to improve the final outcome. In these discussions, many urgent questions will be brought up from the patient and their family concerning functional deficits that might influence the patient's life for a long time or permanently. Since the final result of many neurosurgical complications (surgical errors) may not be predictable early on in the course of a disease, the answers should weigh the possibility of a major deficit yet mitigate this perspective by pointing to the potential for natural healing, especially improvement via rehabilitation.

These ethical guidelines are considered helpful in similarly difficult situations and might be used irrespective of the specific situation of malpractice liability. A good and individualized doctor–patient relationship should be preserved even in a busy neurosurgical practice in a large department structure, and this will help to ensure the best possible patient care.

Many arbitration processes, court rulings, and unsatisfactory clinical courses resulting in unhappy patients could be prevented by following an appropriate preoperative informed consent process where the information is given in nonmedical language. This way, the patient has an idea of what might happen and what might be expected without scaring them. Spending considerable time talking to the patient before surgery is definitely better than sitting in court.

Furthermore, a doctor incurs quite a psychological burden by sitting in court in front of a patient whom that doctor wanted to help yet failed to achieve the best possible outcome for—e.g., by not considering and discussing the possibility of making the patient paraplegic with a procedure in spine surgery. Every possible step needs to be taken before surgery to professionally address such concerns to prevent patients or relatives from finding reasons to sue doctors for an outcome that was not anticipated or discussed.

References

1. Dagi TF. Seven ethical issues affecting neurosurgeons in the context of health care reform. Neurosurgery. 2017;80(4S):S83–91. https://doi.org/10.1093/neuros/nyx017.
2. Nassiri F, Li L, Badhiwala JH, Yeoh TY, Hachem LD, Moga R, Wang JZ, Manninen P, Bernstein M, Venkatraghavan L. Hospital costs associated with inpatient versus outpatient awake craniotomy for resection of brain tumors. J Clin Neurosci. 2019;59:162–6. https://doi.org/10.1016/j.jocn.2018.10.110. Epub 2018 Nov 7.
3. Mehdorn HM, Hoffmann B, Grote W. Erfahrungen einer "Gutachterkommission für Ärztliche Behandlungsfehler" mit Behandlungsfehlern im neurochirurgischen Fachgebiet. Adv Neurosurg. 1990;18:317–23.

Internal Carotid Artery Injury During the Endoscopic Transsphenoidal Surgery of Pituitary Adenoma: Case Illustration, Introspection, and Systematic Review

Rakesh Mishra, Subhash Kanti Konar, and Dhaval P. Shukla

Abstract

Advances in endoscopic technology have made the endoscopic transsphenoidal approach the preferred approach for most surgeries of pituitary adenoma. The goal of these surgeries is to achieve cure, efficacy, and safety. Ample research has deliberated on the complications of cerebrospinal fluid (CSF) leak, meningitis, visual deterioration and nasal crusting after endoscopic transsphenoidal surgery. Among these, injury to the internal carotid artery (ICA) is not common in transsphenoidal pituitary surgery and has an incidence that ranges from 0.1% to 1%. Though it is rare, the effects are devastating and associated with a high risk of mortality and morbidity. As a result, iatrogenic ICA injury is every neurosurgeon's nightmare. Available literature primarily consists of case reports on these injuries. The literature is lacking on preventive and management options. We present an unusual case of a patient who had a nonfunctioning pituitary macroadenoma and an unexpected injury to the internal carotid artery (ICA) during endoscopic transsphenoidal surgery. We share our successful experience with its management via emergency endovascular treatment with parent vessel occlusion for an iatrogenic ICA injury. We present the article to address the pragmatic questions and challenges faced by neurosurgeons experiencing this complication for the first time.

R. Mishra (✉)
Department of Neurosurgery, National Institute of Mental Health and Neurosciences, Bangalore, India

Department of Neurosurgery, All India Institute of Medical Sciences, Bhopal, Bhopal, India

S. K. Konar · D. P. Shukla
Department of Neurosurgery, National Institute of Mental Health and Neurosciences, Bangalore, India
e-mail: dhavalshukla@nimhans.ac.in

Keywords

Iatrogenic ICA injury · Transsphenoidal surgery · Pituitary adenoma · Endosinus surgery · Endoscopic pituitary surgery · Endovascular management · Parent vessel occlusion

Introduction

An iatrogenic injury of the ICA is one of the most dreaded complications of endoscopic pituitary surgery. ICA injury leads to mortality and significant morbidity. Careful preoperative planning and meticulous surgical techniques are essential to avoid this complication. Iatrogenic ICA injury in endoscopic pituitary surgery can have an early or delayed manifestation. Such an injury can lead to overwhelming blood loss, creating an imminent risk to life as well as pseudoaneurysm formation, vasospasm, thrombosis, embolism with subsequent cerebral insult, the formation of carotid-cavernous fistula, and haematoma formation in the tumour cavity with subsequent vision compromise [1–4].

We present a patient with a nonfunctioning pituitary macroadenoma who had an unexpected injury to the internal carotid artery (ICA) during endoscopic transsphenoidal surgery. The senior author has operated on more than 800 consecutive large or giant pituitary adenomas (PAs). This article describes our successful experience with using parent vessel occlusion as an emergency endovascular treatment for an iatrogenic ICA injury and the clinical course, and the article retrospectively analyses the critical management issues that could have reduced the unexpected prolonged hospital stay. Additionally, we systematically searched the literature to inform our discussion on avoidable and unavoidable causes and other responsible factors as we review the management options for ICA injury during transsphenoidal surgery for PA.

K. Turel, E. M. Kasper (eds.), *Complications in Neurosurgery II*, Acta Neurochirurgica Supplement 133,
https://doi.org/10.1007/978-3-031-61601-3_15

Clinical Scenario

A 55-year-old male patient presented with complaints of decreased vision in the left eye and nonspecific headaches for 1 year. He had no pre-existing medical or surgical comorbidities. General and systemic examination was within normal limits. His preoperative visual acuity was 6/9 in the right eye and 6/12 in the left eye, with bitemporal visual field defects. The rest of the neurological examination was normal. No abnormalities were noted in the laboratory investigations at admission. MRI showed a pituitary macroadenoma about 2 cm × 1.7 cm × 2.2 cm in size. The lesion extended bilaterally into the cavernous sinus with the encasement of the ICA on each side (180° for the right ICA and 90° for the left ICA). The clinical and radiological working diagnosis was nonfunctional pituitary macroadenoma, Knosp grade 4 and Hardy grade 4 E (Fig. 1).

Surgery

We planned an endoscopic endonasal transsphenoidal approach for the excision of the lesion. We encountered brisk arterial bleeding while making a cruciate opening on the left-side dura mater at the level of the sellar floor. As we were able to visualize the bleed site and identify rent in the ICA, we alerted the anaesthetist immediately, and blood transfusion was started. We attempted carotid artery compression at the neck to prevent exsanguination; however, the bleeding was not significantly reduced. We could reduce the bleeding and achieve adequate intraoperative haemostasis by using oxidized regenerated cellulose to directly pack the sphenoid sinus and nasal cavity. We hemodynamically stabilized the patient and immediately moved him out of the operating room to the neurointerventional suite as the blood continued to ooze out from the access site. Total blood loss was approximately 2.5 L at this time.

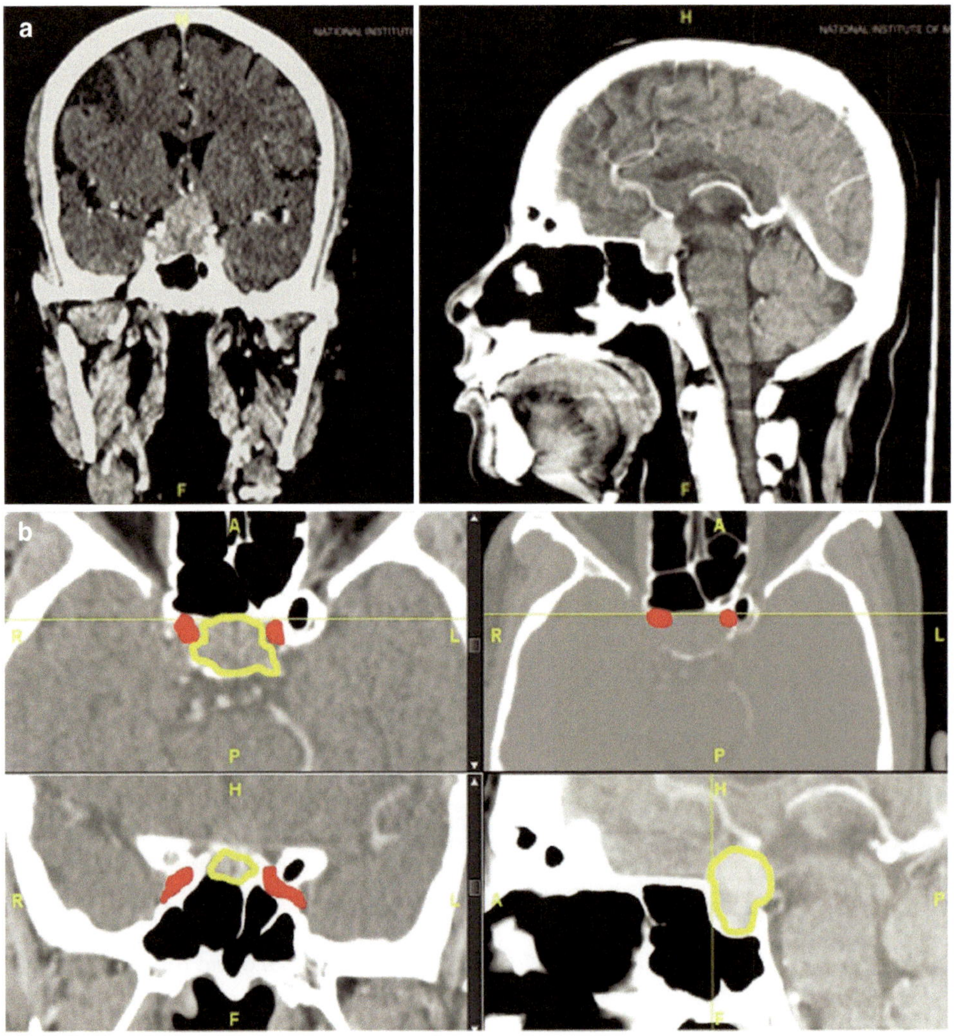

Fig. 1 (**a**) Coronal and sagittal CT brain contrast images depicting sellar hyperdense sellar suprasellar lesion. (**b**) Showing tumour margin in yellow and proximity to artery outline in red

Neurointervention

Digital subtraction angiography (DSA) was performed, which revealed that the left ICA injection showed active contrast extravasation from the cavernous segment of the ICA at the anterior genu (Fig. 2). Good crossflow was seen involving the left posterior communicating (PCOM) artery, left ACA and MCA (Fig. 3). We deployed two coils in the left cavernous ICA across the rent site. An immediate postprocedure angiogram showed a lack of antegrade flow in the left ICA with the normal filling of the left MCA and ACA. No contrast leak appeared on the right ICA and left vertebral artery (VA) angiogram. No perfusion deficit was in the left ACA and MCA territory. The retrograde filling of the left ophthalmic artery with patent left ophthalmic choroidal blush was seen on the left VA angiogram.

Follow-Up Course

After the intervention, a delayed computed tomography (CT) brain scan was obtained, which showed no ischaemic changes or infarcts (Fig. 4). The patient then underwent surgical re-exploration, including nasal pack removal and the near-total removal of the lesion 3 days later. Histopathology was consistent with nonfunctioning pituitary macroadenoma.

Condition at Discharge

At discharge, he was conscious, alert and active and had no limb weakness. However, his vision had deteriorated to complete blindness in the left eye, whereas no deteriora-

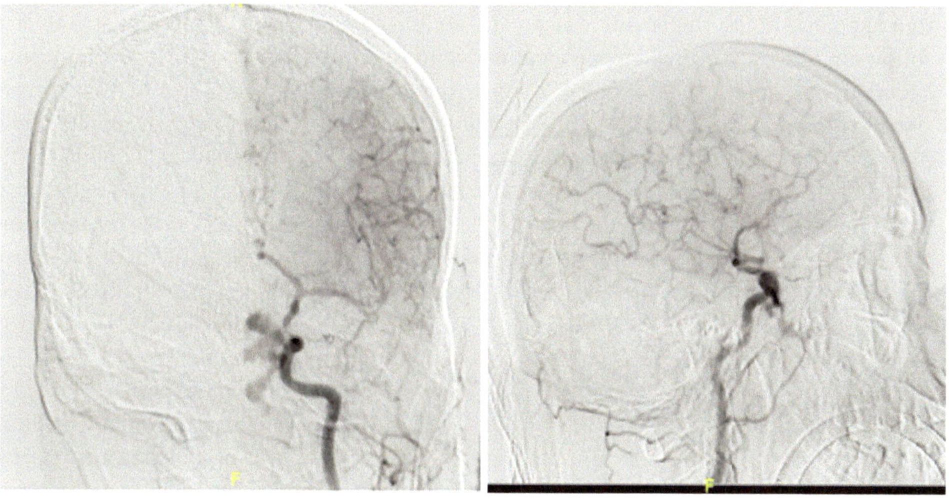

Fig. 2 AP and lateral projection of left ICA angiogram showing the site of rent in cavernous segment of left ICA and extravasation of dye

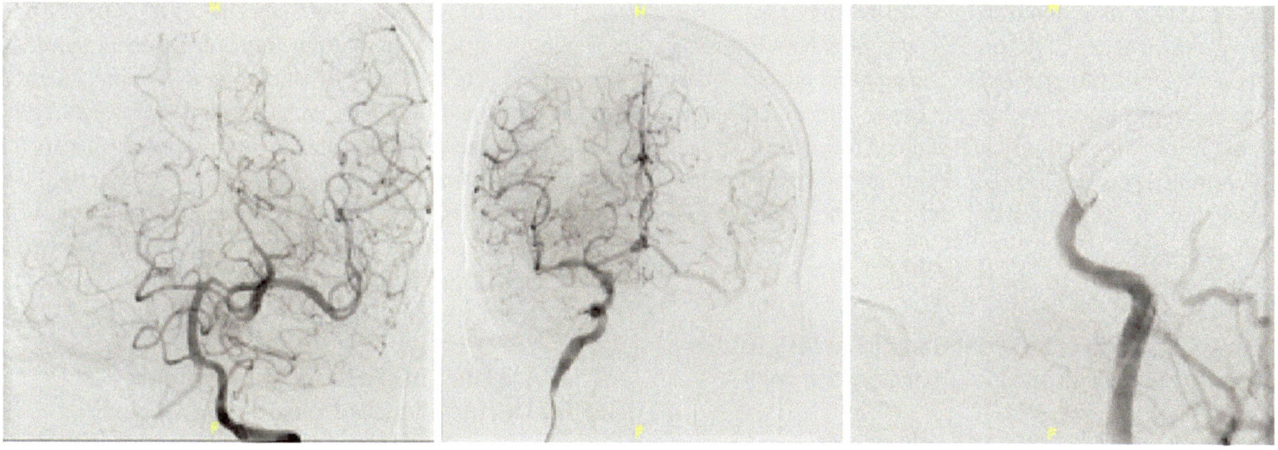

Fig. 3 Showing good cross circulation from PCOM, poor crossflow from contralateral ICA, and post-coiling; left ICA angiogram showing parent vessel occlusion

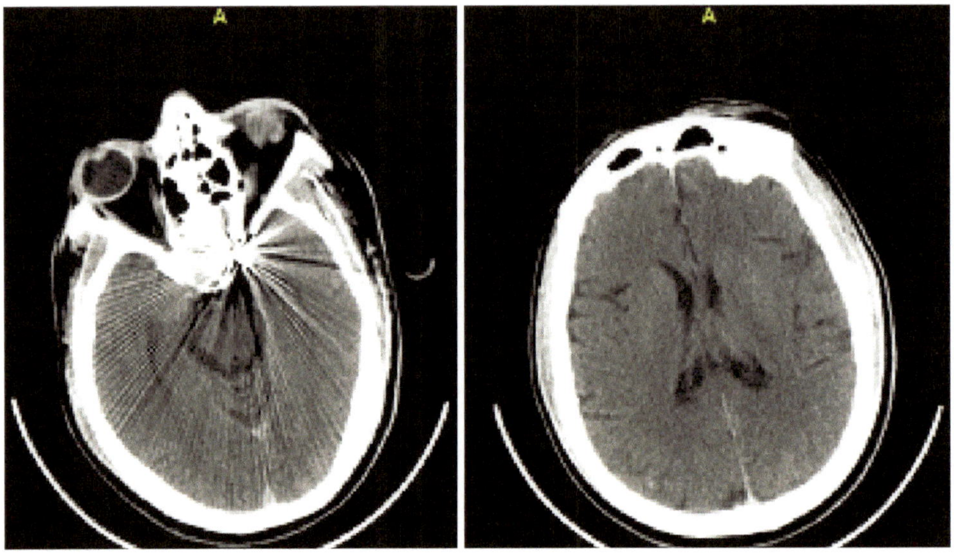

Fig. 4 Delayed postoperative CT brain scan showing no infarcts or haematomas

tion appeared in the right eye's vision. At the eight-month follow-up, the patient was independent and able to do his occupational work and activities of daily living with persistent blindness in the left eye. He showed no change in his functional status during the last follow-up, at 20 months. Deterioration in vision in the left eye could have been due to the inadvertent sacrifice of the ophthalmic artery during the parent vessel occlusion given that a native postoperative CT brain scan revealed no haematoma or tumour bleed.

Discussion

A pituitary adenoma is one of the most familiar pathologies treated by neurosurgeons and ear, nose and throat (ENT) surgeons. Over time, the technological advances in neurosurgery have made PA surgery much safer. Endoscopic transsphenoidal surgery (ETS) has replaced microscopic and transcranial surgery in most the cases. Though ETS is considered a routine and very safe surgical procedure, iatrogenic ICA injuries during endoscopic pituitary macroadenoma surgery do occur at times and are the most dreaded complication.[1]

How Common Is Internal Carotid Artery Injury During Transsphenoidal Pituitary Surgery?

ICA injury during transsphenoidal pituitary surgery is very infrequent. However, it is challenging and potentially disabling and may have fatal consequences [1]. Injury to the ICA may be shown by a torrential haemorrhage that occurs intraoperatively or that manifests later as a pseudoaneurysm due to a vessel spasm or an infarct due to thrombosis. In endoscopic endonasal pituitary surgeries, the incidence of injury to the ICA is estimated to be between 0.2% and 2.0%, according to available studies [2, 5, 6]. The incidence appears to vary depending on the type of surgery. This complication seems to be rare in endoscopic sinus surgery (only 29 cases reported, with higher numbers in transsphenoidal pituitary surgery), with an incidence of 1.1%, and this incidence is higher in extended endonasal surgeries—e.g., procedures for craniopharyngiomas, clival chordomas and chondrosarcomas—at 5–9% [5, 7, 8].

May et al. [9] reported only one patient with an intraoperative ICA injury in their institutional experience, which was a pooled series of 2108 cases that was combined with 2583 patients from another 11 series—a total of 4691 cases. Among the 16,000 endoscopic sinus surgeries conducted over a span of 30 years, Weidenbecher et al. [10] had four encounters of ICA injury following sphenoidectomy. These figures indicate the rarity of iatrogenic ICA injury in endoscopic sinus and transsphenoidal surgeries. However, when we look at the mortality and severe disability due to this complication, we realize that it merits more attention. The mortality rate of iatrogenic ICA injury in endoscopic skull base surgeries is up to 14%, and the incidence of severe disability among survivors is up to 24% [5].

What Are the Risk Factors of Iatrogenic ICA Injury During Transsphenoidal Surgeries?

Many factors increase the risk of inadvertent ICA injury. Two subgroups of patients are at increased risk [11, 12]. The first group consists of patients with pre-existing vascular malformations hidden by an intact mucosa of the sphenoid sinus. ICA injuries in these cases have been fatal in all published cases [13]. The second group consists of cases featuring the direct penetration of the vessel. The chance of survival is higher in this subgroup of patients than in the first [14]. The risk factors for ICA injury have level 4, grade C evidence for anatomic relationships that are predisposed to surgical difficulties. These structural features include carotid dehiscence, sphenoid septal attachment to ICA, midline ICA, revision surgery, prior radiotherapy, prior bromocriptine treatment and acromegaly [12, 14–19].

Nonmodifiable Risk Factors

Nonmodifiable risk factors include tumour characteristics and anatomical variation in the sella or in the ICA course. Important tumour characteristics are the location, nature, consistency and functional status of the lesion. Large and invasive PAs often invade the cavernous sinus or ICA and increase the risk of ICA injury. Our patient had a higher Knosp and Hardy grade of PA. The functional status of the PA also affects the risk of ICA injury, with a higher risk in cortisol- and GH-secreting PAs [15, 18]. Liu et al. [20] reported a patient with prolactinoma on bromocriptine therapy who had an injury of the A1 emanating from a left ICA during transsphenoidal surgery. The authors attributed the injury to the firmness and adhesion of the tumour secondary to fibrosis induced by bromocriptine. The risk of ICA injury is more significant in recurrent PA because previous surgery creates anatomical variation in the sellar region, which may predispose the region to injury [21, 22].

Modifiable Risk Factors

Modifiable risk factors include inadequate preoperative planning and surgical expertise. The occurrence of ICA injury has been linked to intraoperative experience. For surgeries performed in the sphenoid sinus, the rate of ICA injury was inversely proportional to the surgeon's experience: an ICA injury rate of 1.4% for the least experienced surgeons (200 cases of TSS), 0.6% for intermediately experienced surgeons (200–500 cases) and 0.4% for the most experienced surgeons (> 500 cases) [23].

Which Segment of ICA Is Vulnerable to Injury?

Knowing which segment of ICA is most vulnerable to injury during PA transsphenoidal surgery is crucial for decision-making. This knowledge helps in deciding on the course of action to take and how to appropriately manage the neurosurgical intervention. The ICA, which is at most risk during surgery on the paranasal sinuses, is the rostral wall of the infraophthalmic cavernous segment [3, 24]. Interestingly, some studies have reported that injury occurred more frequently on the cavernous segment of the left ICA than on the right side in endoscopic procedures [7, 24]. In our case, we also had an injury on the cavernous segment of the Left ICA. Renn and Rhoton found ICA bulges into the sphenoid sinus in 71% of cases, and these authors observed that the artery may be as close as 4 mm from the midline [25]. Table 1 shows the anatomical landmarks of ICA segments from the endoscopic perspective, which are crucial in preventing these injuries.

Table 1 Anatomical landmarks for various segments of the internal carotid artery [26, 27]

Anatomic landmarks for various segments of the internal carotid artery	
Segment	Anatomic landmark
Paraclinoid	Medial clinoid
Anterior genu	Medial pterygoid
Horizontal segment	Vidian nerve
Ascending carotid	Eustachian tube

What Are the Immediate Challenges in the Management of Iatrogenic ICA Injury?

Significant vessel injury may create panic in operating room (OR) staff, resulting in rapid blood loss that may result in the exsanguination of the patient. Controlling bleeding via vigorous packing with a variety of materials requires a calm mind set and tremendous technical ability. Haemostasis is difficult because of the ample space created during surgical exposure in the endonasal transsphenoidal approach. We faced this challenge and found controlling the bleeding to be very difficult. We used multiple manoeuvres like compression on the external carotid at the neck and the injection of a haemostatic agent (Floseal) at the bleeding site. However, the bleeding reduced only after the complete packing of the sinus with oxidized cellulose. Crossflow from the VA rendered the compression of the external carotid at the neck ineffective.

Because the endoscope has its viewing port on the very tip of the instrument, Cavallo et al. [28] have recommended withdrawing the endoscope to the level of the middle turbinate and inserting cottonoids or haemostatic substances into the sella and the sphenoid sinus [28]. Important steps for surgical field control include two-surgeon techniques working as a team; endoscope navigation to keep the tip free from the jet of blood is a key element at this stage of the procedure [13]. Haemostatic agents like Surgicel and Floseal were ineffective against high-flow, high-pressure leaks and are effective against high-flow, low-pressure leaks.

What Is the Role of Preoperative Neuroimaging in Preventing Iatrogenic Injury?

A detailed study on neuroimaging helps to prevent iatrogenic ICA injuries. Preoperative CT evaluation can show whether the bony wall of the canal of the cavernous carotid artery is very thin or completely dehiscent. A high-resolution spiral CT on the paranasal sinuses revealed a bony septum inserting into the canal wall in 16.3% of cases and an ICA protrusion of >50% of its diameter into the sphenoid sinus in 18.8% of cases [29]. The part of the ICA that is at most risk during surgery on the paranasal sinuses is the rostral wall of the infraophthalmic cavernous segment [3, 24, 29]. Fujii and colleagues demonstrated that the bony wall overlying the ICA is not sufficient to protect the artery if it is less than 0.5 mm thick [30]. Additionally, in 4–22% of cases, the lateral sphenoid wall is dehiscent over the carotid, where only the dura and the sphenoid sinus mucosa separate the ICA from the sphenoid [30]. On axial computed tomography (CT), the protrusions of the ICAs into the sphenoid often resemble teddy bears, according to Vescan et al. [31] In cases with an absent "teddy bear sign" or "grade O teddy bear sign," these authors have suggested using navigation systems or Doppler ultrasound for the intraoperative localization of ICA [31].

What Is the Role of Adjuncts in Preventing Iatrogenic ICA Injury?

Dusick et al. [4] have suggested using in-field Doppler explorations to identify the location of the ICA before opening the dura of the sellar floor. Damage to the internal carotid artery may be associated with the wrong orientation in the surgical wound or excessively aggressive manipulations in the cavernous sinus [32]. The surgeon must remain in the midline and accurately localize the ICA by using a neuronavigation system and Doppler ultrasound.

What Are the Surgical Options for the Management of Iatrogenic ICA Injuries?

The following options are available after an accidental injury to the ICA:

1. Suturing appears time-consuming and ineffective to us and can lead to more blood loss
2. Bipolar coagulation is suitable for perforator injuries, injuries to the sphenopalatine artery and minor lacerations in the ICA (measuring 2–3 mm) [7].
3. Vessel ligation is a viable option.
4. Although vessel reconstruction is theoretically an option, it has never been successfully performed endoscopically.
5. Surgical packing is the first step to immediately control bleeding [33]. It is the most effective method to control acute bleeding and maintain hemodynamic stability. Donaldson et al. [34] reported a case featuring the complete occlusion of contralateral ICA thanks to sphenoid packing in the setting of a pseudoaneurysm. However, this is a rare complication with surgical packing.

What Emergency Endovascular Treatment Options Are Available?

Sacrificing the ICA by using endovascular coiling is the most durable and definite option for management in cases of acute uncontrolled bleeding [5]. The decision to perform DSA for ICA sacrifice is determined primarily on the basis of good collateral filling demonstrated via angiography. Because torrential blood loss occurred during surgery in our case and because we found good cross circulation from PCOM, we decided to go ahead with ICA sacrifice at the region of ICA rent. Covered stents in such cases are not desirable, because of the tortuosity of the anterior genu of the ICA and because surgeons to avoid any occlusion of the branch vessels. A pipeline embolization device (PED) was also not desirable as a solution to the problem, because packing material needed to be removed after a few days, and the patient planned for a re-exploration for definite tumour excision. We have proposed an algorithm based on our clinical experience to manage accidental ICA injury during transsphenoidal pituitary surgery, which is shown in Fig. 5. Romero et al. reported that the safest way to manage arterial injury is vessel sacrifice, and the authors argued that the incidence of pseudoaneurysm formation is too high to recommend any approach other than vessel sacrifice [5].

Lessons Learned

The difficulties that we faced in our case management were due to a number of factors affecting the situation: We used the uninostril approach, we had difficulty maintaining adequate visualization because of the significant rent in ICA, and we found that the pressure on the cervical carotid was inadequate because of good collateral flow. In our case, the contributing factors for the ICA injury included a deviation from normal anatomy in the midline due to the bony septum, the honeycomb configuration of the oblique sphenoid septum, the anatomical variation in the ICA, and a lateral to medial trajectory for the incision of the dura, with our incision lateral to the cavernous sinus.

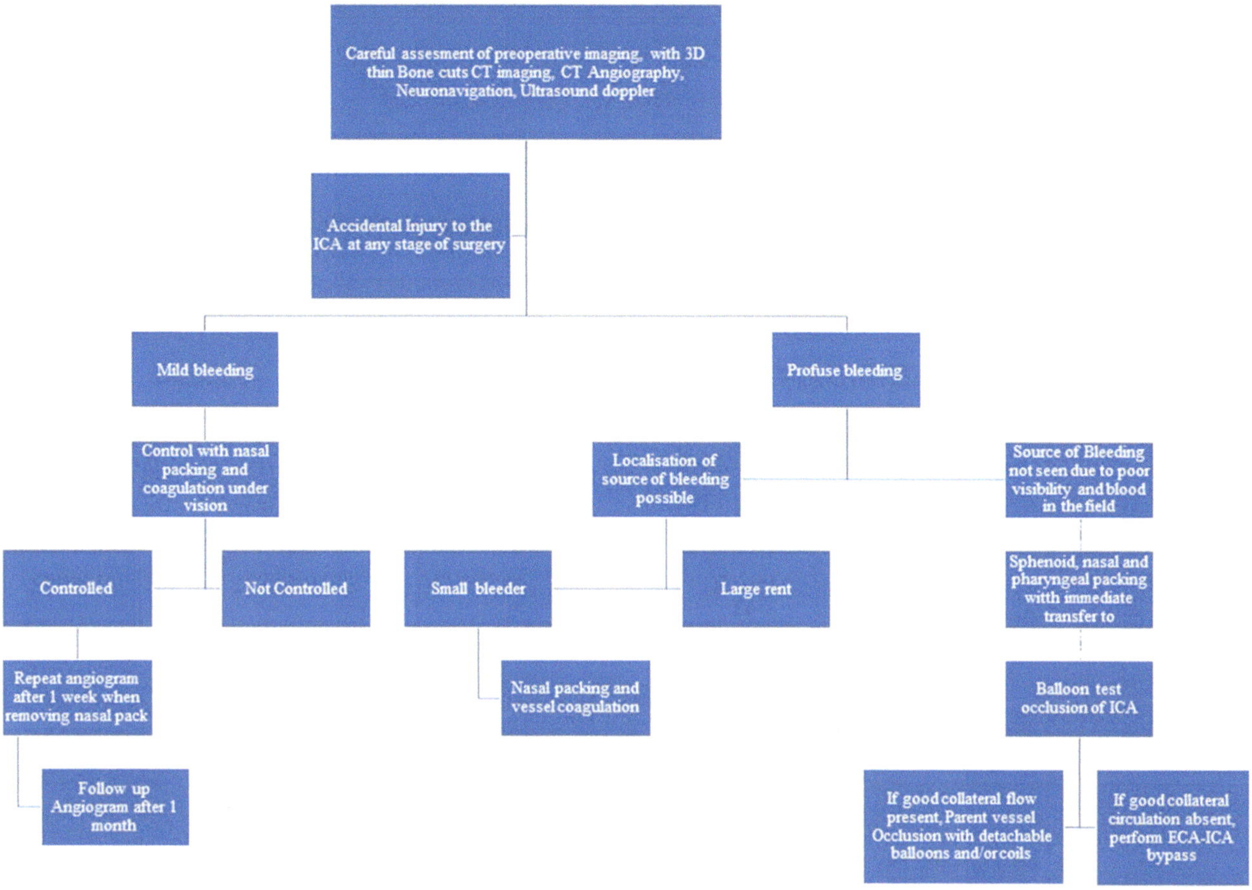

Fig. 5 Proposed algorithm for the management of accidental ICA injuries in transsphenoidal pituitary surgery

The use of a Doppler ultrasound can locate the presence of the ICA and prevent its injury. Having control of the surgical field with two surgeons working as a team is essential. The expeditious bilateral packing of the nose and epipharynx is the primarily life-saving step of treatment. Carotid ligation at the neck is also not feasible, because it will remove all the possible therapeutic options for neurointervention. The management options for ICA injury at different stages of surgery are essentially the same and consist of the same steps in the algorithm depicted earlier. We provide an algorithm for the management of iatrogenic ICA injury during endosinus surgery, as shown in Fig. 5.

Conclusion

Iatrogenic ICA injury is a severe and catastrophic complication that occurs at a low incidence in endoscopic pituitary surgeries. The successful management of these injuries requires careful preoperative planning and meticulous surgical skills. Dynamic two-surgeon/two-handed techniques with an extra suction devise are essential to maintain visibility. Coordination between the neurosurgery suite and the neurointervention suite is critical to the successful management of these injuries. Lastly, all centres should have all forms of endovascular treatment modalities available to manage such an unexpected event.

Acknowledgements We thank the patient for agreeing to permit us to use clinical details Patient Consent Obtained for publication of the clinical details and radiological images.

Disclosure Nothing to disclose.

Conflicts of Interest None.

References

1. Berker M, Aghayev K, Saatci I, Palaoğlu S, Onerci M. Overview of vascular complications of pituitary surgery with special emphasis on unexpected abnormality. Pituitary. 2010;13:160–7. https://doi.org/10.1007/s11102-009-0198-7.
2. Berker M, Hazer DB, Yücel T, Gürlek A, Cila A, Aldur M, Önerci M. Complications of endoscopic surgery of the pituitary adenomas: analysis of 570 patients and review of the literature. Pituitary. 2012;15:288–300.

3. Çinar C, Bozkaya H, Parildar M, Oran I. Endovascular management of vascular injury during transsphenoidal surgery. Interv Neuroradiol. 2013;19:102–9.
4. Dusick JR, Esposito F, Malkasian D, Kelly DF. Avoidance of carotid artery injuries in transsphenoidal surgery with the Doppler probe and micro-hook blades. Operative. Neurosurgery. 2007;60:ONS-322–9.
5. Romero A, Lal Gangadharan J, Bander ED, Gobin YP, Anand VK, Schwartz TH. Managing arterial injury in endoscopic Skull Base surgery: case series and review of the literature. Oper Neurosurg (Hagerstown). 2017;13:138–49. https://doi.org/10.1227/neu.0000000000001180.
6. Sylvester PT, Moran CJ, Derdeyn CP, Cross DT, Dacey RG, Zipfel GJ, Kim AH, Uppaluri R, Haughey BH, Tempelhoff R. Endovascular management of internal carotid artery injuries secondary to endonasal surgery: case series and review of the literature. J Neurosurg. 2016;125:1256–76.
7. Gardner PA, Tormenti MJ, Pant H, Fernandez-Miranda JC, Snyderman CH, Horowitz MB. Carotid artery injury during endoscopic endonasal skull base surgery: incidence and outcomes. Neurosurgery. 2013;73:ons261–269; discussion ons269–270. https://doi.org/10.1227/01.neu.0000430821.71267.f2.
8. Solares CA, Ong YK, Carrau RL, Fernandez-Miranda J, Prevedello DM, Snyderman CH, Kassam AB. Prevention and management of vascular injuries in endoscopic surgery of the sinonasal tract and skull base. Otolaryngol Clin N Am. 2010;43:817–25.
9. May M, Levine HL, Mester SJ, Schaitkin B. Complications of endoscopic sinus surgery: analysis of 2108 patients—sincidence and prevention. Laryngoscope. 1994;104:1080–3. https://doi.org/10.1288/00005537-199409000-00006.
10. Weidenbecher M, Huk WJ, Iro H. Internal carotid artery injury during functional endoscopic sinus surgery and its management. Eur Arch Otorrinolaringol. 2005;262:640–5. https://doi.org/10.1007/s00405-004-0888-8.
11. Hardy J. Pituitary microadenomas. Brain Surg. 1993:276–95.
12. Hardy JIEM. Pituitary microadenomas. In: Apuzzo MLJ, editor. Brain surgery: complication avoidance and management. New York: Churchill Livingstone; 1992. p. 276–95.
13. Valentine R, Wormald PJ. Controlling the surgical field during a large endoscopic vascular injury. Laryngoscope. 2011;121:562–6.
14. Ciceri E, Regna-Gladin C, Erbetta A, Chiapparini L, Nappini S, Savoiardo M, Di Meco F. Iatrogenic intracranial pseudoaneurysms: neuroradiological and therapeutical considerations, including endovascular options. Neurol Sci. 2006;27:317–22.
15. Ebner FH, Kuerschner V, Dietz K, Bueltmann E, Naegele T, Honegger J. Reduced intercarotid artery distance in acromegaly: pathophysiologic considerations and implications for transsphenoidal surgery. Surg Neurol. 2009;72:456–60.
16. Gondim JA, Almeida JPC, Albuquerque LAF, Schops M, Gomes E, Ferraz T, Sobreira W, Kretzmann MT. Endoscopic endonasal approach for pituitary adenoma: surgical complications in 301 patients. Pituitary. 2011;14:174–83.
17. Kassam AB, Prevedello DM, Carrau RL, Snyderman CH, Thomas A, Gardner P, Zanation A, Duz B, Stefko ST, Byers K. Endoscopic endonasal skull base surgery: analysis of complications in the authors' initial 800 patients: a review. J Neurosurg. 2011;114:1544–68.
18. Oskouian RJ, Kelly DF, Edward R Jr. Vascular injury and transsphenoidal surgery. In: Pituitary surgery-a modern approach, vol. 34. Abingdon: Karger Publishers; 2006. p. 256–78.
19. Raymond J, Hardy J, Czepko R, Roy D. Arterial injuries in transsphenoidal surgery for pituitary adenoma; the role of angiography and endovascular treatment. Am J Neuroradiol. 1997;18:655–65.
20. Liu X, Feng M, Dai C, Bao X, Deng K, Yao Y, Wang R. Internal carotid artery injury in the endoscopic transsphenoidal surgery for pituitary adenoma: an uncommon case and literature review. Gland Surg. 2020;9:1036–41. https://doi.org/10.21037/gs-20-354.
21. Nwosu OI, Rubel KE, Alwani MM, Sharma D, Miller M, Ting JY, Payner T. Use of adenosine to facilitate localization and repair of internal carotid artery injury during Skull Base surgery: a case report and literature review. Ann Otol Rhinol Laryngol. 2021;130:532–6. https://doi.org/10.1177/0003489420956373.
22. Saeger W, Müller M, Buslei R, Flitsch J, Fahlbusch R, Buchfelder M, Knappe UJ, Crock PA, Lüdecke DK. Recurrences of pituitary adenomas or second De novo tumors: comparisons with first tumors. World Neurosurg. 2018;119:e118–24. https://doi.org/10.1016/j.wneu.2018.07.056.
23. Ciric I, Ragin A, Baumgartner C, Pierce D. Complications of transsphenoidal surgery: results of a national survey, review of the literature, and personal experience. Neurosurgery. 1997;40:225–236; discussion 236–227. https://doi.org/10.1097/00006123-199702000-00001.
24. Chin OY, Ghosh R, Fang CH, Baredes S, Liu JK, Eloy JA. Internal carotid artery injury in endoscopic endonasal surgery: a systematic review. Laryngoscope. 2016;126:582–90. https://doi.org/10.1002/lary.25748.
25. Renn W, Rhoton A. Microsurgical anatomy of the sellar region. J Neurosurg. 1975;43:288–98.
26. Kassam AB, Vescan AD, Carrau RL, Prevedello DM, Gardner P, Mintz AH, Snyderman CH, Rhoton AL. Expanded endonasal approach: vidian canal as a landmark to the petrous internal carotid artery. J Neurosurg. 2008;108:177–83.
27. Vescan AD, Snyderman CH, Carrau RL, Mintz A, Gardner P, Branstetter B IV, Kassam AB. Vidian canal: analysis and relationship to the internal carotid artery. Laryngoscope. 2007;117:1338–42.
28. Cavallo L, Briganti F, Cappabianca P, Maiuri F, Valente V, Tortora F, Volpe A, Messina A, Elefante A, De Divitiis E. Hemorrhagic vascular complications of endoscopic transsphenoidal surgery. Minminimally invasive. Neurosurgery. 2004;47:145–50.
29. Koitschev A, Baumann I, Remy C, Dammann F. Rational CT diagnosis before operations on the paranasal sinuses. HNO. 2002;50:217–22.
30. Fujii K, Chambers SM, Rhoton AL Jr. Neurovascular relationships of the sphenoid sinus. A microsurgical study. J Neurosurg. 1979;50:31–9. https://doi.org/10.3171/jns.1979.50.1.0031.
31. Yeung W, Twigg V, Carr S, Sinha S, Mirza S. Radiological "teddy bear" sign on CT imaging to aid internal carotid artery localization in Transsphenoidal pituitary and anterior Skull Base surgery. J Neurol Surg B Skull Base. 2018;79:401–6. https://doi.org/10.1055/s-0037-1615749.
32. Kalinin PL, Sharipov OI, Shkarubo AN, Fomichev DV, Kutin MA, Alekseev SN, Kadashev BA, Iakovlev SB, Dorokhov PS, Bukharin E, Kurnosov AB, Popugaev KA. Damage to the cavernous segment of internal carotid artery in transsphenoidal endoscopic removal of pituitary adenomas (report of 4 cases). Zh Vopr Neirokhir Im N N Burdenko. 2013;77:28–37. discussion 38.
33. Zuo KJ, Xu R, Lai YY, Yang ZQ, Zhang QH, Xu G. Salvage management and subsequent treatment after internal carotid artery injury during transnasal endoscopic surgery. Zhonghua Er Bi Yan Hou Tou Jing Wai Ke Za Zhi. 2012;47:554–8.
34. Donaldson AM, Martinez-Paredes J, Domingo R, Tawk RG. Nasal packing causing occlusion of contralateral internal carotid artery during control of Pseudoaneurysm bleed. World Neurosurg. 2020;138:262–8. https://doi.org/10.1016/j.wneu.2020.02.132.

Avoidance and Management of Complications in Retrosigmoid Approach to Vestibular Schwannomas

Sanjeev Pattankar and Basant K. Misra

Abstract

An experience with two rare complications during surgery of vestibular schwannomas (VSs) is presented, and measures to avoid and manage the complications are discussed.

Case A: Spinal cord ischemia in semi-sitting position: A 47-year-old with a giant vestibular schwannoma (VS) underwent surgery through a retrosigmoid approach in the semi-sitting position. The intraoperative phase was uneventful, except for an episode of moderate hypotension. Postoperatively, the patient woke up with quadriparesis. MRI on the cervical spine revealed restricted diffusion from C4 to C7 suggestive of cord ischemia. Complete neurological recovery occurred over the following 3 months. Awareness of this potential complication, preoperative screening for degenerative spine disease, avoiding excessive intraoperative cervical flexion, using sensory & motor evoked potentials, and diligently avoiding intraoperative hypotension can prevent such occurrences.

Case B: High-riding jugular bulb (HRJB) injury: A 42-year-old male patient underwent a retrosigmoid approach for a right-sided VS in the lateral position. During internal auditory canal (IAC) drilling, there was an injury to the HRJB, resulting in torrential bleeding. It was managed successfully with the sequential application of Gelfoam, fibrin glue, and Surgicel. The drilling was carefully continued by using a diamond drill, and the complete excision of VS was achieved with no injury to cranial nerve 7 (CN7) while maintaining normal facial symmetry. Awareness of an HRJB reduces the risk, and in case of injury, sequential hemostatic measures ensure adequate IAC drilling and the total excision of the tumor.

Keywords

Semi-sitting position · Spinal cord ischemia · High-riding jugular bulb · Vestibular schwannoma

Introduction

The retrosigmoid approach is a "workhorse" in vestibular schwannoma (VS) surgery. However, it is not without its fair share of complications [1, 2]. Cerebrospinal fluid (CSF) leak, meningitis, wound infection, and cranial nerve palsies are commonly encountered complications that neurosurgeons are well versed in managing [3]. The rarer complications are the ones with devastating consequences that pose significant clinical challenges. We report our experience with and insights into avoiding/managing two such complications, namely spinal cord ischemia in the semi-sitting position and high-riding jugular bulb (HRJB) injury during internal auditory canal (IAC) drilling.

One of the earliest reports of spinal cord ischemia in the semi-sitting position in VS surgery was published in 1980 by Hitselberger and House [4]. Several large VS surgical case series have confirmed its incidence to be in the range of 0–1.2% [5–8]. Cervical or upper thoracic segments are most commonly affected, often leading to quadriparesis or paraparesis. The hyperflexion of the cervical spine (positioning related) and intraoperative hypotension (anesthesia related) are the two commonly associated factors [9].

The drilling of IAC is an important step in the surgical excision of VS as it facilitates the complete excision of the tumor and the early identification of the facial nerve. Because the reported incidence of HRJB varies from 6% to 65%, depending on the anatomical landmarks used, the efficient management of HRJB injury while IAC drilling is a skill that every skull base surgeon should possess [10].

S. Pattankar
P. D. Hinduja Hospital and MRC, Mumbai, India

B. K. Misra (✉)
DNB Neurosurgery, Department of Neurosurgery and Gamma Knife Radiosurgery, P. D. Hinduja Hospital and Medical Research Center, Veer Savarkar Marg, Mahim, Mumbai, India
e-mail: dr_bmisra@hindujahospital.com

K. Turel, E. M. Kasper (eds.), *Complications in Neurosurgery II*, Acta Neurochirurgica Supplement 133,
https://doi.org/10.1007/978-3-031-61601-3_16

Case Reports

(A) Spinal Cord Ischemia in Semi-Sitting Position

A 47-year-old female patient presented with complaints of decreased right-sided hearing for 1 year, imbalance while walking for 6 months, and occasional holo-cranial headache for 2 months. On neurological examination, her right ear was functionally deaf, accompanied by severe right-sided cerebellar signs and an absent right corneal reflex. The remaining neurological examination was normal. The clinical picture was suggestive of right cerebellopontine angle (CPA) syndrome. Gadolinium-enhanced MRI brain revealed a heterogeneously enhancing 41.6 mm × 36.8 mm × 41 mm right CPA lesion with IAC extension—suggestive of right giant VS (Fig. 1a).

Following informed consent for microsurgery, a detailed preanesthetic workup and a two-dimensional (2D) echocardiogram (echo)—plus a saline agitation test to rule out patent foramen ovale—confirmed the patient's fitness for surgery in the semi-sitting position. Because the patient did not have any symptoms or signs suggestive of cervical spondylosis, no screening evaluation was carried out for this. Somatosensory evoked potentials (SSEPs)/motor-evoked potentials (MEPs) were not employed in this case. The patient underwent microsurgery via the retrosigmoid approach in the semi-sitting position (Fig. 2), under facial, transesophageal echo, ETCO2, and intra-arterial pressure monitoring. A jugular central 3-lumen intravenous (IV) line was in place. The intraoperative phase was uneventful, except for an episode of moderate hypotension (mean pressure of about 90 mm Hg) lasting for around 5 min. The near total excision of the tumor with IAC drilling was carried out. A sliver of tumor that was stuck to the brainstem was left behind (Fig. 1b). Postoperatively, the patient woke up with right-sided House–Brackmann (HB) grade 2 facial function and, much to our surprise, with quadriparesis (legs 2–3/5 > arms 4/5; left > right). The patient also had approximately 50% sensory loss in their right leg and 20–30% sensory loss in their left leg. The patient underwent an expedited diagnostic MRI of the cervical spine with whole spine screening on postoperative day 1. MRI on the cervical spine revealed a swollen spinal cord with a diffuse

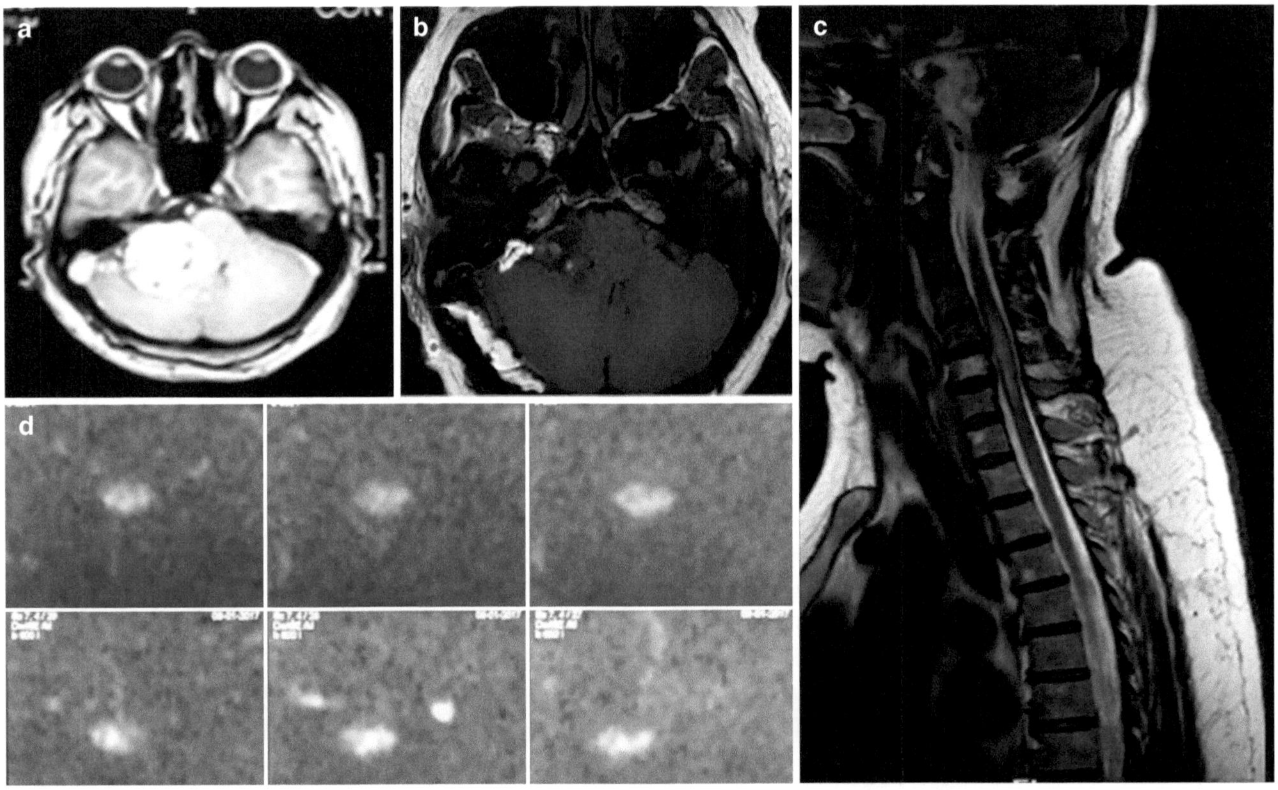

Fig. 1 (**a**) Preoperative contrast T1-weighted axial MRI image showing a giant right-sided vestibular schwannoma with significant compression on the brainstem. (**b**) Postoperative T1-weighted axial MRI image showing the near total excision of the tumor with a sliver of residual tumor stuck to the brainstem. A bright fat graft can also be seen plugging the internal auditory canal. (**c**, **d**) Postoperative T2-weighted sagittal MRI image (**c**) and axial diffusion weighted images (**d**) of cervicodorsal spine showing diffuse signal abnormality with restricted diffusion from C4 to C7. Diffuse posterior disc bulges with the effacement of the anterior subarachnoid space are also noted at the C5/C6 and C6/C7 levels

intrinsic signal abnormality extending from C4 to C7 with restricted diffusion suggestive of ischemia/infarct (Fig. 1c, d). Diffuse posterior disc bulges with an effacement of the anterior subarachnoid space were also noted at the C5/C6 and C6/C7 levels. The patient was managed with a tapering dose of steroids for 3 weeks and simultaneous rigorous physiotherapy. Fortunately, the complete clinical recovery of quadriparesis occurred over the course of the next 3 months. In this particular case, we attributed the spinal cord ischemia to the intraoperative hypotensive episode. Some contribution might also have been made by the degenerative cervical pathology secondarily worsened by cervical flexion during positioning.

(B) High-Riding Jugular Bulb (HRJB) Injury During Internal Auditory Canal (IAC) Drilling

A 42-year-old male patient underwent surgery for his right-sided small VS (Fig. 3a1, a2) through the retrosigmoid approach in the lateral position, under facial nerve monitoring. During IAC drilling, we noticed a bluish discoloration

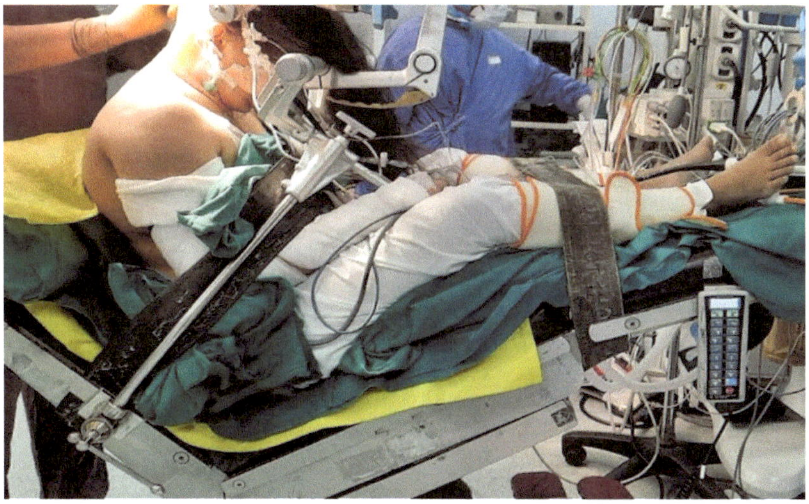

Fig. 2 Photograph from the operating room showing the patient's position in the semi-sitting position. Special care is taken to avoid excessive cervical flexion before fixing the head in Mayfield's clamp. Hips and knees are flexed, with the legs above the heart level, and transesophageal echo monitoring is in place. Care is taken to properly pad the pressure spots

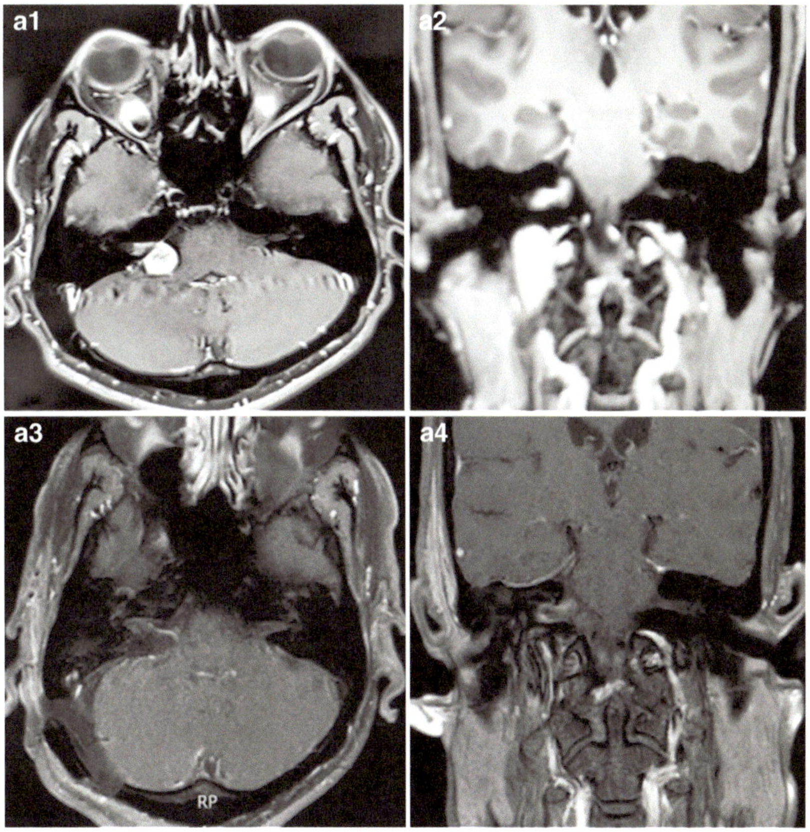

Fig. 3 (**a1**, **a2**) Preoperative contrast T1-weighted axial (**a1**) and coronal (**a2**) images showing a small right-sided vestibular schwannoma with intracanalicular extension. (**b1**, **b2**) Postoperative contrast T1-weighted axial (**b1**) and coronal (**b2**) images showing the complete excision of the right-sided vestibular schwannoma

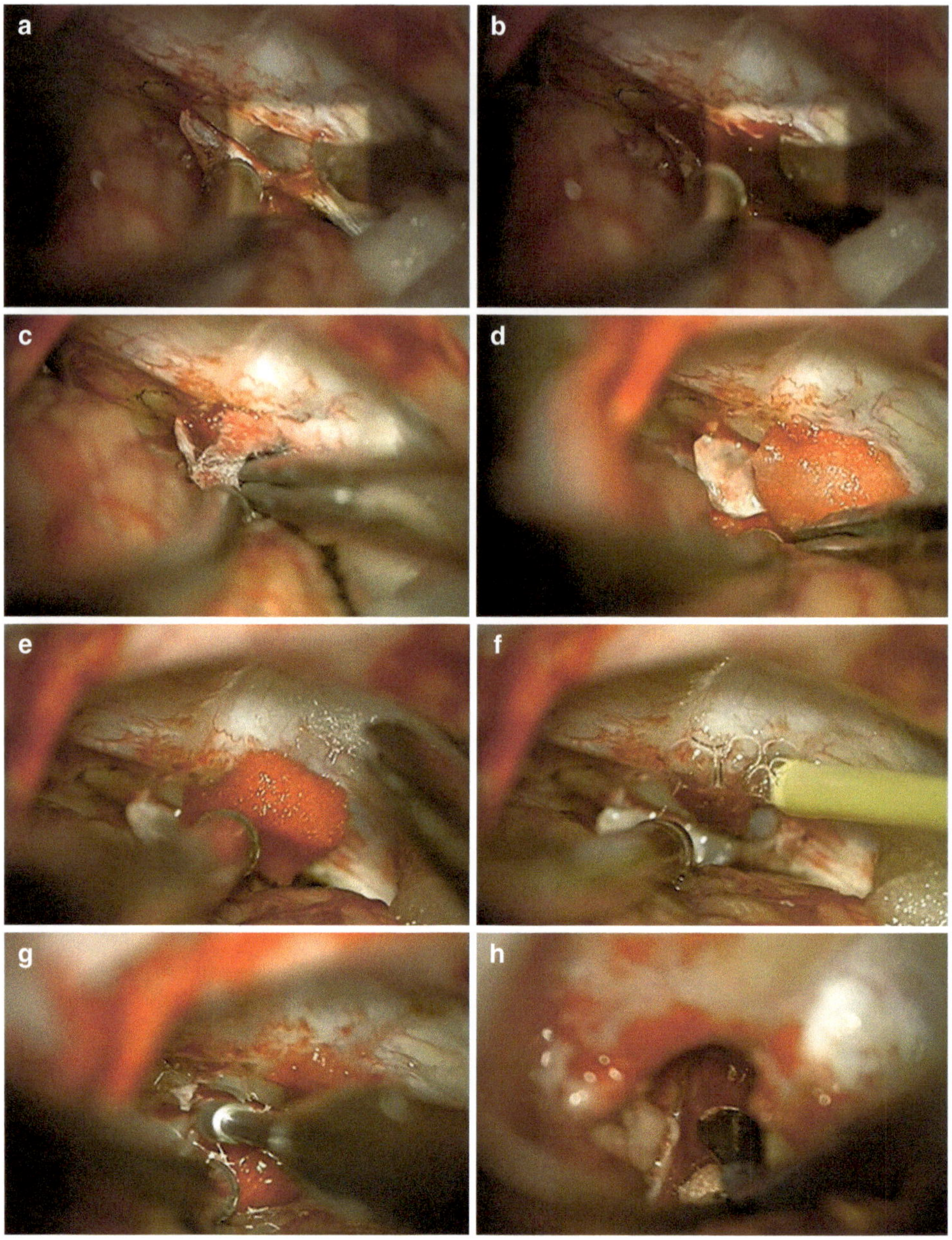

Fig. 4 Sequential intraoperative microscopic images depicting the case of a high-riding jugular bulb (HRJB) injury while drilling the internal auditory canal (IAC). (**a**) The dura over the arcuate eminence incised to expose the posterior wall of the IAC. A suspicious bluish patch is highlighted. (**b**) Trying to explore the bluish patch prior to starting the IAC drilling led to brisk bleeding. (**c**, **d**) Bleeding was first managed with Gelfoam and patty application. (**e**) Surgicel (fibrillar) placed on petrous bone and the excess Gealfoam covering the injured site of HRJB was removed. (**f**) Fibrin glue applied over Surgicel (fibrillar). (**g**) The IAC drilling was carefully continued by using a diamond drill. (**h**) The total excision of the IAC component of the VS can be seen with an intact facial (VII) nerve. Facial (VII) nerve stimulator-dissector is depicted

over the posteroinferior wall of the IAC (Fig. 4a). Tapping on the bluish patch prior to starting the IAC drilling led to brisk bleeding (Fig. 4b). This was because of an HRJB in combination with a bony dehiscence and the inadvertent iatrogenic injury that was caused to the HRJB by probing the dehiscent bone covering it. The bleeding was efficiently managed with a sequential application of Gelfoam pieces on a patty (Fig. 4c, d) and a layer of Surgicel that was enforced with fibrin glue (Fig. 4e, f). The IAC drilling was subsequently carefully continued by using a diamond drill. The complete excision of the VS was achieved while maintaining normal facial symmetry (Fig. 4g, h). In this case, sequential hemostatic measures mitigated the HRJB injury and ensured a chance of completing the IAC drilling. Postoperative gadolinium-enhanced MRI brain showed the complete excision of the tumor, including the IAC component (Fig. 3b1, b2).

Discussion

The retrosigmoid approach remains the most preferred access route for VS surgery by neurosurgeons worldwide. Because VS is a benign tumor and because an acceptable noninvasive alternative treatment modality (stereotactic radiosurgery) is available to the treatment team, there is an ever-increasing emphasis on microsurgery's consistently delivering on its promises (i.e., complete tumor resection and good functional outcomes). The avoidance and effective management of complications are the key steps in achieving this goal.

In this manuscript, we address two rare but potentially serious complications seen in VS surgery that can encounter via a retrosigmoid approach: spinal cord ischemia in the semi-sitting position and HRJB injury during IAC drilling.

The technical advantages provided by using the semi-sitting position (such as a clean surgical field and a better chance of bimanual dissection) is overshadowed by its unique disadvantages, such as the risk of venous air embolism and spinal cord ischemia [5]. Because of its commonality and recognizable intraoperative manifestations, a lot has been written and done to establish protocols to avoid/manage venous air embolisms. However, similar recognition and efforts are lacking in establishing protocols to avoid or manage possible spinal cord ischemia, which is most likely explained by its extreme rarity and missing intraoperative clinical signs. The underlying cause of such a devastating complication could be compressive (the hyperflexion of the cervical spine) and/or vascular (intraoperative hypotension) in origin [9]. Proper awareness of the clinical entity, preoperative screening for degenerative spinal disorders, avoiding excessive cervical flexion while positioning, the intraoperative monitoring of spinal cord function via SSEPs/MEPs in high-risk cases, and avoiding intraoperative hypotensive episodes can help circumvent such occurrences.

IAC drilling in VS surgery helps achieve two goals: decompressing the intracanalicular tumor component and recognizing the facial (VII) nerve early. Hence, it is an equally important step in the microsurgical management of both large and giant VSs (when VII nerve identification takes precedence) and intracanalicular/small tumors (when intracanalicular tumor decompression takes precedence).

The term *HRJB* is suitable when the dome of the jugular bulb lies within 2 mm of proximity to the IAC floor or higher. A cadaveric prevalence study of HRJB in the Indian population by Gupta et al. (2009) reported this configuration in as many as 38.6% of cases [10]. A jugular bulb lying within 1.5 mm below the IAC floor poses a significant risk of causing damage during IAC drilling. The sequential hemostatic measures depicted in Fig. 4 can help mitigate any HRJB injury, ensure a chance of completing the IAC drilling, and achieve both the aforementioned clinical goals, even in patients with an HRJB [11]. Routine preoperative imaging for HRJB in every patient with a VS via computed tomography (CT) venograms may be worthwhile. Unfortunately, economic concerns prevent us from routinely repeating imaging in already radiographically investigated patients who are referred to our tertiary referral center for surgery, especially when the patient has to pay out of pocket for such services.

Conclusion

Both spinal cord ischemia in the semi-sitting position and HRJB injury while IAC drilling can be effectively avoided/managed to achieve the planned microsurgical goals via the retrosigmoid approach for VS. Appropriate clinical knowledge about the entities and having preset protocols to keep a watchful eye on every case will go a long way in avoiding/managing the aforementioned rare yet potentially catastrophic complications.

Conflict of Interest Statement The authors have no conflicts of interest concerning the reported materials or methods.

References

1. Misra B, Purandare H, Ved R, Bagdia A, Mare P. Current treatment strategy in the management of vestibular schwannoma. Neurol India. 2009;57(3):257.
2. Pattankar S, Churi O, Misra BK. Quality of life in patients of unilateral vestibular schwannoma treated with microsurgery: a South-Asian tertiary care hospital experience. J Clin Neurosci. 2021;89:264–70.
3. Heman-Ackah SE, Golfinos JG, Roland JT. Management of surgical complications and failures in acoustic neuroma surgery. Otolaryngol Clin N Am. 2012;45(2):455–70.
4. Hitselberger WE, House WF. A warning regarding the sitting position for acoustic tumor surgery. Arch Otolaryngol-Head Neck Surg. 1980;106(2):69.
5. Breun M, Nickl R, Perez J, Hagen R, Löhr M, Vince G, Trautner H, Ernestus R-I, Matthies C. Vestibular schwannoma resection in a consecutive series of 502 cases via the Retrosigmoid approach: technical aspects, complications, and functional outcome. World Neurosurg. 2019;129:e114–27.
6. McCutcheon BA, Grauberger J, Murphy M, et al. Is patient age associated with perioperative outcomes after surgical resection of benign cranial nerve neoplasms? World Neurosurg. 2016;89:101–7.
7. Samii M, Matthies C. Management of 1000 vestibular schwannomas (acoustic neuromas): surgical management and results with an emphasis on complications and how to avoid them. Neurosurgery. 1997;40(1):11–23.
8. Tonn J-C. Acoustic neuroma surgery as an interdisciplinary approach: a neurosurgical series of 508 patients. J Neurol Neurosurg Psychiatry. 2000;69(2):161–6.
9. Yahanda AT, Chicoine MR. Paralysis caused by spinal cord injury after posterior fossa surgery: a systematic review. World Neurosurg. 2020;139:151–7.
10. Gupta T, Gupta SK. Anatomical delineation of a safety zone for drilling the internal acoustic meatus during surgery for vestibular schwanomma by retrosigmoid suboccipital approach. Clin Anat. 2009;22(7):794–9.
11. Muhammad S, Lehecka M, Sinkkonen ST, Niemelä M. Management of jugular bulb injury during drilling of the internal auditory canal (ICA) for vestibular schwannoma surgery. Am J Otolaryngol. 2019;40(2):341.

Unexpected Complications Following Accidental Petrosal Vein Damage during Standard Retrosigmoid Surgery for a Large Vestibular Schwannoma: Introspection and Lessons Learned

Suresh Nair, Adesh Shrivastava, Anirudh Nair, and Rakesh Mishra

Abstract

We present the case of a patient with a vestibular schwannoma (VS) who developed vascular complications following surgery and discuss the potential mechanisms. Additionally, we systematically searched the literature to identify citations on vascular and brain stem complications following VS surgery. We excluded the articles related to facial and vestibulocochlear nerve–related complications and other complications, such as headache, tinnitus, and ataxia. We also excluded the articles related to recurrent vestibular schwannoma because our article focuses on primary VS surgery–related complications due to vascular injury. We have clearly come a long way in managing vestibular schwannoma (VS) surgery over the past century. In the early twentieth century, VS surgery entailed high morbidity and mortality. The principles of microneurosurgery have improved the outcomes of surgery on VSs to a great extent. The current concept in modern VS surgery is maximal safe resection with minimal complications and minimal cranial nerve deficits. The management of VS has undergone a paradigm shift from reducing mortality to facial nerve preservation and the preservation of hearing. Surgery of the cerebellopontine (CP) angle requires a unique skill set and is a craft in that any iatrogenic damage can have devastating results on the neurovascular structures and brain stem in the vicinity. As with other neurosurgical procedures, the goal of VS surgery is to minimize complications, but complications are always possible, from the positioning of the patient under general anaesthesia to complications during the various steps of VS surgery. In spite of advancements in surgical techniques and better illumination provided by modern high-end microscopes, the surgical removal of large and giant vestibular schwannomas with good preservation of facial nerve function continues to be one of the most challenging operations in modern neurosurgery. The complexity of operating on the vestibular schwannoma is attributable not only to the difficult anatomy in the CP angle but also to the presence of multiple vital neurovascular structures and the brain stem in the vicinity. The various complications arising out of surgery for vestibular schwannomas range from one or more cranial nerve deficits to life-endangering complications associated with vascular and/or brain stem damage. The senior author, who has a personal experience with consecutively operating on 835 such cases of large and giant vestibular schwannoma, describes the clinical course following petrosal vein damage to a patient who underwent a standard retrosigmoid operation for a large vestibular schwannoma. We retrospectively analyse the critical management issues that could have reduced the unexpected morbidity resulting in a prolonged hospital stay.

Keywords

Vestibular schwannoma · Petrosal vein · Retrosigmoid approach · Skull base · Vascular injury

S. Nair (✉)
Sree Chitra Tirunal Institute for Medical Sciences and Technology, Trivandrum, Kerala, India

A. Shrivastava · R. Mishra
Department of Neurosurgery, All India Institute of Medical Sciences, Bhopal, Madhya Pradesh, India

A. Nair
Department of ENT, All India Institute of Medical Sciences, Raipur, Chhattisgarh, India

K. Turel, E. M. Kasper (eds.), *Complications in Neurosurgery II*, Acta Neurochirurgica Supplement 133,
https://doi.org/10.1007/978-3-031-61601-3_17

Introduction

We present the case of a patient with a vestibular schwannoma (VS) who developed vascular complications following surgery and discuss the potential mechanisms. Additionally, we systematically searched the literature to identify citations on vascular and brain stem complications following VS surgery. We excluded the articles related to facial and vestibulocochlear nerve–related complications and other complications, such as headache, tinnitus, and ataxia. We also excluded the articles related to recurrent vestibular schwannoma because our article focuses on primary VS surgery–related complications due to vascular injury. We have clearly come a long way in managing vestibular schwannoma (VS) surgery over the past century. In the early twentieth century, VS surgery entailed high morbidity and mortality. The principles of microneurosurgery have improved the outcomes of surgery on VSs to a great extent. The current concept in modern VS surgery is maximal safe resection with minimal complications and minimal cranial nerve deficits. The management of VS has undergone a paradigm shift from reducing mortality to facial nerve preservation and the preservation of hearing. Surgery of the cerebellopontine (CP) angle requires a unique skill set and is a craft in that any iatrogenic damage can have devastating results on the neurovascular structures and brain stem in the vicinity. As with other neurosurgical procedures, the goal of VS surgery is to minimize complications, but complications are always possible, from the positioning of the patient under general anaesthesia to complications during the various steps of VS surgery. In spite of advancements in surgical techniques and better illumination provided by modern high-end microscopes, the surgical removal of large and giant vestibular schwannomas with good preservation of facial nerve function continues to be one of the most challenging operations in modern neurosurgery. The complexity of operating on the vestibular schwannoma is attributable not only to the difficult anatomy in the CP angle but also to the presence of multiple vital neurovascular structures and the brain stem in the vicinity. The various complications arising out of surgery for vestibular schwannomas range from one or more cranial nerve deficits to life-endangering complications associated with vascular and/or brain stem damage. The senior author, who has a personal experience with consecutively operating on 835 such cases of large and giant vestibular schwannoma, describes the clinical course following petrosal vein damage to a patient who underwent a standard retrosigmoid operation for a large vestibular schwannoma. We retrospectively analyse the critical management issues that could have reduced the unexpected morbidity resulting in a prolonged hospital stay.

Clinical Scenario

A 47-year-old female patient presented with complaints of decreased hearing in her right ear for 1 year, diplopia for 8 months, gait unsteadiness (swaying to the right side) for 6 months, and choking while drinking for 3 months. She had no other medical or surgical comorbidities. General and systemic examination was within normal limits. On neurological examination, the patient had bilateral papilledema, bilateral horizontal gaze-evoked nystagmus, and a Weber test lateralizing to the left, with right bone conduction (BC) better than air conduction (AC) and left AC better than BC. She also had impaired tandem walking and a decreased and impaired palatal gag reflex on the right side. She was investigated in the referral hospital with an MRI scan, which revealed a 4 × 3 cm right vestibular schwannoma extending into the internal acoustic meatus (IAM).

As for the radiographic assessment, on T2-weighted images, the lesion was mixed hypo-/isointense with peripheral areas of hyperintensity and showed heterogeneous contrast enhancement as well as irregular borders. It showed a widening of the ipsilateral cerebellomesencephalic cistern, where the necrotic component was in the centre of the lesions, blooming on susceptibility weighted imaging (SWI) images with a mass effect and a distortion of the brain stem (Fig. 1). When the patient came to our tertiary hospital for definitive

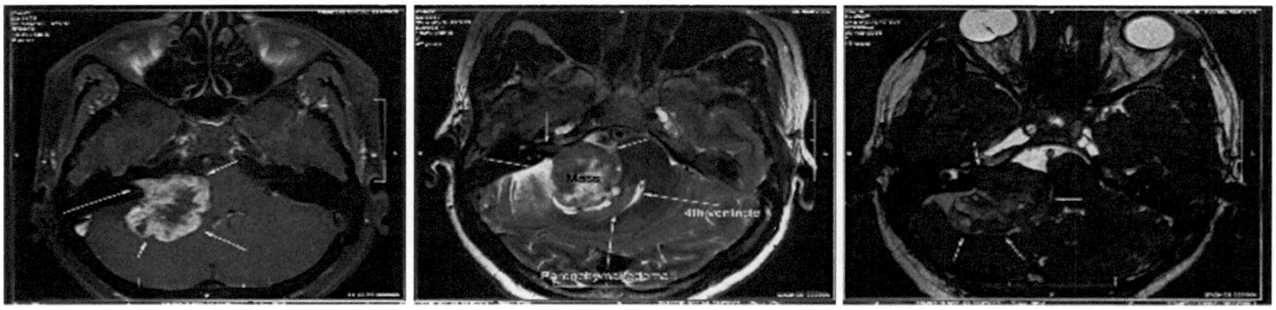

Fig. 1 Contrast-enhanced MRI of the brain showing tumour in the right cerebellomesencephalic cistern with central necrosis. There is a mass effect causing a distortion of the brain stem

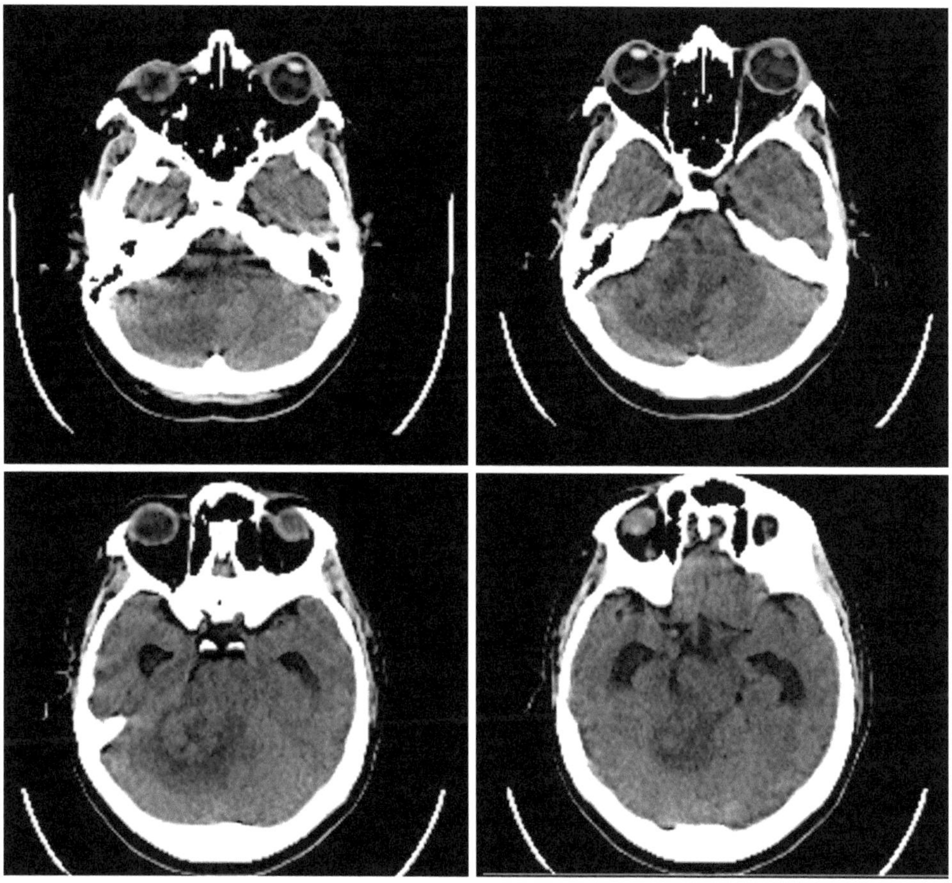

Fig. 2 Noncontrast CT scan of the patient showing a tumour in the right cerebellopontine angle, causing a mass effect over the brain stem

surgery 6 months after her initial detection of a tumour on MRI, a plain computed tomography (CT) scan (Fig. 2) was performed only to look for hydrocephalus. A repeat MRI was not performed at that time because MR remains an expensive investigation in our country. This CT showed mild hydrocephalus, but unusual hypodensity was seen around the tumour that was suggestive of perilesional oedema.

Surgery

The patient was positioned in the left lateral position with adequate padding and underwent a right retrosigmoid suboccipital craniotomy and an excision of the lesion with intraoperative brain stem potential and cranial nerve monitoring. After opening the dura, cerebrospinal fluid (CSF) was released, and after peeling away the double layer of invested arachnoid over the tumour in the standard way, internal debulking was performed by using the Cavitron ultrasonic aspirator. The tumour was vascular and soft to mildly firm in consistency, and after sufficient debulking, the capsule could be dissected from the surrounding cerebellum by employing stainless steel (SS) forceps under irrigation and mild suction. Once the capsule started folding into the decompressed tumour cavity, lesional tissue was progressively cut away and removed. Surface coagulation was kept to a minimum to avoid missing the inner investing arachnoid layer. During continued tumour decompression, the petrosal vein got snapped inadvertently, and torrential bleeding ensued, which was controlled with Gelfoam and local pressure. The complete excision of the tumour could be achieved, but we were surprised to see engorged veins over the brain stem bed after total removal. The tumour bed was carpeted with Surgicel, and the anaesthetist was asked to raise the blood pressure to confirm haemostasis. We also performed a Valsalva manoeuvre. Upon the removal of the retractors, the cerebellum was found to be full, and we decided to remove the lateral third of the swollen cerebellum. The dura was closed with a lax duroplasty, and the wound was closed after leaving the bone flap off. Additionally, through a burr hole at the right Frazier point, an external ventricular drain (EVD) was placed to release CSF, and we could then successfully canulate the ventricle on our first attempt. As notable cerebellum swelling was of concern, we decided to continue to electively ventilate the patient to perform a CT scan. This CT performed immediately after surgery (Fig. 3) showed gross total tumour resection with a lax cerebellum and a CSF pocket at the level of the bone flap, with only two minor specks of blood in the operative bed. A decision to continue ventilation overnight was made, and in the morning of the next day, a repeat CT

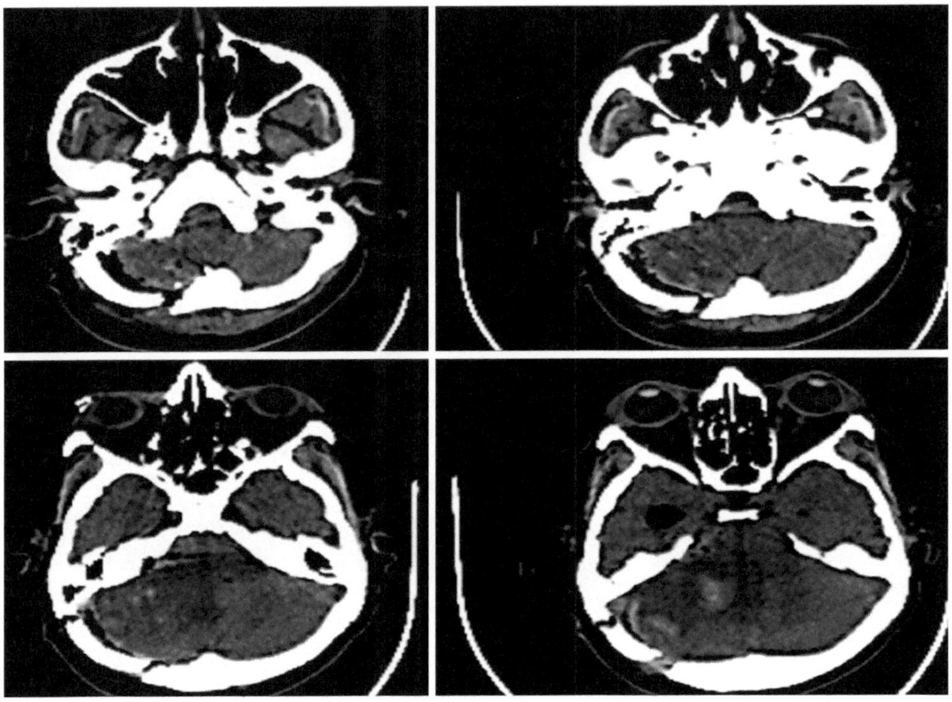

Fig. 3 Postoperative day 1 CT scan images showing total tumour resection and CSF in the subdural space at the operative site

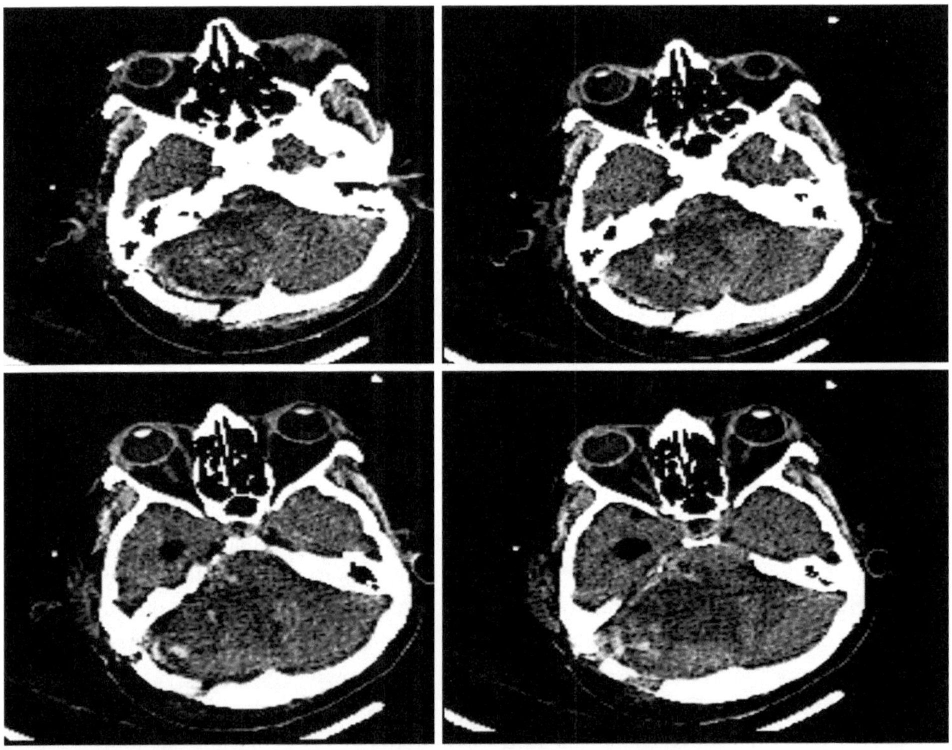

Fig. 4 Postoperative day 2 CT scan showing reduced subdural CSF space with the effacement of fourth ventricle

(Fig. 4) was carried out prior to considering the planned extubation. However, this CT showed a significant decrease in subdural space under the bone flap with an effacement of the fourth ventricle, so we decided to continue ventilation for another 24 h. There was no evidence of any increase in the blood on the surgical bed, which had been noted on the previous scan the evening prior. We decided to assess the neurological status and sensorium of the patient on the second postoperative day. The patient was taken off sedation to assess her responses, and given that she displayed no eye, verbal, or motor responses, we decided to perform a repeat MRI to look for any new infarct or possible hydrocephalus.

The MR was carried out expeditiously (Fig. 5) and showed large areas of SWI blooming with patchy restricted diffusion and T2 hyperintensity involving the right cerebellar hemisphere, right middle cerebellar peduncle and right and central regions of the pons. The basal cisterns were effaced, and sulcal flair hyperintensity was seen diffusely in the bilateral cerebral hemispheric subarachnoid space. A T2 flair hyperintense oedema was also seen in the right side of the midbrain region extending into the right thalamus and posterior limb of the right internal capsule (Fig. 6). Ascending transtentorial herniation was noted, resulting in the effacement of the suprasellar cisterns. We noted additional evidence of downward tonsillar herniation. An external ventricular shunt tip was localized to the right lateral ventricle, but the dilatation of both the lateral ventricles was seen. As the MRI findings were suggestive of extensive haemorrhagic venous infarct, the patient was continued on ventilator support with intermittent CSF drainage and antioedema measures. Since we noticed slow neurological status recovery over the next several hours, an elective tracheotomy was performed on the third postoperative day, and we decided to assess the patient's sensorium and neurological status every other day. On the seventh postoperative day, while weaning the sedation off for a formal assessment, the patient displayed posturing episodes of the left upper and bilateral lower limbs. The EVD was therefore kept in place and converted to the left ventriculoperitoneal shunt by using a medium pressure shunt. During a further course in the hospital, the patient had septicaemia from multidrug-resistant Klebsiella as well as a significant number of other complications: altered liver function, chest infiltrates, the segmental collapse of right upper lobe of lung, the consolidation of the left lung, ascites, lower gastrointestinal bleeding, nonoliguric drug-induced kidney damage, and status epilepticus, and she went through multiple episodes of shunt malfunction that required shunt revision, which led to an iatrogenic intraventricular bleed. This set of complications required that the patient be managed in the hospital for a total of 5 months. The patient could be weaned off the ventilator three and a half months after the initial surgery. From the time of discharge to rehabilitation, the patient was afebrile and nonambulatory; she underwent an exam that consisted of opening her eyes and moving her lower left limbs spontaneously, occasionally following objects and obeying simple commands. She was discharged to her native local hospital on room air with tracheostomy, nasogastric tube feeds, and a bladder catheter in situ.

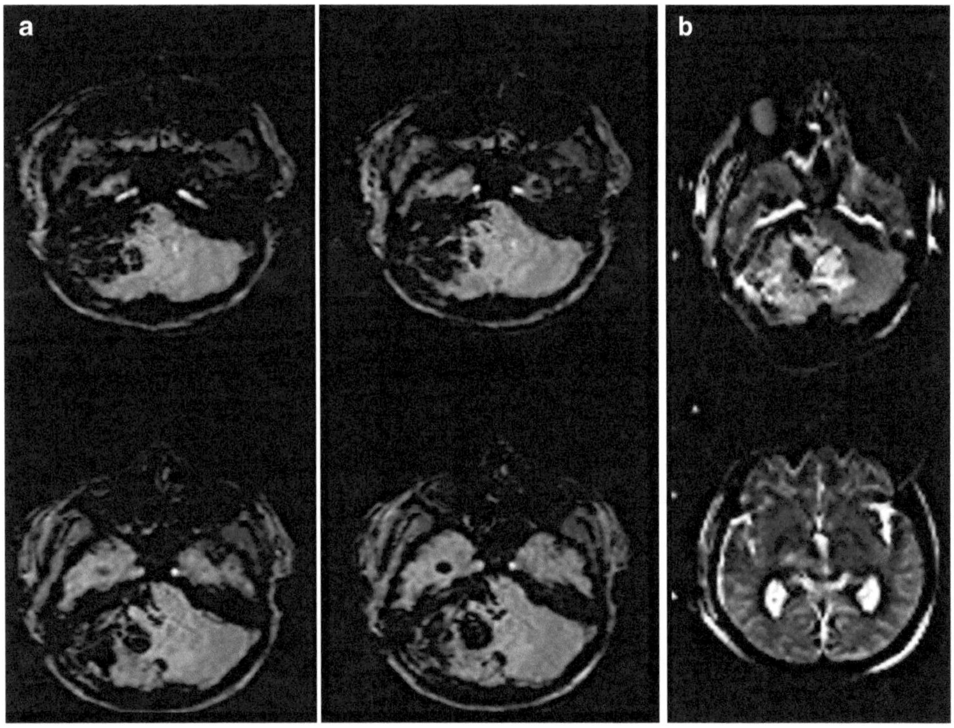

Fig. 5 MRI on the second postoperative day showing large areas of SWI blooming (**a**) with patchy diffusion restriction (**b**)

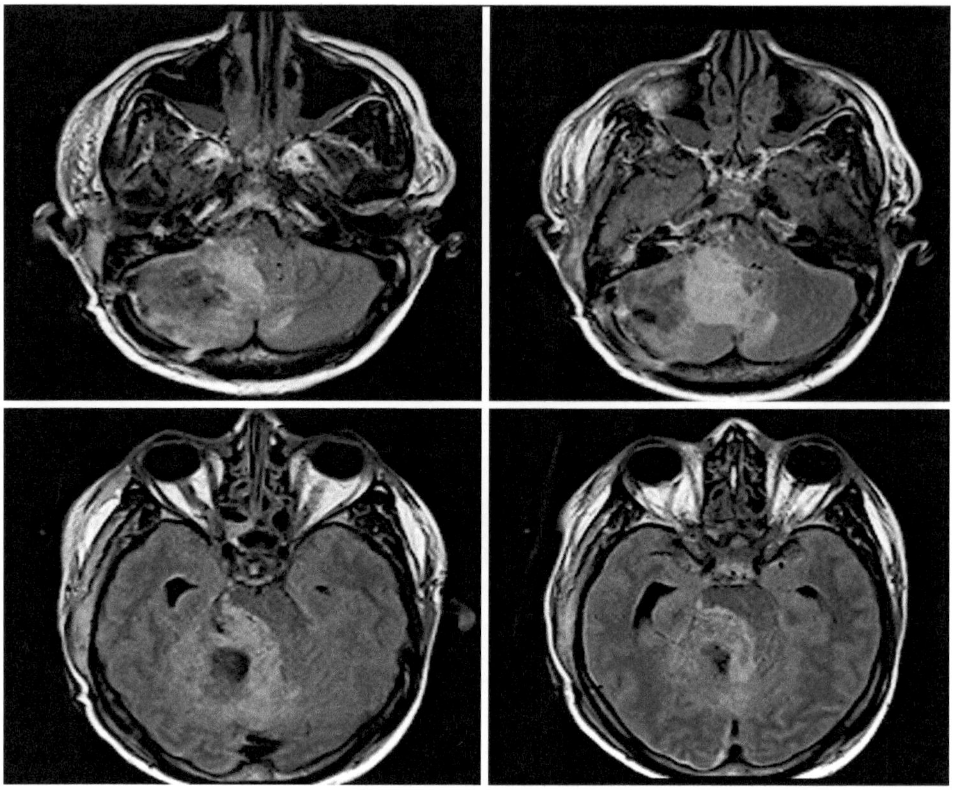

Fig. 6 Postoperative MRI showing T2 hyperintensities involving the right cerebellar hemisphere, the right middle cerebellar peduncle, and the right and central regions of pons. Basal cisterns were effaced, and sulcal flair hyperintensity was seen diffusely in the bilateral cerebral hemisphere subarachnoid space

Introspection

We looked at the possible intraoperative and radiological factors that might have led to this very unfortunate hospital course for our patient and discussed the following key points:

1. Can superior petrosal vein (SPV) damage alone lead to such a massive venous infarct? Theoretically, the closure of superior petrosal vein is expected to cause a massive venous outflow obstruction in the area, which may lead to infarction, but the rich amount of venous anastomosis, especially in the anterior portion of brain stem, makes this occurrence quite rare. Given the low rate of serious complications related to microvascular decompression procedures and the frequently established practice of coagulating the vein to achieve a better exposure in cases of upper-CP-angle surgery, the dramatic venous infarction seen in our case on a postoperative MRI scan was totally unexpected. The extent of the infarction into the supratentorial compartment with the involvement of the posterior thalamus and the posterior limb of the internal capsule was difficult to attribute to the closure of the petrosal vein alone since those areas are usually drained by the internal cerebral veins and the basal vein of Rosenthal.
2. Was any preoperative venous anomaly (like a nondominant transverse sinus) on the operative side with or without poor collateral flow to the opposite side? This may have resulted in the intra–/postoperative secondary thrombosis of the sigmoid sinus, which would have further contributed to our patient's adverse outcome. This complication is known to occur rarely in vestibular schwannoma surgery.
3. Another possibility that came to mind was whether the unusual peritumoural oedema that was seen on the immediate preoperative scan could have contributed to the adverse outcome.
4. Another factor that we looked at was the contribution of upward transtentorial herniation from the placement of the external ventriculostomy. This was noted on the postoperative MRI, and it might well have contributed to the patient's prolonged coma.
5. Was any microtrauma sustained by the small vessels at the tumour–brain stem interface? After all, we know that vestibular schwannoma is subarachnoid in origin and not epiarachnoid as previously thought.
6. Could the intraoperative venous engorgement seen after tumour removal be due to a venous breakthrough phenomenon seen after the sudden decompression of chronically compressed veins?

Reflection: Can Petrosal Vein Damage Alone Cause Poor Outcomes? Pros and Cons

Venous drainage is an important consideration when operating on CP-angle tumours and selecting suitable operative approaches, and stressing the importance of preserving the venous outflow while performing any skull base approach is crucial.

The sacrifice of veins that limit operative exposure may result in postoperative venous complications, which are difficult to predict because of the pattern of anastomoses that may develop in the presence of large tumours. However, significant variations are found in the configuration of the venous system. The superior petrosal vein is usually the major venous outflow vessel of the cerebellar hemisphere in the posterior cranial fossa. The veins that drain the cerebellum and brain stem merge to form three draining groups: galenic, tentorial, and petrosal. The superior petrosal veins, which drain into the superior petrosal sinus, may actually be duplicated—commonly one to three bridging veins, which are the major draining veins forming the petrosal group. These veins, known collectively as the "petrosal vein," or "Dandy's vein," comprise one of the largest and most constant venous complexes in the posterior fossa. This complex is located in proximity to the trigeminal nerve, below the tentorial edge, and it runs anteriorly and laterally from the upper portion of cerebellopontine angle, towards the petrous bone, and into the superior petrosal sinus. It often blocks access to the upper cerebello pontine angle (CPA) during a standard retrosigmoid approach. It acts as a significant anatomical landmark, though it can become a hindrance for the retrosigmoid approach in the sense that it limits the extent of cerebellar retraction and the visualization of the supratrigeminal corridor, especially while dealing with petroclival tumours.

The tributaries of the superior petrosal veins can be subdivided in four subgroups: (1) the petrosal subgroup, with tributaries draining the fourth ventricle, lateral medulla, middle cerebellar peduncle, and petrosal cerebellar surface facing the posterior surface of the temporal bone, such as the veins of the cerebellopontine fissure and the middle cerebellar peduncle; (2) the posterior mesencephalic subgroup, with tributaries draining the walls of the cerebellomesencephalic fissure, located between the posterior surface of the midbrain and the opposing surface of the cerebellum, such as the pontotrigeminal and lateral mesencephalic veins; (3) the anterior pontomesencephalic subgroup, with tributaries draining the anterior portion of the midbrain and pons, such as the transverse pontine veins; and (4) the tentorial subgroup, with tributaries draining the lateral part of the cerebellar surface that faces the tentorium and the petrosal cerebellar surface that faces the posterior surface of the temporal bone, such as the anterior lateral marginal vein [1, 2].

Whether sacrificing the vein of Dandy, which limits cerebellar retraction when it is in the line of the approach while operating on upper-CP-angle areas, is permissible remains controversial. While many surgeons believe that sacrificing this vein at such a juncture is justified [3], strong contrary views argue that petrosal vein preservation is desirable in all surgical posterior fossa cases [4]. Studies have described the almost negligible side effects of petrosal vein sacrifice in posterior fossa surgeries: Samii et al. and Mizutani et al. reported minimal effects after sectioning the vein of Dandy in their large series of patients with petrous apex tumours [5, 6] They hypothesize that in cases when the SPV is significantly displaced or compressed by a tumour, this constellation leads to the development of collateral veins. McLaughlin et al. described in their extensive series of 4400 microvascular decompression (MVD) surgeries that SPV can be sacrificed in the vast majority of cases without major morbidity or mortality [7]. Gharabaghi et al. also reported that the obliteration of the petrosal vein during surgery for petrous apex meningioma (PAM) did not have any major influence on the postoperative outcome. In their series of 55 patients with PAM, the vein of Dandy was sacrificed in 27 (49%) patients. While 11% patients in whom the vein was sacrificed developed minor deficits, a similar deficit was also noted in the cohort in which the vein was preserved [8]. Padmanabhan et al. [9] published their own experience of 184 patients with coagulation and the division of the SPV during MVDs. The overall rate of venous complications in this study was 2.7%; however, no case of venous infarction was noted in 184 patients who had the obliteration of the SPV. The study also reported that the incidence of venous infarction after SPV obliteration in MVD surgeries was <0.5% [9]. Elhammady and Heros mentioned sacrificing the SPV while performing MVD surgery in their large cohort of patients with trigeminal neuralgia (TN), and they did not attribute any morbidity directly to it [10]. In an excellent review of the safety profile of superior petrosal vein sacrifice in neurosurgical procedures by Narayan et al., [11] the incidence of operative complications at their centre in 32 out of the 50 MVD surgeries in whom petrosal vein was sacrificed was 6.2%, as opposed to none in the remaining 18 cases with a preserved SPV. Several cases of major complications after sacrificing the superior petrosal veins have been reported. In a report by Koerbel et al., [12] approximately 30% of patients had postoperative complications after petrous apex meningioma removal with superior petrosal vein sacrifice. Watanabe et al. also reported complications in 31% of operations for the removal of CPA meningiomas in which at least one petrosal vein was occluded, and they emphasized that other bridging veins could play critical roles in providing drainage if the superior petrosal vein were occluded by a tumour [13]/ While Zhong and colleagues mentioned that the diameter of the petrosal vein is an important factor, they found that a vein with a diameter of less than 2 mm could be coagulated and cut without risk [14]. Koerbel et al. suggested that the sacrifice of any vein more than 1.3 mm in diameter is a significant predictor of venous complications. Elhammady et al. [10] postulated that differences in the outcome may ensue when sectioning petrosal veins, which is based on the underlying pathology. While normal anatomy is usually seen in MVD surgery, the anatomy gets distorted in the presence of tumours because of the encasement of tributaries, leading to potential damage to these vessels during surgery. According to these authors, the obliteration of the petrosal veins in MVD surgery may be safe thanks to the intact compensatory venous outflow—as opposed to tumour pathologies, where it can be altered, resulting in dangerous complications [10]. Some authors have suggested that the intraoperative transient obliteration of the main trunk of the petrosal vein with simultaneous brain stem and auditory evoked potential or even an assessment of collateral venous drainage by using indocyanine green prior to the obliteration of these vessels may help in predicting the occurrence of venous hypertension in the intra-/postoperative period [12, 15, 16].

On the basis of the above discussion, we strongly conclude that the obliteration of the bridging vein on the tentorial cerebellar surface should be avoided in operative manoeuvres in CP-angle surgeries unless it is absolutely warranted to again access to deeper areas. We highly recommend that extreme care be taken to avoid its accidental avulsion, to minimize potential complications.

Role of Cerebral Venous Sinus Thrombosis (CVST)

Patients undergoing surgery for cerebellopontine-angle tumours are at an increased risk for developing cerebral venous sinus thrombosis (CVST). Transverse and sigmoid sinuses are the most commonly involved structures in CVSTs that occur after posterior fossa surgery. Postoperative sinus thrombosis occurs in about 4.7–11.6% of patients undergoing posterior fossa surgeries, yet it is infrequent after vestibular schwannoma surgery [17–19]. The incidence of CVST after surgery for VS was 6% in the most extensive series of 116 patients [20]. Intra- and postoperative CVST likely occurs mainly because of dural desiccation (when the sinus is overexposed), sinus injury, sinus manipulation, tumour infiltration, retraction over the sinus, intracranial hypotension, dehydration, and pre-existing hypercoagulable states. Studies have noted that the exposure of the transverse sinus in suboccipital craniotomy and prolonged retraction during surgery are the most significant factors in transverse sinus thrombosis [17, 18]. In the series reported by Couldwell's group [20], patients who underwent vestibular schwannoma surgery via the retrosigmoid route or the translabyrinthine route were at risk of developing this complication, and all cases of transverse/sigmoid sinus thrombosis occurred in their series in patients who had a codominant or nondominant sinus and not in patients who had a dominant sinus. They postulated that higher blood flow in the dominant sinus decreases the risk of venous stasis and thrombus formation and its propagation after surgery. These authors have stressed minimizing thermal injury not only from drilling and but also from illumination via the operative microscope and have stressed that all efforts should be made to minimize sinus exposure and its manipulation. They further suggested that drilling always be performed under constant irrigation and that the exposed sinus be protected with moist neurosurgical patties. Finally, they recommended that sinus retraction be frequently released to prevent intraluminal venous stasis. Such per-/postpostoperative CVST is different from spontaneous CVST, which is a systemic disorder of the hypercoagulable state. Per-/postoperative CVST is primarily due to the local causes already described above. Understanding this difference is important because spontaneous CVST requires aggressive anticoagulation with an inherent risk of postoperative haematoma formation. Most patients with a peri-/postoperative CVST are asymptomatic, and therefore, this problem is considered a less aggressive pathology than that of spontaneous CVST. Collateral venous circulation explains the individual differences in tolerating CVST. However, symptomatic postoperative CVST patients present a unique challenge to neurosurgeons. The surgeon needs to find a balance between haematoma due to venous hypertension and the risk of bleeding in the tumour cavity. Because of the rarity of postoperative CVST in vestibular schwannoma surgery, its natural course, pathophysiology, and management options have not been well elucidated.

The thrombosed sinus may undergo recanalization, and the patient may remain asymptomatic; however, some patients develop progressive symptoms with cerebellar swelling, raised intracranial pressure, and neurological deterioration. Although the occlusion of the nondominant transverse or sigmoid sinus is believed to be well tolerated, Keiper et al. [18] reported five patients with a thrombosis of the nondominant transverse sinus during posterior fossa surgery who later with with features of raised intracranial pressure. When the thrombosis of the transverse sinus becomes symptomatic and when it is apparent on neuroimaging remains unclear. Dehydration due to the preoperative use of mannitol, the poor intraoperative optimization of hydration status, and intracranial hypotension due to CSF release from an EVD were the causative factors of remote CVST [21]. Strategies to prevent CVST development following VS surgery include minimizing bone removal over the transverse and sigmoid sinus, retraction, and sinus injury; the judicious use of both mannitol and CSF release; and adequate hydration [18]. Copious saline irrigation during drilling and using wet cotton patties prevents the dural desiccation from causing a thermal injury. Because of the higher risks of operative site haematoma with the postoperative use of anticoagulation, no clear consensus on its use has been reached. While some have suggested that asymptomatic patients are best treated with a conservative approach and that anticoagulation be reserved only for symptomatic patients or those with severe cerebellar swelling [19], Couldwell and colleagues suggested anticoagulation with heparin even for asymptomatic patients with evidence of CVST on MRI/CT scans unless the involved sinus is diminutive in comparison to the contralateral patent sinus and unless the sinuses communicate at the torcula [20]. Another area lacking evidence is how many patients with CVST after surgery will develop severe cerebellar oedema. Whether cerebellar swelling developing in the absence of CVST is due to some other causes or to inadequate detection because of the varying protocols of postoperative MRI at different centres remains unclear. Therefore, whether anticoagulation should be given at all is mainly unknown.

We suggest that all patients of VS requiring surgery be evaluated with an MR venogram to assess the patency of the transverse and sigmoid sinus. Sawarkar et al. [21] reported a patient with vestibular schwannoma who developed a thrombosis of the superior sagittal sinus and torcula after surgery. The authors did not find the thrombosis of the transverse and sigmoid sinus in the hypercoagulable state, and that patient had no prolonged retraction or sinus injury. Dehydration due to the preoperative use of mannitol, the poor intraoperative optimization of hydration status, and intracranial hypotension due to CSF release from an EVD were the causative factors of remote CVST. Sawarkar et al.'s strategies to prevent CVST development following VS surgery also included adequate hydration and the judicious use of both mannitol and CSF release.

We did not suspect sinus occlusion in our case presented above, because no obvious injury to the sigmoid sinus occurred during exposure and because this patient had petrosal vein avulsion at surgery. Thus, we assumed that the venous infarct was secondary to this insult. Our case was not investigated with a presurgical MR venogram. Retrospectively considering the massive venous infarct with extension to the supratentorial compartment that our patient developed, we presume there would have been some element of sinus thrombosis that could have contributed to the adverse outcome because we know that some of the routine intraoperative steps—such as retraction, overwaxing the exposed sigmoid–transverse junction to obliterate the opened mastoid air cells, and parenchymal damage (the lateral third of the cerebellum was removed before dural closure)—can add to the insult.

Arterial Complications

Microvascular complications in VS surgery have not been well described owing to the inconsistency in the clinical features, the nonspecific symptoms, and the variable protocols for pre- and postoperative MRI scans [22]. The parafloccular space is a critical triangular area between the superior and inferior cerebellopontine fissure and contains an anterior inferior cerebellar artery and its perforators [23]. The anterior inferior cerebellar artery (AICA) vascular territory includes the inferolateral pons, the middle cerebellar peduncle, and the flocculus/para floccular region. With advanced neuroimaging and routine postoperative MRI, researchers have found that many a time worsening in the postoperative period could be due to microvascular brain stem ischaemia. Recurrent perforator arteries initially course towards IAM and in due course supply the posterolateral brain stem, making the brain stem vulnerable to microvascular ischaemia. Injury to the proximal AICA results in a devastating infract of the pons, whereas injury to the distal AICA and perforators results in a middle cerebellar peduncular infarct. Proximal AICA injury usually produces a devastating infarct of the pons, whereas distal AICA injury may be clinically rather benign. Distal AICA may not be salvageable in some cases, because of its adherence to the tumour capsule. Contrary to the old belief, now we know that vestibular schwannoma is not extra-arachnoid in origin at the far lateral end of the internal auditory canal, as proposed by Yasargil [24], but instead, it arises in the subarachnoid space inside the canal, close to the site of Scarpa's ganglion. These tumours—as they extend towards the cerebellopontine angle in the acoustic-facial cistern—have no arachnoid layer that separates the capsule, which is formed by the perineurium of the vestibular nerve, from the seventh auditory nerve and the anterior inferior cerebellar artery and its perforating branches [25–28]. Also, sometimes the anatomical variation in AICA makes it susceptible to injury during surgical removal [29]. Typically, AICA is inferiorly displaced by the tumour during the retrosigmoid approach and can be preserved via a meticulous, sharp dissection of the vessel from the slack capsule of an internally debulked tumour. Contrary to the old concept of the extra-arachnoid origin, where one expects an arachnoid layer to be separating the capsule from neurovascular structures of the acoustic-facial cistern, we now know that such an arachnoid layer does not exist and that the surgeon comes in direct contact with AICA and its branches during the surgical dissection of the decompressed folded capsule.

One should understand that a tumour/arachnoid plane is always above the lesion between the vestibular schwannoma and the fifth cranial nerve and superior cerebellar artery, which are in the adjacent trigeminal cistern and also below the lower cranial nerves and posterior inferior cerebellar arteries, which are in the cerebellomedullary cistern.

Our patient did not have any overt injury to AICA or its perforating branches during surgery.

Contributing Factors of Preoperative Oedema

The preoperative scan performed on our patient a few days prior to definitive surgery showed extensive perilesional oedema. As opposed to intracranial meningiomas, which sometimes present with peritumoural oedema, its occurrence in vestibular schwannoma has been reported only occasionally, and its correlation with intrinsic tumour features found during surgery, like the presence of a pseudocapsule, adhesion, and vascularity, was reported by Samii et al. [30] In a recent publication by the same authors, peritumoural oedema in vestibular schwannomas was described in one or more of the following areas: the brachium pontis (88%), the cerebellum (60%), or the brain stem (12%) [31]. They categorized oedema extension as mild if one region was involved, moderate if two of these areas were involved, and severe if all three regions were involved. However, they could not find a relation between tumour volume and oedema volume, though this has often been noticed in meningiomas [32]. They also observed that the peritumoural oedema seen in vestibular schwannoma is not exclusively located in the main area of compression, which is usually perpendicular to the major axis of tumour growth, and this finding contradicts a compressive mechanism that was proposed for meningiomas. It is quite intriguing to understand why prelesional oedema is less often seen even in larger vestibular schwannomas, which we now understand is a subarachnoid tumour, as opposed to its more frequent occurrence in similar-size meningiomas, which are extra-arachnoid tumours. Guo et al. reported that the presence of preoperative peritumoural oedema on imaging is associated with an increased risk of postoperative haematoma in patients, and the authors even stressed that the venous anatomy should be evaluated in detail in all such cases [33]. Our patient had a significant peritumoural oedema on a preoperative CT. However, we could not find any abnormal venous malformation during surgery. The engorged veins seen over the tumour bed after the surgical extirpation of the schwannoma could be a reflection of raised venous pressure from damage to the major petrosal draining vein during surgery, compounded by raised intracranial pressure.

Role of Reverse Herniation in the Postoperative Period from External Ventricular Drainage

Hydrocephalus is an important factor influencing the outcome of surgery in posterior fossa tumours. Preresection ventricular drainage comes with a risk of upward herniation, though this complication is rare for extra-axial tumours. CSF diversion procedures can disrupt the critical equilibrium maintained between the CSF pathways and the tumour that preserves the diencephalic and brain stem functions, thus increasing morbidity and the potential for mortality. Supratentorial ventriculomegaly associated with an increased CSF pressure allows the tumour to be confined within a specified space, and external ventriculostomy should be kept closed until tumour exposure has been accomplished to prevent any disruption to this equilibrium [34]. In a previous publication from our centre [35], out of the 95.2% of the posterior fossa tumour patients who presented with symptomatic hydrocephalus, 29.8% required a CSF diversion procedure in the postoperative period. We reported that the symptom duration had an inverse relation with the likelihood of CSF diversion and midline tumours in comparison to laterally placed lesions, which are more likely to need CSF diversion. All the patients who are brought in moribund from hydrocephalus used to be treated with a preoperative CSF diversion procedure in our institute. If the patient with hydrocephalus is not sick and not symptomatic from hydrocephalus, our policy was to perform an external ventriculostomy, keeping the ventricular catheter closed and removing it only after few days if the CSF pressure was not raised. We now realize that the engorged veins seen in the surgical bed after tumour removal and the cerebellar bulge at the time of closure were from persistent intracranial pressure. The postoperative MRI performed on the second postoperative day showed evidence of reverse herniation, which also could have contributed to the poor outcome for our patient.

Lastly, we are not sure whether the intraoperative venous engorgement seen after tumour removal in this patient was due to a venous breakthrough phenomenon seen after a sudden decompression of chronically compressed veins in large and giant tumours.

Summary: Lessons Learned

We have no doubt that our patient had a poor outcome most likely from the avulsion of the petrosal vein. Another factor that could have contributed to this adverse outcome is the preoperative perilesional oedema along with a continuous external ventricular drain that led to reverse herniation. Furthermore, the replacement of the bone flap after surgery would have increased posterior fossa pressure. We are not sure whether this patient in the presence of peri-lesional oedema had any pre-existing venous anomaly or a nondominant transverse sigmoid sinus on the operated side. This constellation is known for occlusion with excessive dural flap retraction and heat-induced injury from the drill and operating microscope, even in the absence of any direct operative injury. We certainly agree strongly with the comments of others that the superior petrosal vein complex should be treated with respect and that every effort must be taken to avoid its accidental avulsion, which can occur after good intra-tumoural decompression, leading to the inward folding of the slack tumour capsule into the decompressed tumour cavity, itself leading to the stretching of the petrosal vein and its avulsion.

The variability in the anatomy and function of the veins, especially in the face of pathology, is well known. No one knows how many collaterals are present and functioning or which one can be taken without consequence. The old neurosurgical principle, stressed by the great vestibular schwannoma surgeon Leonard Malis, stated that "no structure should be taken unless necessary," and this notion applies to vessels that are as seemingly well collateralized as the superior petrosal vein [36]. CSF drainage and the insertion of an external ventricular or ventriculoperitoneal shunt should be carried out with caution because of the increased risk of reverse herniation in these patients with high pressure in the posterior fossa. If the cerebellum is full after surgery, performing a resection of the lateral third of the cerebellar hemisphere and closing with a lax duroplasty are prudent, both of which were carried out for our patient, and in these instances, not positioning the bone flap back in the craniectomy site is better.

Disclosure of Funding None.

Conflicts of Interest None.

References

1. Matsushima K, Matsushima T, Kuga Y, Kodama Y, Inoue K, Ohnishi H, Rhoton AL Jr. Classification of the superior petrosal veins and sinus based on drainage pattern. Neurosurgery. 2014;10 Suppl 2:357–367; discussion 367. https://doi.org/10.1227/NEU.0000000000000323.
2. Matsushima T, Rhoton AL Jr, de Oliveira E, Peace D. Microsurgical anatomy of the veins of the posterior fossa. J Neurosurg. 1983;59:63–105. https://doi.org/10.3171/jns.1983.59.1.0063.
3. Xia Y, Kim TY, Mashouf LA, Patel KK, Xu R, Casaos J, Choi J, Kim ES, Hung AL, Wu A, Garzon-Muvdi T, Bender MT, Jackson CM, Bettegowda C, Lim M. Absence of ischemic injury after sacrificing the superior Petrosal vein during microvascular decompression. Oper Neurosurg (Hagerstown). 2020;18:316–20. https://doi.org/10.1093/ons/opz163.
4. Bhatoe HS. Letter: absence of ischemic injury after sacrificing the superior Petrosal vein during microvascular decompression. Oper Neurosurg (Hagerstown). 2021;20:E258–9. https://doi.org/10.1093/ons/opaa432.
5. Samii M, Tatagiba M, Carvalho GA. Retrosigmoid intradural suprameatal approach to Meckel's cave and the middle fossa: surgical technique and outcome. J Neurosurg. 2000;92:235–41. https://doi.org/10.3171/jns.2000.92.2.0235.
6. Mizutani K, Toda M, Yoshida K. The analysis of the Petrosal vein to prevent venous complications during the anterior Transpetrosal approach in the resection of Petroclival meningioma. World Neurosurg. 2016;93:175–82. https://doi.org/10.1016/j.wneu.2016.06.018.
7. McLaughlin MR, Jannetta PJ, Clyde BL, Subach BR, Comey CH, Resnick DK. Microvascular decompression of cranial nerves: lessons learned after 4400 operations. J Neurosurg. 1999;90:1–8. https://doi.org/10.3171/jns.1999.90.1.0001.
8. Gharabaghi A, Koerbel A, Lowenheim H, Kaminsky J, Samii M, Tatagiba M. The impact of petrosal vein preservation on postoperative auditory function in surgery of petrous apex meningiomas. Neurosurgery. 2006;59:ONS68–74 discussion ONS68-74. https://doi.org/10.1227/01.NEU.0000219821.34450.59.
9. Pathmanaban ON, O'Brien F, Al-Tamimi YZ, Hammerbeck-Ward CL, Rutherford SA, King AT. Safety of superior Petrosal vein sacrifice during microvascular decompression of the trigeminal nerve. World Neurosurg. 2017;103:84–7. https://doi.org/10.1016/j.wneu.2017.03.117.
10. Elhammady MS, Heros RC. Cerebral veins: to sacrifice or not to sacrifice, that is the question. World Neurosurg. 2015;83:320–4. https://doi.org/10.1016/j.wneu.2013.06.003.
11. Narayan V, Savardekar AR, Patra DP, Mohammed N, Thakur JD, Riaz M, Nanda A. Safety profile of superior petrosal vein (the vein of Dandy) sacrifice in neurosurgical procedures: a systematic review. Neurosurg Focus. 2018;45:E3. https://doi.org/10.3171/2018.4.FOCUS18133.
12. Koerbel A, Gharabaghi A, Safavi-Abbasi S, Samii A, Ebner FH, Samii M, Tatagiba M. Venous complications following petrosal vein sectioning in surgery of petrous apex meningiomas. Eur J Surg Oncol. 2009;35:773–9. https://doi.org/10.1016/j.ejso.2008.02.015.
13. Watanabe T, Igarashi T, Fukushima T, Yoshino A, Katayama Y. Anatomical variation of superior petrosal vein and its management during surgery for cerebellopontine angle meningiomas. Acta Neurochir. 2013;155:1871–8. https://doi.org/10.1007/s00701-013-1840-8.
14. Zhong J, Li ST, Xu SQ, Wan L, Wang X. Management of petrosal veins during microvascular decompression for trigeminal neuralgia. Neurol Res. 2008;30:697–700. https://doi.org/10.1179/174313208X289624.
15. Liebelt BD, Barber SM, Desai VR, Harper R, Zhang J, Parrish R, Baskin DS, Trask T, Britz GW. Superior Petrosal vein sacrifice during microvascular decompression: perioperative complication rates and comparison with venous preservation. World Neurosurg. 2017;104:788–94. https://doi.org/10.1016/j.wneu.2017.05.098.
16. Matsushima K, Ribas ES, Kiyosue H, Komune N, Miki K, Rhoton AL. Absence of the superior petrosal veins and sinus: surgical considerations. Surg Neurol Int. 2015;6:34. https://doi.org/10.4103/2152-7806.152147.
17. Apra C, Kotbi O, Turc G, Corns R, Pages M, Souillard-Scemama R, Dezamis E, Parraga E, Meder JF, Sauvageon X, Devaux B, Oppenheim C, Pallud J. Presentation and management of lateral sinus thrombosis following posterior fossa surgery. J Neurosurg. 2017;126:8–16. https://doi.org/10.3171/2015.11.JNS151881.
18. Keiper GL Jr, Sherman JD, Tomsick TA, Tew JM Jr. Dural sinus thrombosis and pseudotumour cerebri: unexpected complications of suboccipital craniotomy and translabyrinthine craniectomy. J Neurosurg. 1999;91:192–7. https://doi.org/10.3171/jns.1999.91.2.0192.

19. Moore J, Thomas P, Cousins V, Rosenfeld JV. Diagnosis and Management of Dural Sinus Thrombosis following resection of Cerebellopontine angle Tumours. J Neurol Surg B Skull Base. 2014;75:402–8. https://doi.org/10.1055/s-0034-1376421.
20. Abou-Al-Shaar H, Gozal YM, Alzhrani G, Karsy M, Shelton C, Couldwell WT. Cerebral venous sinus thrombosis after vestibular schwannoma surgery: a call for evidence-based management guidelines. Neurosurg Focus. 2018;45:E4. https://doi.org/10.3171/2018.4.FOCUS18112.
21. Sawarkar DP, Verma SK, Singh PK, Doddamani R, Kumar A, Sharma BS. Fatal superior sagittal sinus and Torcular thrombosis after vestibular Schwannoma surgery: report of a rare complication and review of the literature. World Neurosurg. 2016;96:607 e619–24. https://doi.org/10.1016/j.wneu.2016.09.075.
22. Sade B, Mohr G, Dufour JJ. Vascular complications of vestibular schwannoma surgery: a comparison of the suboccipital retrosigmoid and translabyrinthine approaches. J Neurosurg. 2006;105:200–4. https://doi.org/10.3171/jns.2006.105.2.200.
23. Sosa P, Dujovny M, Onyekachi I, Sockwell N, Cremaschi F, Savastano LE. Microvascular anatomy of the cerebellar parafloccular perforating space. J Neurosurg. 2016;124:440–9. https://doi.org/10.3171/2015.2.JNS142693.
24. Yaşargil MG, Smith RD, Gasser JC. Microsurgical approach to acoustic Neurinomas. In: Advances and technical standards in neurosurgery. Advances and technical standards in neurosurgery. Vienna: Springer; 1977. p. 93–129. https://doi.org/10.1007/978-3-7091-7073-1_5.
25. Kohno M, Sato H, Sora S, Miwa H, Yokoyama M. Is an acoustic neuroma an epiarachnoid or subarachnoid tumour? Neurosurgery. 2011;68:1006–1016; discussion 1016-1007. https://doi.org/10.1227/NEU.0b013e318208f37f.
26. Ohata K, Tsuyuguchi N, Morino M, Takami T, Goto T, Hakuba A, Hara M. A hypothesis of epiarachnoidal growth of vestibular schwannoma at the cerebello-pontine angle: surgical importance. J Postgrad Med. 2002;48:253–258; discussion 258-259.
27. Sudhir BJ, Nair S. Lilliputian nuances of giant vestibular schwannomas. Neurol India. 2016;64:373–5. https://doi.org/10.4103/0028-3886.181562.
28. Shrivastava A, Nair S. Commentary: "save the nerve": technical nuances for hearing preservation and restoration in vestibular Schwannoma surgery: 2-dimensional operative video. Oper Neurosurg (Hagerstown). 2021;21(4):E328–9. https://doi.org/10.1093/ons/opab250.
29. Yamakami I, Kubota S, Higuchi Y, Ito S. Challenging anterior inferior cerebellar artery in Retrosigmoid vestibular Schwannoma removal. World Neurosurg. 2019;121:e370–8. https://doi.org/10.1016/j.wneu.2018.09.111.
30. Samii M, Giordano M, Metwali H, Almarzooq O, Samii A, Gerganov VM. Prognostic significance of Peritumoural edema in patients with vestibular Schwannomas. Neurosurgery. 2015;77:81–85; discussion 85-86. https://doi.org/10.1227/NEU.0000000000000748.
31. Giordano M, Gerganov V, Metwali H, Gallieni M, Samii M, Samii A. Imaging features and classification of peritumoural edema in vestibular schwannoma. Neuroradiol J. 2020;33:169–73. https://doi.org/10.1177/1971400919896253.
32. Lee KJ, Joo WI, Rha HK, Park HK, Chough JK, Hong YK, Park CK. Peritumoural brain edema in meningiomas: correlations between magnetic resonance imaging, angiography, and pathology. Surg Neurol. 2008;69:350–5; discussion 355. https://doi.org/10.1016/j.surneu.2007.03.027.
33. Guo X, Zhu Y, Wang X, Xu K, Hong Y. Peritumoural edema is associated with postoperative hemorrhage and reoperation following vestibular Schwannoma surgery. Front Oncol. 2021;11:633350. https://doi.org/10.3389/fonc.2021.633350.
34. Habib HAM. Intraoperative precautionary insertion of external ventricular drainage catheters in posterior fossa tumours presenting with hydrocephalus. Alex J Med. 2019;50:333–40. https://doi.org/10.1016/j.ajme.2013.11.001.
35. Gopalakrishnan CV, Dhakoji A, Menon G, Nair S. Factors predicting the need for cerebrospinal fluid diversion following posterior fossa tumour surgery in children. Pediatr Neurosurg. 2012;48:93–101. https://doi.org/10.1159/000343009.
36. Strauss C, Neu M, Bischoff B, Romstock J. Clinical and neurophysiological observations after superior petrosal vein obstruction during surgery of the cerebellopontine angle: case report. Neurosurgery. 2001;48:1157–1159; discussion 1159-1161. https://doi.org/10.1097/00006123-200105000-00043.

Complications in Occipitocervical Surgery

Ali Fahir Ozer

Abstract

The occipitocervical junction is formed by the foramen magnum (FM) and the adjacent anatomical structures of the C1 and C2 vertebrae. The FM is formed anteriorly by the basilar part of occipital bone. Anterolaterally, it borders the occipital condyles and hypoglossal canal as well as the jugular foramen. Posteriorly, the FM is formed by the squamous part of the occipital bone with the internal occipital crest. In the midline, named landmarks at the anterior margin are the basion and, at the posterior margin, the opisthion. Vital anatomic structures are located in the FM or pass through. Among these are the medulla oblongata, meninges, anterior and posterior spinal arteries, vertebral arteries, and spinal roots of the accessory nerve. The FM is firmly anchored to the cervical canal via strong ligamentous support.

Pathologies in this area can be of congenital, acquired, traumatic, neoplastic, or infectious origin, with the respective surgical indications and approaches depending on the nature and location of the pathology. If the pathology is occipitoatlantal, the occiput is usually involved in surgery. On the other hand, if the pathology is only at the level of C1-C2, surgery may be limited to these two vertebrae.

In this section, we present the surgical management of exemplary congenital cases, and we discuss the complications and what needs to be done to deal with them.

Keywords

Occipitocervical anatomy · Occipitocervical measurements · Occipitocervical complications · Occipitocervical surgery

A. F. Ozer (✉)
Department of Neurosurgery, Koc University School of Medicine, Istanbul, Turkey

Part 1: Congenital Pathologies

Introduction

The occipitocervical region is a complex region with characteristic anatomical structures. Conceptually, as a spherical mass, the rigid head is attached to a long mobile cylindrical structure, the cervical region. This layout shows that the specific architectural features and musculoskeletal anatomy is very solid. To this end, the cervical region is firmly attached to the cranium via strong ligamentous support. The connective tissue in this area is much stronger than that connecting vertebrae in other parts of the spine. For this reason, occipitocervical stabilization carries significance when this structural relationship is weakened or compromised.

What is the common problem in occipitocervical region pathologies? The answer to this question is important: If the occipitocervical connection is disrupted, instability develops, neural tissue damage can occur, a severe neurological deficit may develop, and the patient might ultimately die. The aim of surgery is thus to restore normal structural integrity in a way that protects the critical structures of the cervicomedullary junction (CMJ). Because this region contains vital anatomical contents, even minor procedural mistakes or carelessness in management can result in high morbidity and mortality. Attention has to be paid from the very beginning to the patient's position. The surgeon who performs the operation often has to position the patient in rigid skeletal fixation and carefully adjust alignment. Radiographic control is mandatory. For example, in cases of occipitoatlantal or atlantoaxial shifts resulting in an anterior deformity, the spinal canal opens when the patient has been brought into extension. Conversely, if the head is fixed in flexion, the spinal canal will be narrowed and the CMJ compressed. If the head position remains misaligned during surgical decompression, fusion and instrumentation may be difficult and insufficient.

The safest and easiest way to reach the pathology should be chosen, and all available technology should be used.

K. Turel, E. M. Kasper (eds.), *Complications in Neurosurgery II*, Acta Neurochirurgica Supplement 133,
https://doi.org/10.1007/978-3-031-61601-3_18

Surgery should be performed with neuromonitoring, navigation, and real-time radiographic control (e.g., O-arm) as indicated [1–8].

Sufficient experience, correct planning, and choosing the most appropriate approach are necessary for surgical success. Most of the complications are due to a lack of expertise, incomplete surgical approaches, or overtreatment. While unnecessary surgery increases the risk of complications, incomplete surgery eliminates the chance of success.

Congenital Anomalies

Congenital pathologies of the occipital bone can be due to developmental anomalies (e.g., hypoplasia or agenesis) or segmentation disorders. Developmental anomalies include hypoplastic disorders of the occipital area, basioccipital hypoplasia, and occipital condyle hypoplasia. Basioccipital hypoplasia is the formation defect of four occipital sclerotomes. It results in a hypoplastic or short clivus and/or basilar invagination. This anomaly is best measured with the Chamberlain line. Occipital condyle hypoplasia results in a short and flat condyle, leading to limited movement and basilar invagination. Although the deformity is mostly bilateral, it can be seen unilaterally.

Segmentation Anomalies

Atlas Assimilation Segmentation disorders are the most caudal elements of the skull base and C1 can lead to atlanto-occipital assimilation. In this scenario, the atlas adheres to the skull base at the level of the foramen magnum. Adhesion may be complete or partial and often occurs with basilar invagination. Restrictions to the range of motion between C0 andC1 can lead to instability at C1-C2. Of those patients with such atlantooccipital assimilation, 50% develop C1-C2 instability and myelopathy, which usually occurs around the third decade of life.

Congenital Anomalies of the Atlas Except for atlantooccipital assimilation, atlas anomalies do not compromise the anatomical relations of the occipitocervical region and do not result in basilar invagination.

Congenital Anomalies of the Axis Most congenital anomalies of the axis are dens related and lead to basilar invagination. However, they can also cause atlantoaxial instability. Atlas anomalies are occasionally mistaken as fractures. Axis ossification centers allow us to understand the pathogenesis of these anomalies: The axis has three ossification centers, of which two are columnar centers that ossify, prenatally forming the dens body, and the last one is located in the tip of the dens (apex).

Os Odontoideum (Persistent Ossiculum Terminale or Bergman Ossicle) This characteristic radiographical feature occurs as a result of the nonunion of the terminal ossification center of the odontoid and the remaining part of the dens. It may be confused with a high-riding type I odontoid fracture. However, it has little clinical significance. The dentocentral synchondrosis normally fuses at about the age of 6 years. Os odontoideum hence develops as a result of the fusion failure of the dental synchondrosis line. Although os odontoideum is often radiologically confused with an odontoid fracture, the thick and round upper cortex of C2 and the round anterior arch of C1 allow us to distinguish these two entities. Os odontoideum may cause atlantoaxial instability. This condition is frequently seen in individuals with Down syndrome, spondylo-epiphyseal dysplasia, Morquio syndrome, and some other congenital connective tissue diseases. The total aplasia of the odontoid is very rare. Os odontoideum, which is seen clearly above the arch of the atlas on an anterior to posterior (AP) open-mouth radiograph, is rarely confused with odontoid aplasia [9–13] (Fig. 1).

Atlantoaxial Facet Joint Anomalies This category is divided into type I and type II.

Type I: Here, the atlas facets slide on the axis, and spondylolisthesis develops because of sagittal malalignment. In this type of basilar invagination, the odontoid migrates upward and backward and compresses the brainstem. Neurological deficits may develop. It is mostly seen in young patients with acute and severe clinical symptoms. By pulling the odontoid with traction or by using distraction with an inter-facet spacer, normal alignment can be re-established, and stabilization is accomplished via C1-C2 fixation (Fig. 2).

Type II: Type II is defined by central facet dislocation. Over time, changes in bone and soft tissue result in instability. The odontoid is pushed toward the clivus together with the atlas at the level of the foramen magnum. Over time, the atlas assimilates into the occiput and the bones fuse. Consequently, the atlas disappears, almost becoming an extension of the occiput. In Type II invagination, the atlantodental interval (ADI) remains normal. Chiari malformation and syringomyelia may develop secondarily. Traction and intra-facet maneuvers may be insufficient to restore alignment in Type II abnormalities. Anterior decompression and posterior occipitocervical fusion and instrumentation may be required [14–19] (Fig. 3).

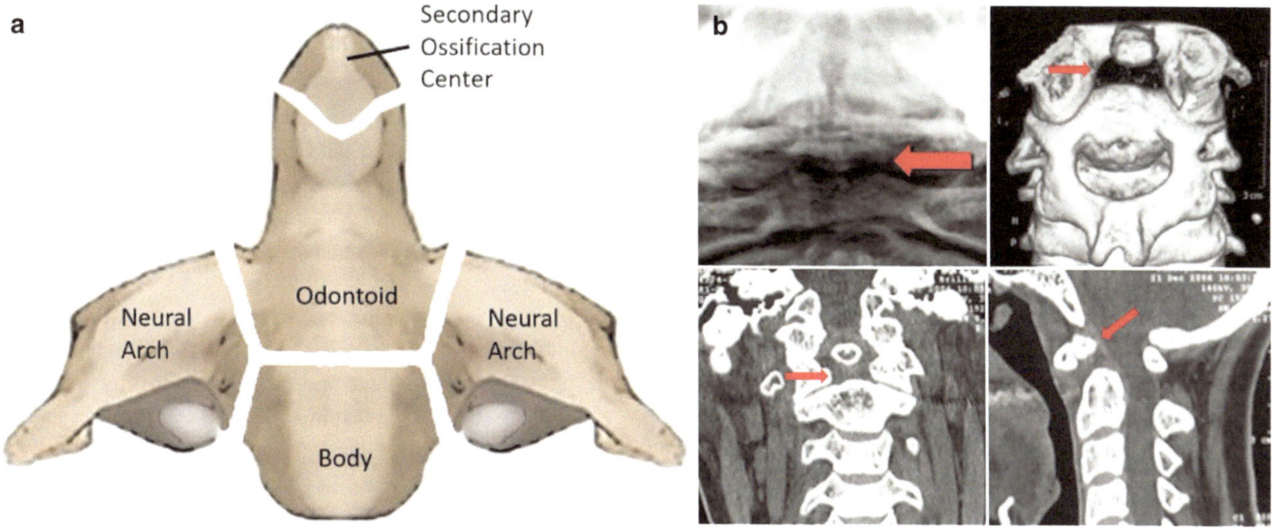

Fig. 1 (**a**) Ossification centers in the odontoid, (**b**) os odontoideum. The latter is a congenital anomaly, often confused with odontoid fractures as the most important cause of atlantoaxial instability

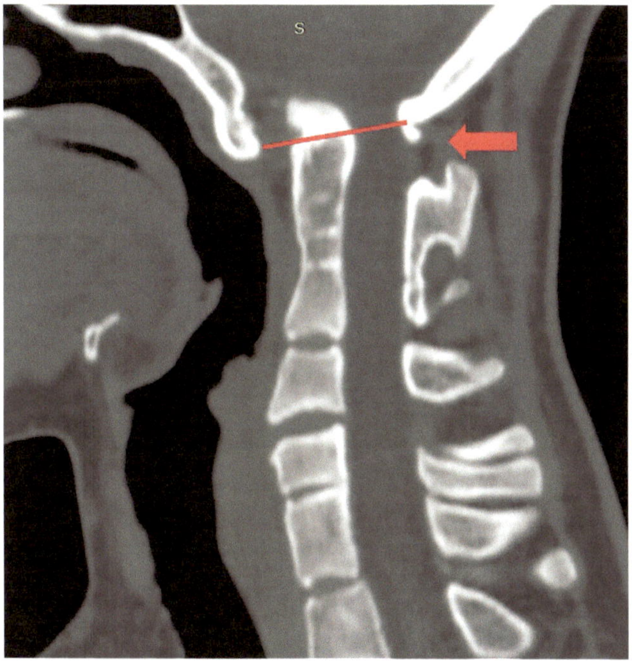

Fig. 2 Goel type I basilar invagination with atlas assimilation

If we look at the treatment complications that occur in patients with congenital anomalies, the most common one is related to atlas assimilation.

Case Study A 57-year-old female patient presented with complaints of an inability to use both her hands, numbness, gait instability, and difficulty walking (Fig. 4). The patient underwent decompressive surgery for spinal cord compro-

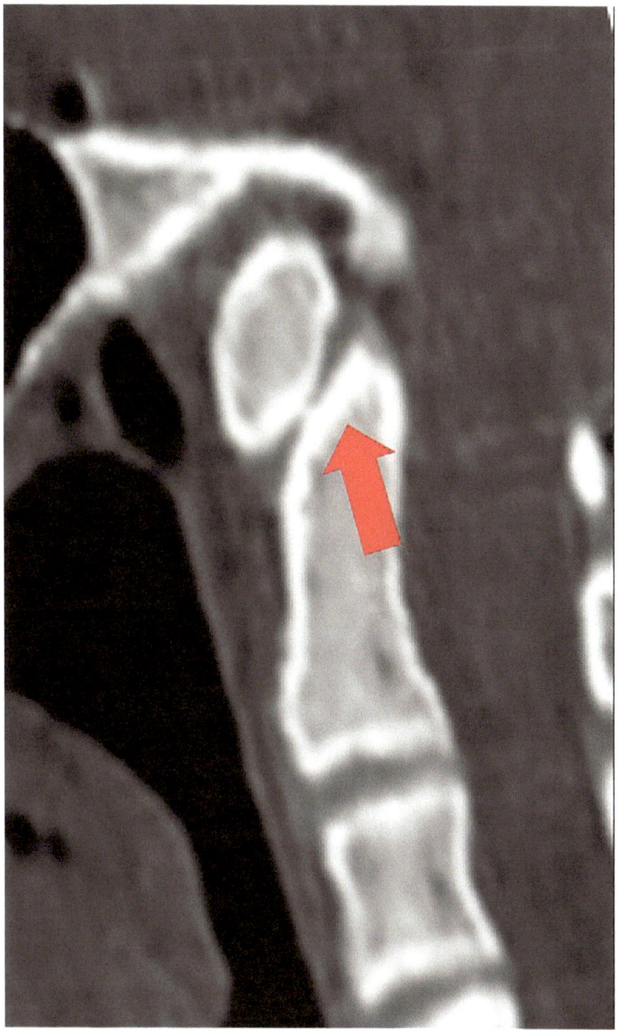

Fig. 3 Goel type II basilar invagination. The odontoid pushes on the clivus, and both compromise the neurocranium at the level of the foramen magnum

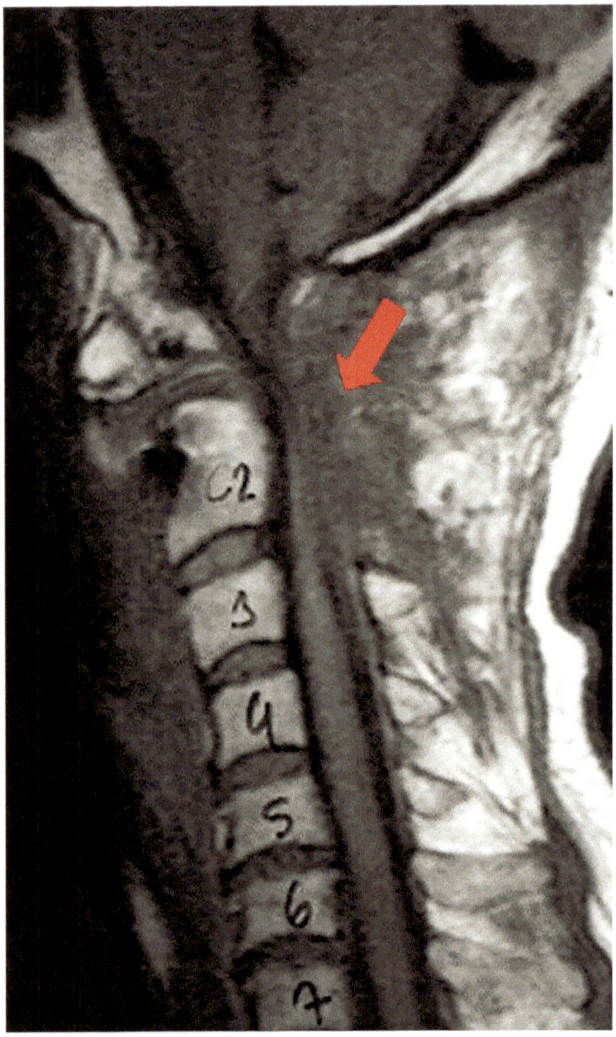

Fig. 4 Spinal cord compression caused by anterior shift (translational instability) due to os odontoideum. This scenario was further destabilized by a C1-C2 laminectomy, which led to the formation of fibrous tissue and the development of the postlaminectomy membrane

mise at C1, but the patient became worse after the operation and then could not walk at all. She was bedridden and largely unable to move her hands or arms. According to the post-OP magnetic resonance imaging (MRI), the patient had an os odontoideum. What had happened? The unnoticed os caused spinal cord compression since the C1 vertebra and the os odontoideum shifted forward during surgery, and the posterior arch of the atlas compressed the spinal cord. The removal of the C1 and C2 laminae caused increased instability. The already-unstable C1-C2 joint showed an increase in mobility with the destruction of the posterior tension band, and a reactive membrane formed at the laminectomy site. There was excess connective tissue production to keep the alignment tight, resulting in compression. Unfortunately, this patient did not accept any revision surgery.

The right intervention here would have been to stabilize the C1-C2 junction with the Goel-Harms or Magerl methods or at least by placing graft material between C1-C2. Since this stabilization includes retracting C1, already effectively widening the canal, further laminectomy may not have been necessary.

Another complication occurring in the setting of an os odontoideum is related to the stabilization technique. A 40-year-old male patient presented to a hospital with complaints of weakness and numbness in his arms and legs for about 3 months. On examinations, he was diagnosed with atlantoaxial dislocation due to the fracture of the dens, and stabilization surgery was recommended. The patient underwent surgery, where the C1-C2 spinous processes were tied with wires. The C1-C2 posterior laminae were fused by placing an interposition bone graft between them. At the time of a follow-up examination 1 year later, the wires were loose, and revision surgery was recommended. While stabilizing C1 and C2 according to Magerl's technique, fusion was performed by placing a new bone graft between the laminae. At postoperative controls, C1-C2 had fused well, and there were no problems at the 10-year follow-up (Fig. 5).

No real mistake was made during the primary surgery in this case, but stabilization with wires only is known to be biomechanically weak. Goel-Harms or Magerl techniques of rigid occipitocervical fixation should be preferred in such cases [3, 20, 21].

Another case represents the overtreatment of an os odontoideum. This patient was a 32-year-old man with complaints of numbness, clumsiness in both hands, and balance problems, which had been increasing over 6 months. On clinical assessment, mild quadriparesis was found. Radiographic examination showed atlantoaxial dislocation, possibly due to dens fracture, and myelomalacia was detected in the spinal cord. Surgery was performed elsewhere. Occipitocervical stabilization was performed. The patient's neurological status improved considerably, but he stated that his quality of life deteriorated because he could no longer move his head properly (Fig. 6).

In this case, the occiput was unnecessarily included in the fusion surgery, resulting in a loss of all head movement. The original pathology was at the C2 level, and as a result, only the C1-C2 relationship had been impaired. Fixating the C1-C2 by using the Goel-Harms or Magerl transarticular technique would have been an adequate surgical method. In addition, extended surgery carried a higher risk, including potential pseudoarthrosis and the risk of infection since surgery was prolonged. Most importantly, though, an unnecessary loss of range of motion was inflicted on the patient.

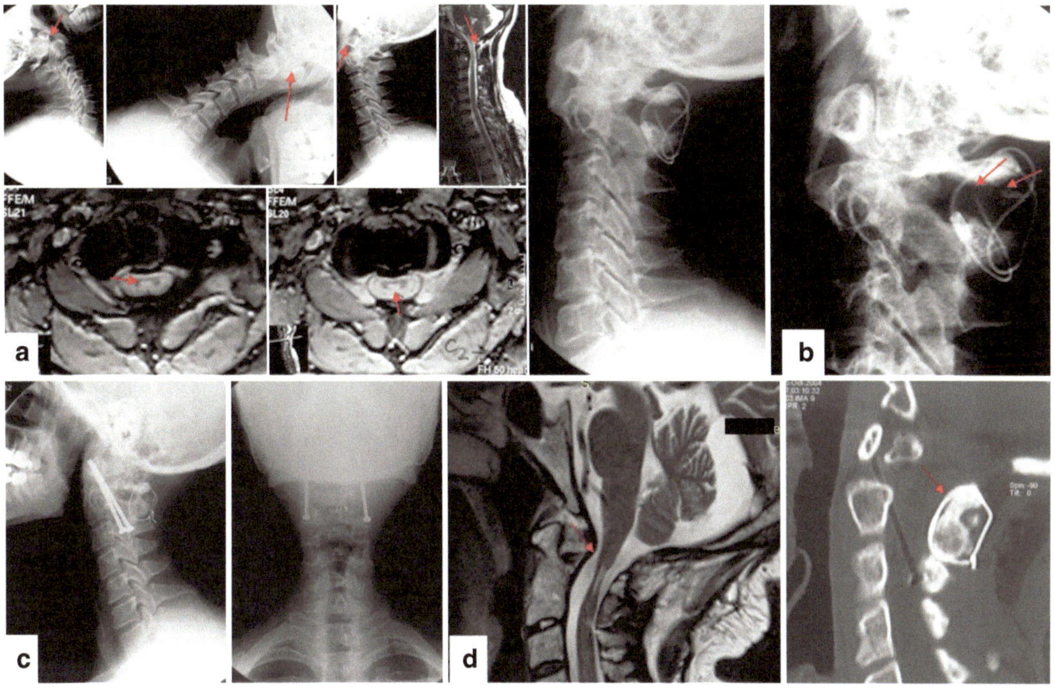

Fig. 5 (**a**) Patient with atlantoaxial dislocation due to the os odontoideum. Signal changes indicate myelomalacia of the spinal cord due to chronic compression. This patient underwent stabilization with C1-C2 wires. (**b**) The wire construct at C1-C2 failed over time as seen in the control radiographs performed after 14 months. Comparison of XR obtained immediately after the first surgery to X-rays displaying the findings after 14 months, (**c**) status after C1-C2 stabilization (Magerl) and bone graft placement, (**d**) posterior fusion is observed at 4 years. The old myelomalacia of the spinal cord remains visible with the canal effectively enlarged

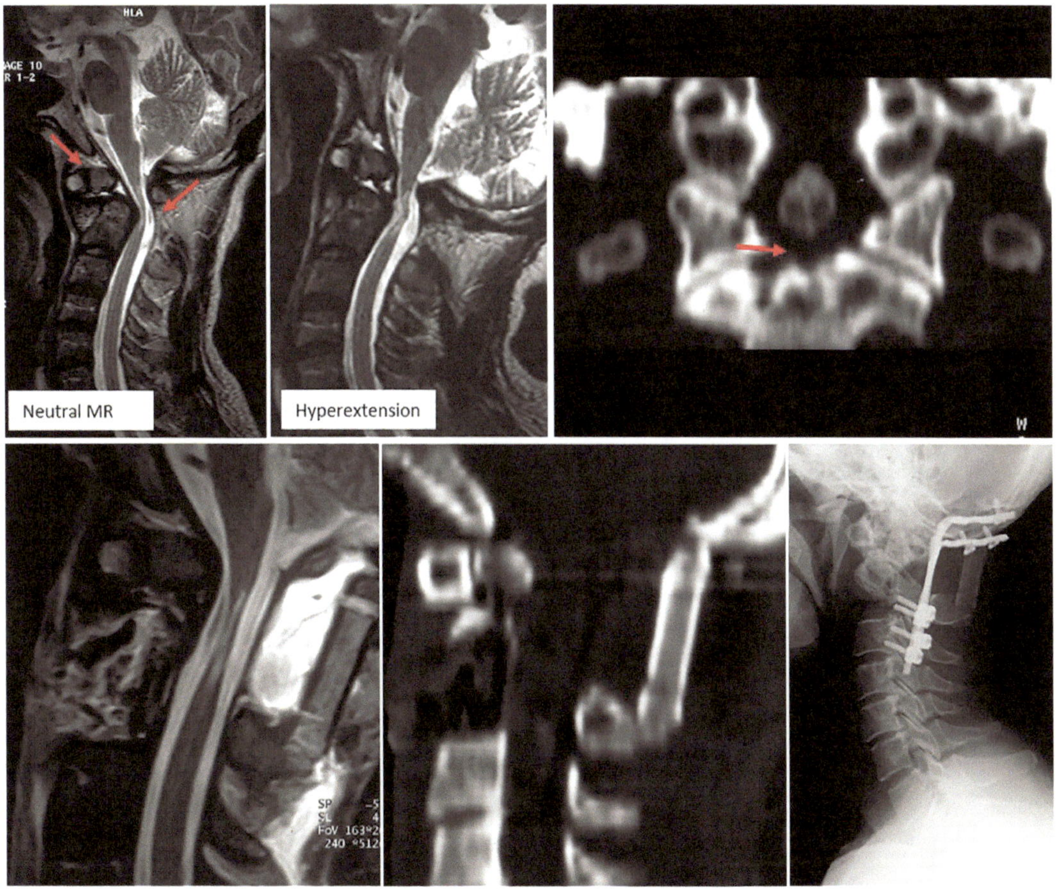

Fig. 6 In this patient, C1 was anteriorly dislocated over C2 due to Os Odontoideum fracture. The resulting problem is C1-C2 instability which requires fixation. In this case, the occiput was used to place bone graft and occiput-C3 fixation was performed. The odontoid was removed transorally and effective expansion of the spinal canal was achieved

Another Case Study A 35-year-old female patient presented with imbalance, dizziness, and dysphagia for 6 months. Chiari malformation with impaired CSF circulation and mild hydrocephalus were detected during the MRI examination (Fig. 7). C1 laminectomy and suboccipital craniectomy were performed with duraplasty to re-establish normal CSF flow. However, the patient became worse after surgery, to the point of impaired consciousness. Emergency computed tomography (CT) and MRI revealed obstructive hydrocephalus, including an enlarged fourth ventricle, due to the further descensus of the tonsils blocking CSF passage. An urgent ventriculoperitoneal shunt was placed. The patient recovered slowly, and she was discharged 3 weeks later.

An important error in management occurred here: The mistake was to not evaluate the patient well preoperatively. First, hydrocephalus could have been treated with a ventriculoperitoneal shunt from the beginning. Then, while decompressing the craniocervical junction (CCJ), too much bone was removed, which resulted in the sagging of the posterior fossa contents, leading to complete obstruction. Performing too wide a craniectomy is a technical mistake.

This complication teaches us another important lesson: Surgeons have to make sure that the CSF passage is open. In our institution, after opening arachnoid adhesions around the cerebellar tonsils, we routinely place silicone tubes bilaterally to ensure CSF flow from the cerebellar cisterns to the cervical subarachnoid space. This technique can also be used for other clinical pathologies, such as traumatic syringomyelia [22].

Finally, we have another case study of a CCJ complication occurring in a patient with a congenital anomaly: The patient, a 33-year-old man, presented to us with complaints

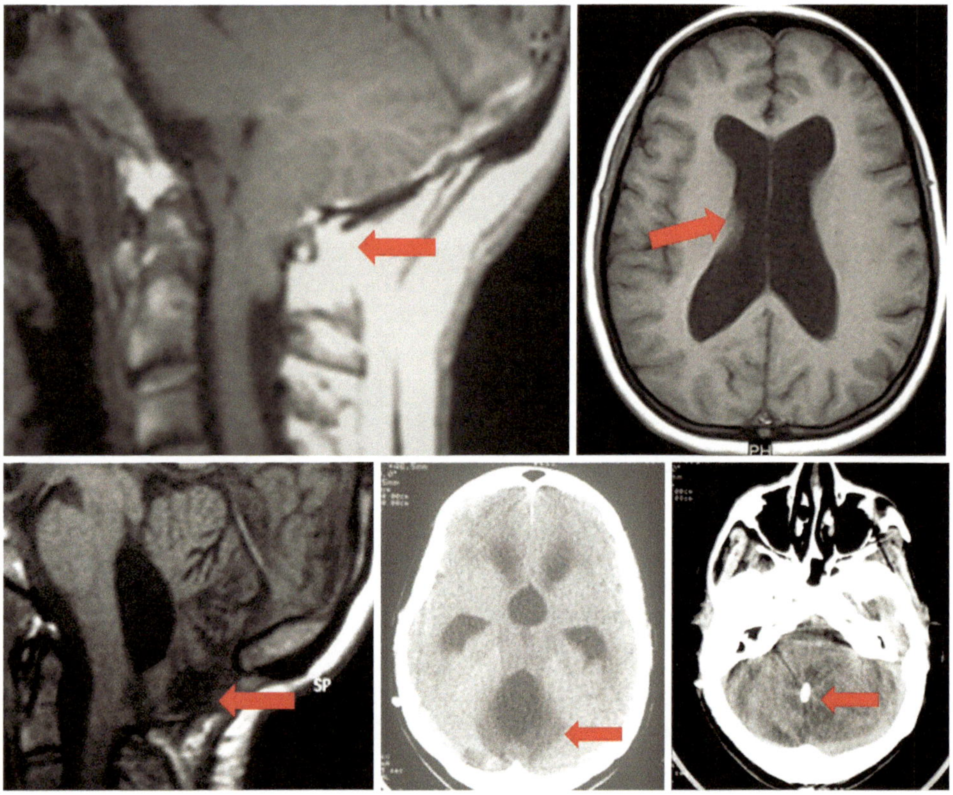

Fig. 7 A 30-year-old female had problems with imbalance, dizziness, and dysphagia for the last 6 months. Chiari malformation and mild hydrocephalus were detected in the MRI examination. Due to extensive suboccipital craniectomy, the cerebellar tonsils drooped and completely blocked the passage of CSF in the foramen magnum. The patient developed acute hydrocephalus and the enlargement of the ventricle was remarkable due to the discharge of CSF trapped in the fourth ventricle. The patient entered the herniation process. She was treated with emergency VP and fourth ventricle shunts

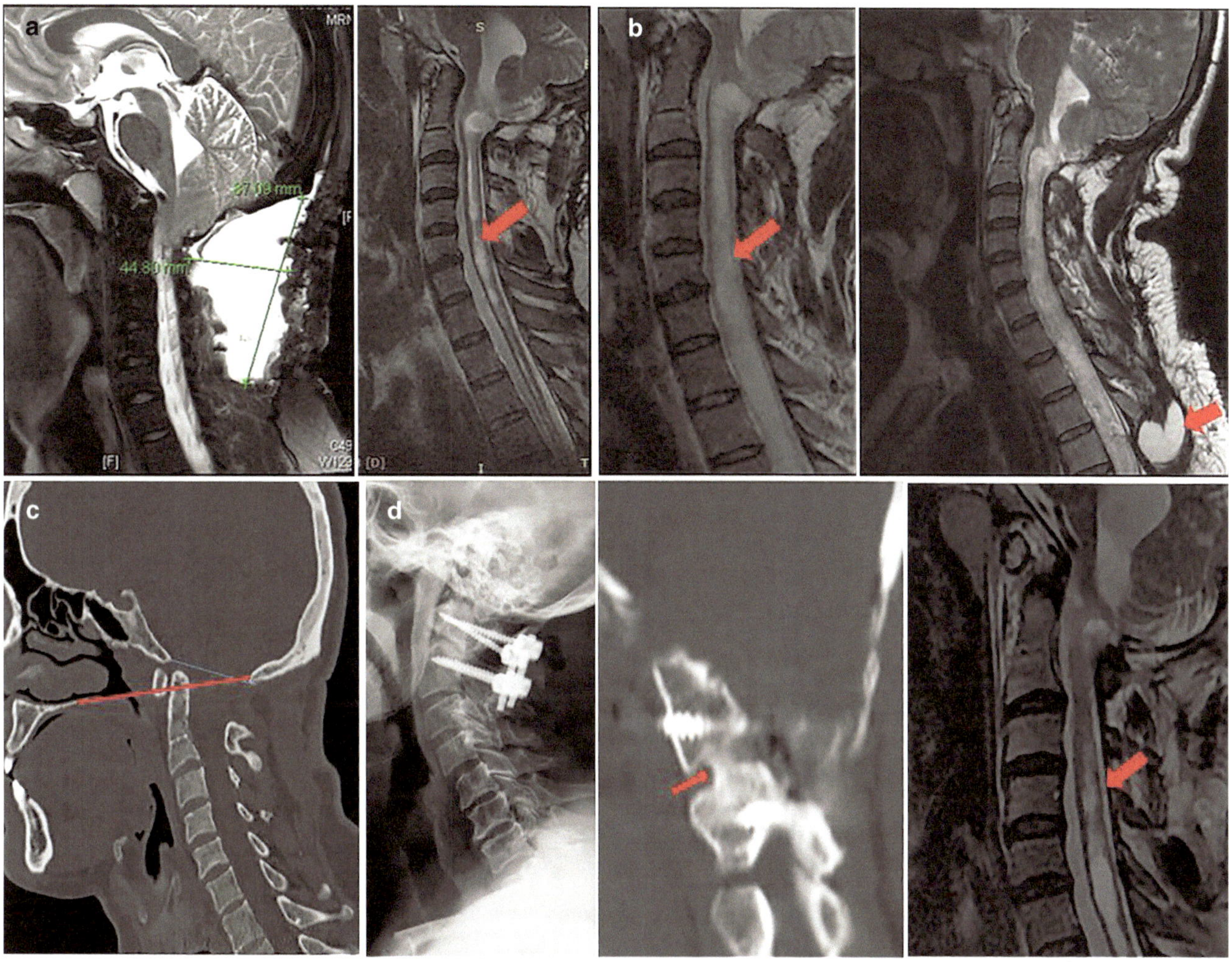

Fig. 8 The patient, who was diagnosed with syringomyelia and Chiari malformation in 2012, underwent posterior decompression surgery in 2013. Suboccipital craniectomy and duraplasty were performed. Pseudomeningocele developed in the early period, but it resolved spontaneously. The patient's syringomyelia improved after the operation. In the MRI examination performed in 2016, the syringomyelia, which had initially disappeared in the early period, recurred. (**a**) Shows the pseudomeningocele that had transiently formed postoperatively. (**b**) Shows the recurrent syringomyelia that had formed in a delayed fashion after initial improvement as seen in the panel to the left of the top row. (**c**) After reevaluation, it was determined that the patient had Goel type 1 basilar invagination. The condition was stabilized with screw and rod system. C1-C2 facet joint was distracted with small bone grafts in both sides. The canal was widened by performing duraplasty in craniovertebral junction. (**d**) In the last control of the patient in 2020, the syringomyelia had recovered, the subarachnoid space was opened, and the patient had recovered neurologically, and he was able to do his daily work independently

of weakness in his hands and feet, difficulty walking, and feeling unsteady when standing for the last 3 months (Fig. 8). The patient displayed clinically mild quadriparesis and radiographically extensive syringomyelia from the upper cervical to the thoracic spinal cord. In this case, suboccipital craniectomy, C1 laminectomy, and duraplasty were performed. Three years later, the syringomyelia had reformed, and a syringopleural shunt was performed, leading to the resolution of his symptoms. Repeat MRI after an interval revealed that the syrinx had recurred. However, when all imaging was reviewed carefully, type I basilar invagination was noted. A third operation was undertaken to pull the odontoid away from the foramen magnum. It was planned to revise the duraplasty and to put a bone graft between C1 and C2. Following this, C1 and C2 were stabilized with screws. This strategy succeeded, where the syrinx nearly resolved after the operation. No high-pressure fluid collection formed. The patient gradually returned to normal neurological status, and MR has remained stable since surgery.

An error in judgment was made here by initially overlooking the basilar invagination, which led us to treat the patient inadequately (assuming a simple Chiari malformation). The syringomyelia could have been corrected with suboccipital decompression alone in simple cases, but the added complexity of an odontoid in the foramen magnum from the basilar invagination made this a complex scenario preventing the passage of normal CSF flow.

Lastly, we mention the anatomical variant of a high-riding vertebral artery, which is an important pathology in this region. In fact, it can be encountered in healthy people and can be found

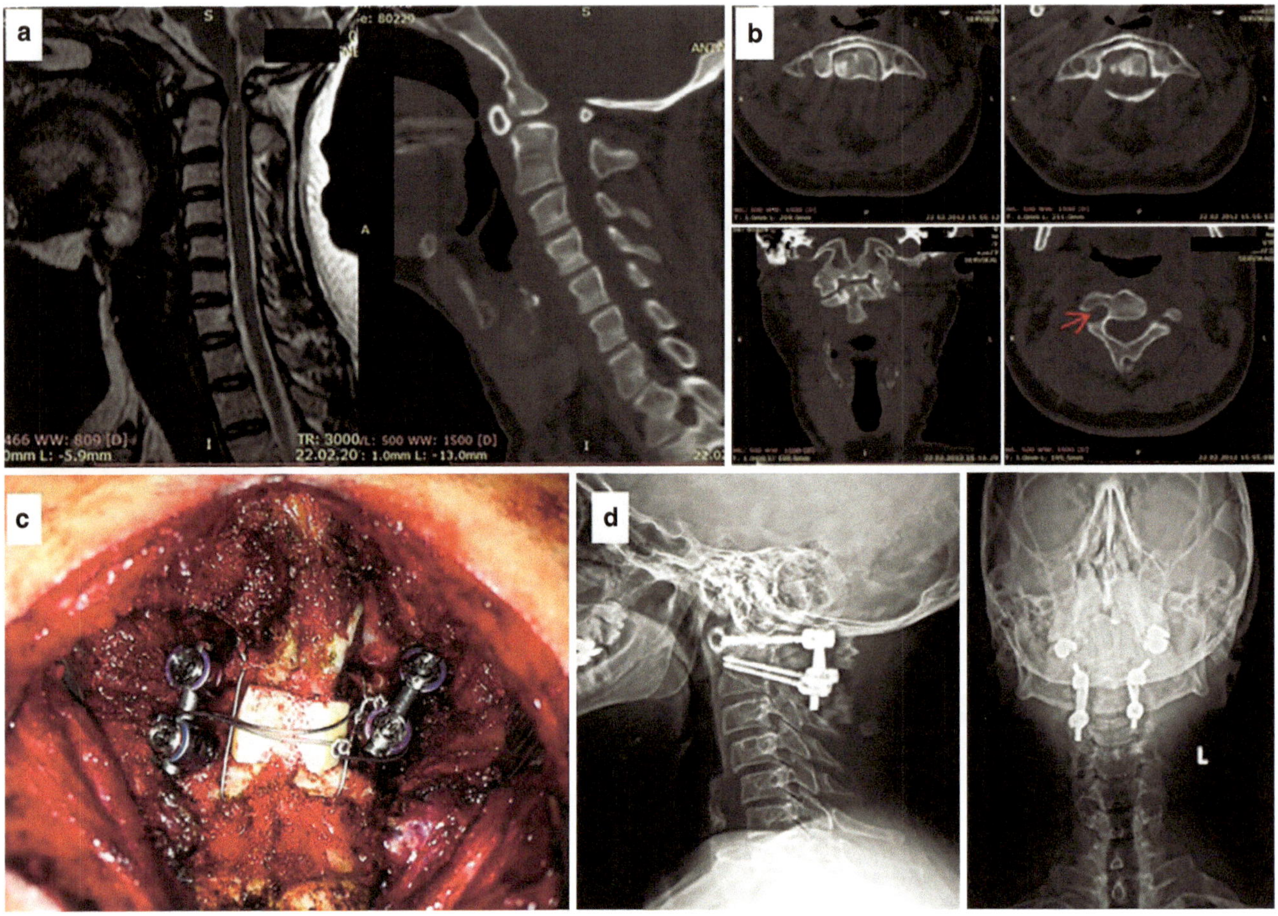

Fig. 9 (**a**) Atlantoaxial instability due to os odontoideum as seen on T2 MR images and CT with myelomalacia on MR and narrowing in the canal on CT. (**b**) On the right, it is seen that the highly located vertebral artery enters the C2 corpus (high riding vertebral artery). (**c**) The bone graft placed during the surgery. (**d**) C1-C2 stabilization was performed using the Goel-Harms technique with navigation

in the treatment of other pathologies, such as trauma and tumors. It should come to light in presurgical imaging examinations.

The patient, a 25-year-old male worker, felt tired and weak while working. The patient displayed neurologically mild quadriparesis, and he was also diagnosed with atlas assimilation and C1-C2 dislocation at the time of the preliminary examinations. The right vertebral artery was noted as having taken a variant medial course (high-riding vertebral artery) on CT angiogram (Fig. 9). Navigation and an O-arm were used during surgery. Screws were placed using the Goel-Harms technique. During screw placement at C2, the trajectory aimed at the isthmus of C2 by assessing the course of the vertebral artery and using navigation. Navigation and an O-arm are recommended in such cases to prevent injury to the high-riding vertebral artery.

Conclusion

Surgery in the occipitocervical region requires particular diligence to preserve vital nerve tissue. Carefully examining each patient is necessary to identify and apply the appropriate treatment. A surgical procedure should be pursued only after a complete examination and after a comprehensive assessment of radiological studies, to prevent complications. The treatment of these regional pathologies should be carried out with sufficient technology and expertise.

Part 2: Acquired Pathologies

In this article, we discuss the surgical management of craniocervical pathologies caused by acquired disorders, traumas, tumors, and infections and give case studies of complications. This group of patients constitutes the major group of craniocervical region pathologies that require special treatment.

Acquired Disorders

Paget's disease, osteomalacia, rickets, osteogenesis imperfecta, rheumatoid arthritis, and neurofibromatosis are frequently seen among the acquired diseases that soften and disrupt the bone and soft tissue structures at the skull base.

The upward migration of the odontoid as a result of the softening of the skull base results in basilar impression.

Diseases that disrupt the ligamentous structure of the occipitocervical region, such as rheumatoid arthritis, can also cause the upward migration of the dens, called cranial settling. Rheumatoid arthritis and psoriatic arthritis are chronic, systemic inflammatory diseases that disrupt the synovial layer, leading first to synovitis and subsequently to the destruction of the articular cartilage and postinflammatory ankylosis. In rheumatoid arthritis, inflammatory pannus formation is seen in the synovial joints. Supporting ligamentous structures are also damaged as a result of cytokine release. Psoriatic arthritis is observed in 1–2% of patients with psoriasis, and it disrupts the synovial joints via the same mechanism. In these diseases, both the occipitocervical region and the subaxial cervical spine are affected, and damage to the ligaments results in atlantoaxial instability. The atlantodental interval (ADI) is a very important measure for assessing this pathology. With the progression of the disease, erosions of the occipital condyles, C1 lateral masses, and C2 facets are observed. This erosion causes the head to further misalign, causing CCJ obstruction with myelopathy and even increased intracranial pressure and other neurological deficits. In patients with advanced rheumatoid arthritis (RA), the dens impales the neurocranial space even higher as vertical subluxation increases, leading to compression on the brain stem and vertebrobasilar system, which can lead to sudden death. Once patients present with an ADI > 10 mm, complete neurological recovery is unlikely even after surgery [22–25].

Case Study Rheumatoid Arthritis A patient presented to our hospital complaining of difficulty walking, gait instability, and numbness in his hands and feet for about 20 years. MRI showed no significant compression on the brain stem, but the dens was completely transformed into an inflammatory pannus, and atlantoaxial instability was demonstrated. Neurologically, the patient displayed mild quadriparesis. No remaining osseus odontoid was seen on CT. Occipitocervical fusion was indicated and performed with a horseshoe plate connecting the occipital bone to the cervical lateral mass. However, at radiographic follow-up 1 year later, the screws had loosened and pulled out. At revision surgery, a different horseshoe construct design was used, one that added wires to the vertebral laminae. No problems were detected in subsequent control studies. The technical mistake in the first operation was that the lateral mass screws that were used turned out to be too short. Importantly, the inflamed bone quality is often not good in patients with rheumatoid arthritis. A diligently employed

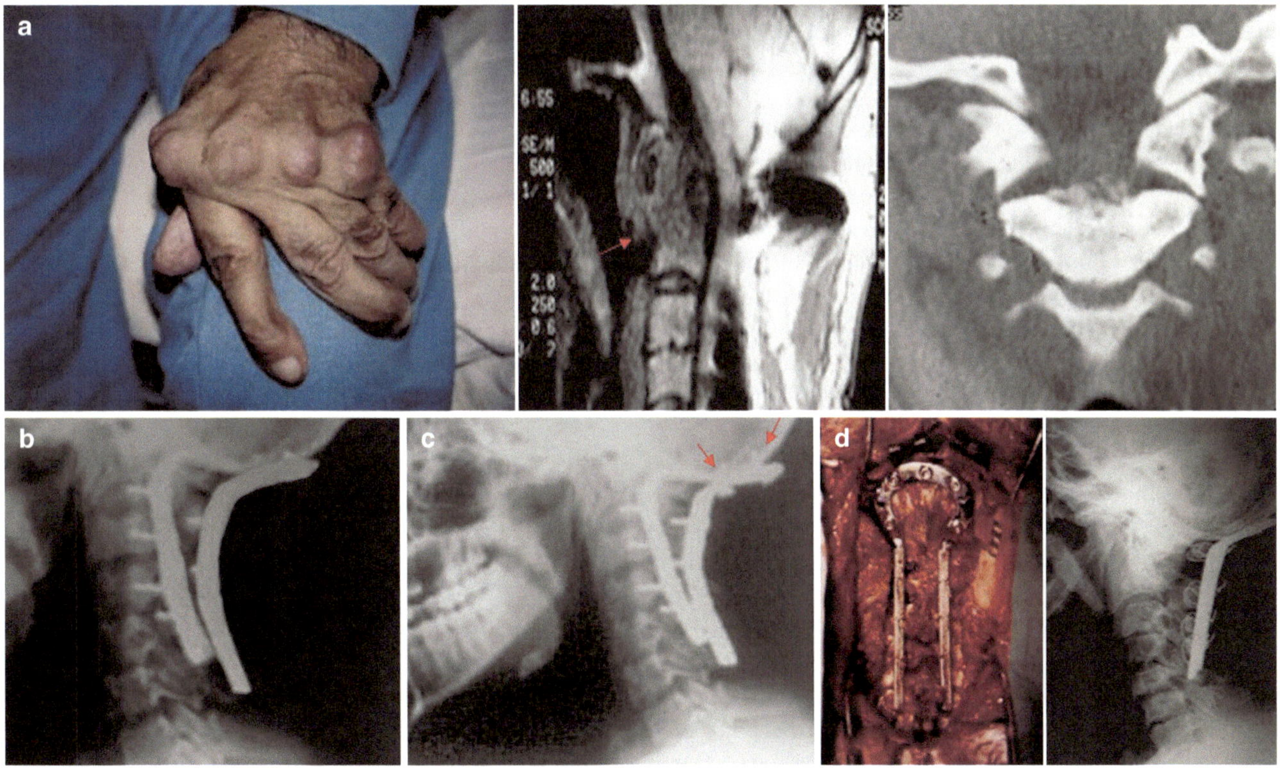

Fig. 10 A patient with rheumatoid arthritis who was treated 20 years ago: (**a**) C2 pannus formed, and spinal cord compression formed; he also had C1-C2 instability. (**b**) The patient underwent occipitocervical stabilization surgery. (**c**) The screws were removed after 1 year. (**d**) The patient was taken to surgical intervention again; occipitocervical stabilization was achieved by attaching the occipital bone with screws and more tightly connecting it to the cervical region with wires

sublaminar wiring technique may be more advantageous in such cases than screws alone (Fig. 10).

Trauma

Cervical spine injury has been observed in as many as 2.4% of blunt trauma patients, and 34% of these injuries occur in the occipitocervical region. Any ADI > 5 mm in an adult patient should be considered as pathological indicative of atlantoaxial instability. A highly sensitive measurement to determine atlantooccipital compromise is the "Harris rule of 12" method. In this assessment technique, the basion–dens measure (BDM) and the basion–axis measure (BAM) are carefully measured (see Appendix). According to Harris and colleagues, 95% have a BDM and 98% a BAM value that does not exceed 12 mm in adults. Any such interval >12 mm is considered abnormal and indicates instability deserving stabilization.

Occipital Condyle Fracture This is a rare injury type and was first described in victims who died after trauma. These fractures are classified according to the degree of damage to the ligaments or bone. Fractures with large bone fragments are more stable and have a better chance of healing with conservative treatment. CT with parasagittal and coronal reconstructions is useful in identifying occipital condyle fractures.

Atlas Traumas Jefferson was the first to describe a characteristic burst fracture of C1 after axial load injuries. Stability in this setting can be determined through open-mouth dens X-rays. According to Spence and colleagues, a simple rule applies in this setting: If the lateral displacement of both lateral masses of C1 are (combined) more than 7 mm apart above the matching joint surfaces of C2, the fracture is considered unstable because of transverse ligament damage, and surgical stabilization is required.

Axis Traumas After blunt trauma, C2 fractures occur in as many as 24% of cervical fractures, and among these, one-third show an odontoid fracture. The location, separation, and angulation of the fracture elements are important prognostic factors for healing and for treatment algorithms. The displacement of the fractured dens segment is measured from the anterior margin of the fractured part to the anterior break-off point at the C2 base. The D'Alanso classification into three dens fracture types remains popular today. Type I is an apical fracture, type II is a dens fracture at or above odontoid base, and type III is a C2 corpus fracture. In type IIA, additional corpus fragments are found at the base of the odontoid. Many displaced type II and IIA injuries require surgical intervention.

Traumatic Spondylolisthesis of the Axis The management of this classic injury type (Hangman's fracture, which was first described in executed death-row prisoners). It was well described by Levine and Edwards in 1985 (*Levine AM, Edwards CC. The management of traumatic spondylolisthesis of the axis. (1985) The Journal of bone and joint surgery. American volume. 67 (2): 217–26*). The alignment to the adjacent level bones is disrupted by pars interarticularis fractures. Some of these fractures are unstable and require surgery, whereas others can recover with conservative treatment [26–28].

Clinical Study of C2 Traumatic Spondylolisthesis A 32-year-old female patient sustained a traffic accident, after which she complained of severe and constant neck pain. Her neurological status was normal, but on radiographic examination, she was found to have an unstable type II C2 fracture, which was stabilized at C1-C2 with the Goel-Harms technique. One month later, another ligamentous disruption was identified at the C3-C4 level. The patient was taken back to surgery, and her lateral mass screws were extended to C5 (Fig. 11).

This case teaches us an important lesson: If a very prominent major pathology (C2 fracture) is present in the first trauma assessment, it may cause us to overlook other injuries. For this reason, all initial radiographic trauma studies should be carefully reviewed again without time pressure, and the possibility of multitrauma should be kept in mind.

Another case was seen in a young university student, who also had a traffic accident and experienced severe neck pain, for which she was taken to a local hospital. The patient was neurologically intact but was diagnosed with a minimally displaced type II odontoid fracture. Conservative treatment was recommended. A halo brace was fitted, and the patient was discharged with instructions for follow-up (Fig. 12). After an unremarkable initial period, the patient was admitted 8 months later to our department with neck pain and a noticeable limitation in her neck movements. Radiological examinations revealed that the dens fragment was anteriorly displaced, with the atlas and half of the odontoid fused with the vertebral body of C2. Over time, the fracture had healed in misalignment. However, a different problem was caused by the slip since the distance between the occiput and the

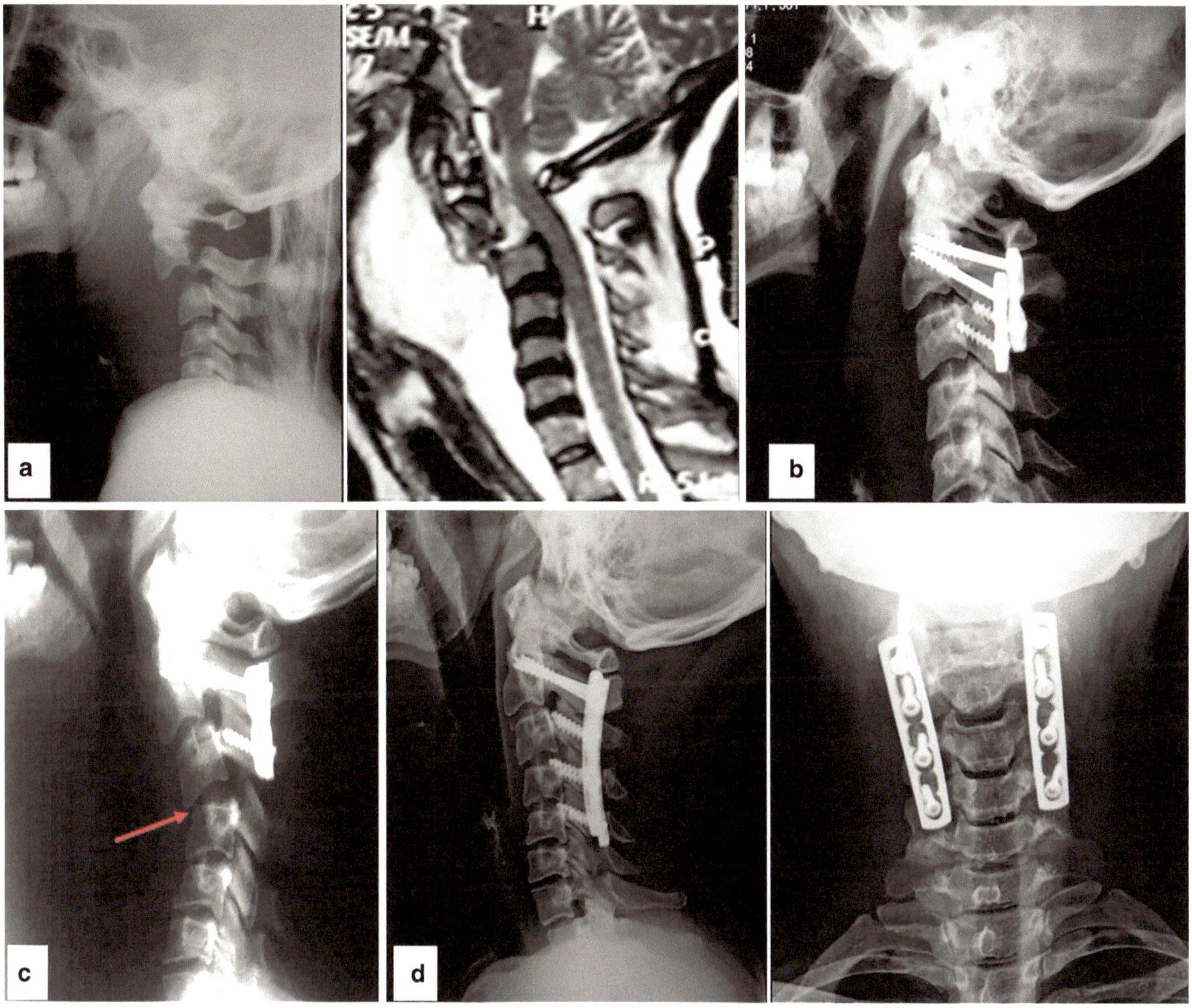

Fig. 11 The patient was a 32-year-old woman who had a traffic accident. She had severe and constant neck pain after the accident. It was evaluated as neurologically normal. (**a**) She had an unstable Levine–Edwards type IIII fracture on her radiological examinations, (**b**) we stabilized C1-C2 with the Goel-Harms technique, and the patient was discharged happily. (**c**) We found that there was a dislocation. (**d**) The patient was reoperated, and lateral mass plates lowered the plate in C2-C3 to C4 and C5

body of C2 had narrowed, causing spinal cord compression. We successfully addressed this by simply performing an occipital craniectomy, and no further intervention was needed for the misaligned odontoid, which had already fused. The lesson to be learned here is that some complications can be corrected by timely intervention. If the patient had represented in the first 6 weeks after the accident and before complete fusion, she still could have had a chance for an anterior approach [29]. A better initial solution could have been the placement of an anterior screw for the odontoid fracture, which should be performed under fluoroscopic alignment. This way, neck movement could have been preserved in this young patient.

Tumors

Occipitocervical region tumors either originate from bone structures or neural or soft tissues in the region or arise from a secondary spread to this region. These lesions are often divided into extradural, intradural-extraaxial, and intradural-intraaxial pathologies. The most common extradural tumors are metastases and chordomas. Other pathologies include primary bone tumors, such as chondromas, chondrosarcomas and osteoblastomas, plasmacytomas, eosinophilic granulomas, giant cell tumors, and aneurysmal bone cysts.

The most frequent intradural-extraaxial tumors in this region are schwannomas and meningiomas. Intradural parenchymal tumors are rare and include ependymomas, gliomas,

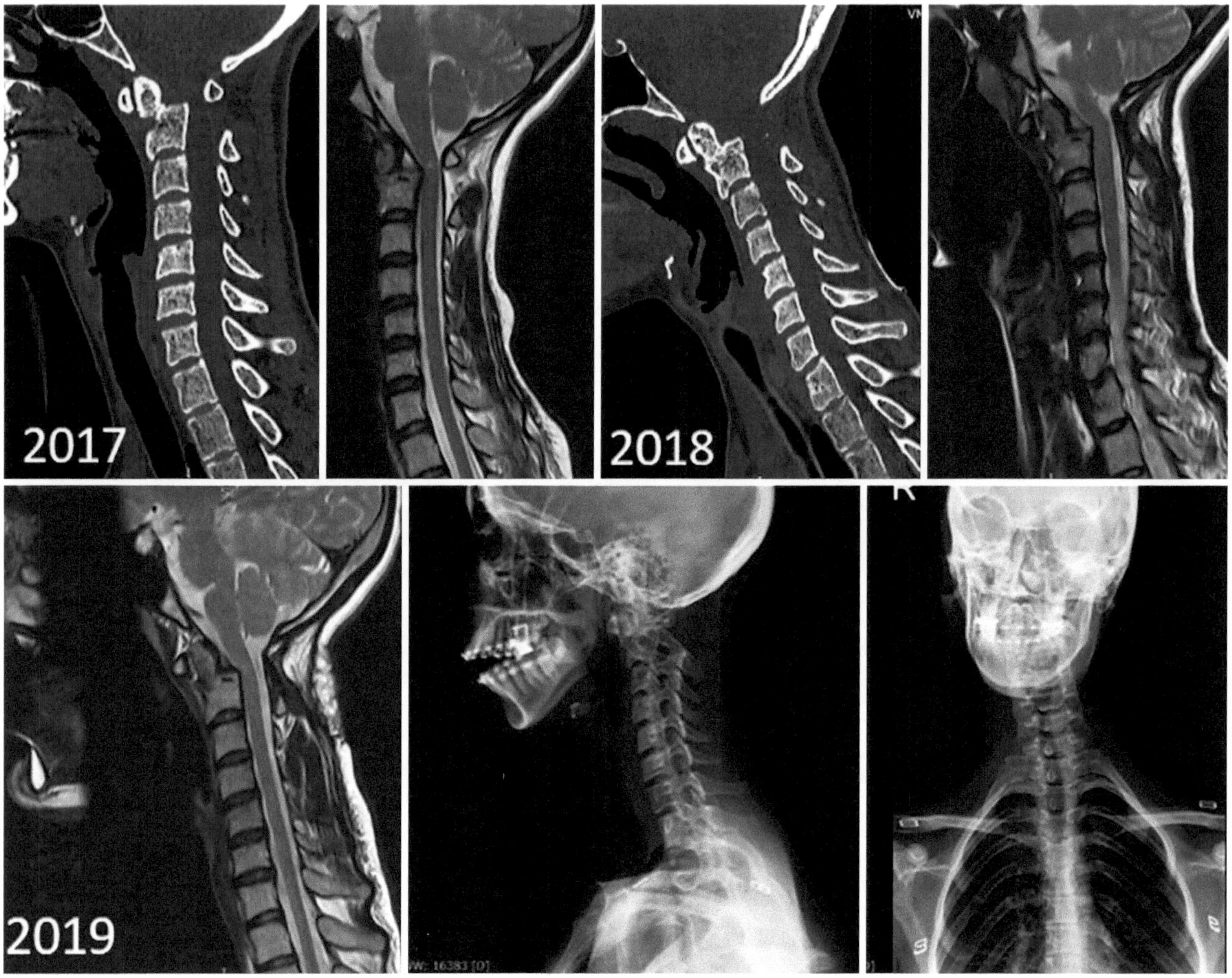

Fig. 12 This patient came after a traffic accident with a Type II fracture that was conservatively treated. At follow-up 1 year later, CT detected that the odontoid fused incorrectly and on MRI, there was narrowing of the foramen magnum. Suboccipital craniectomy was performed, but there was nothing to be done for the impaired odontoid and the cervical deformity

hemangioblastomas, dermoids, epidermoids, Wilms tumors, plexus papillomas, lipomas, metastases, and mixed tumors. Most of the latter originate from glial cells, ependymas, or astrocytes. Tumors originating from the fourth ventricle or the lower part of the cerebellar hemisphere or vermis may also secondarily extend into the occipitocervical region, but their origins exceed the scope of this manuscript [30].

A rare case with an important anatomic variant that was noticed only during surgery is now presented. This patient was a 48-year-old woman who complained of neck pain, early fatigue, and gait instability. On radiological examination, an intradural, extraaxial mass was detected at the level of the foramen magnum, resulting in left-sided compression on the spinal cord (Fig. 13). The working diagnosis was a possible neuroma at the C1-C2 level, and the left vertebral artery that entered through the foramen magnum was pushed over to reside exactly in the midline, which can be an anatomical variant or secondary to the mass effect of the tumor. Identifying this scenario is crucial because the aberrant vertebral artery (VA) in the midline can suffer iatrogenic damage during surgery. In tumor surgery in this region, vascular topography should thus be studied via CT angiography or ordinary angiography.

Infections

Surgical site infection is one of the most feared postoperative complications since it leads to higher morbidity and mortality and, subsequently, increased healthcare costs. It is associated with longer hospital stays and worse patient outcomes. Researched have reported that the incidence of infection in spine surgery is between 0.65% and 12%, depending on the type of surgery and the target population [4, 31, 32]. Numerous studies have attempted to identify the risk factors

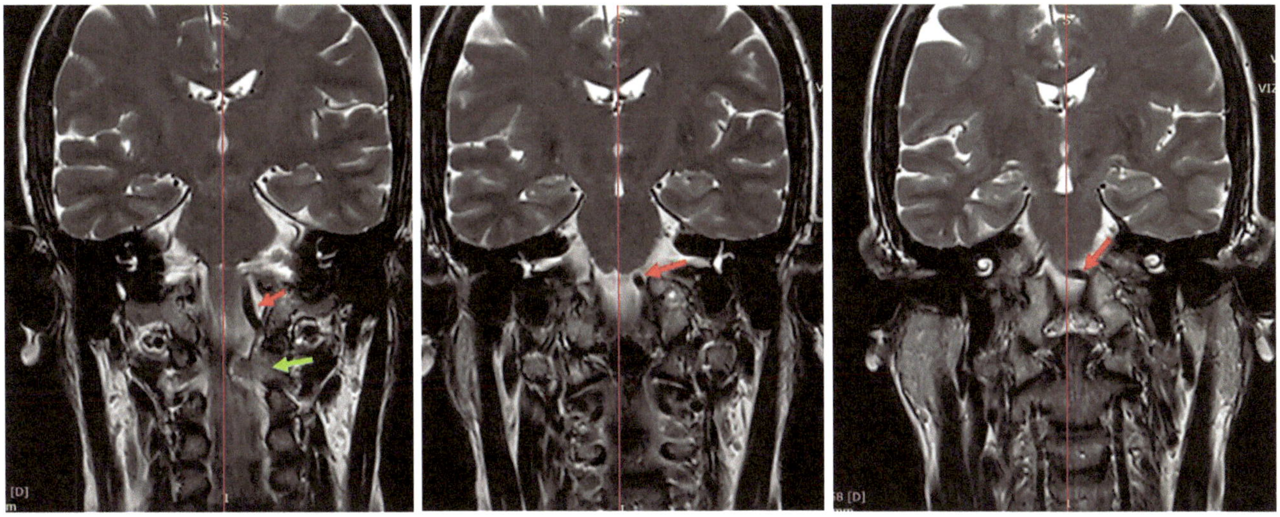

Fig. 13 Vertebral artery anomaly in the midline. Normally, the vertebral artery is not this medial, which puts it at considerable risk at surgery. Lower left neuroma progressing towards the foramen is seen (*green arrow*)

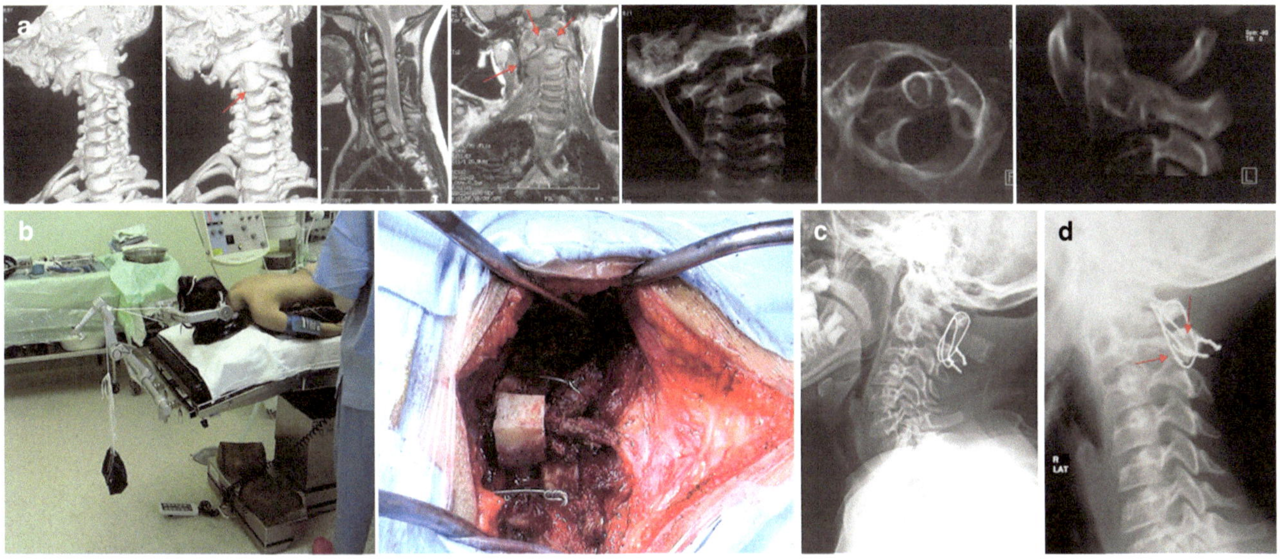

Fig. 14 A 9-year-old girl who had a bend in her neck. The last time she showed such a bent, she did not recover. (**a**) Atlanto axial rotatory dislocation and related torticollis were observed (Cock-robin position of head). (**b**) Stabilization was performed with wire and bone graft placed between C1-C2 vertebrae under traction. (**c**, **d**) Postoperative X-ray showing bone graft and wires holding C1-C2. At examination 6 months later, the bone graft has been resorbed and the wires are broken and loosened

for infection in this setting to develop strategies to reduce the incidence. Advanced age, high body mass index (BMI), diabetes, revision status, smoking, American Society of Anesthesiologists (ASA) score, chronic corticosteroid use/immunosuppression, and prior spinal instrumentation have all been reported as significant contributing factors. Beyond this, other factors may influence surgery, which affects outcomes: Active rheumatoid arthritis, dural tear, significant intraoperative bleeding, and prolonged surgical time are all high-risk factors for the development of an infection. If such a complication occurs, important clinical findings include redness, swelling, purulent discharge, and pain at the wound site. High fever, malaise, and weakness dominate the clinical picture. CRP, ESR, a complete blood cell count, and the differential will be informative, and a Gram stain of a wound swab and cultures are important steps to be taken. If an abscess is radiologically detected in a symptomatic patient, it should be drained. Limiting pharmacotherapy to targeted antibiotics and basing it on culture results with the use of broad-spectrum antibiotics are important until the culture results are available [33–37].

Case Study (Fig. 14) A 9-year-old girl repeatedly developed a "bulge in her neck" over the past 3 years without any other clinical issues and returned to normal status within a few weeks each time. At presentation, she had this problem for 3 months without returning to normal. Antibiotic treatment was given, and some traction therapy was applied, but these had no success, and instead, she continued to complain of constant pain and had an abnormal neck posture. This patient had developed a secondary torticollis caused by a deep neck infection known as Grisel syndrome [38, 39], first described in 1930. Although its pathophysiology has not been fully understood, it appears that the nontraumatic dislocation of the atlantoaxial joint and rotational distortion (torticollis) occurs because of an infection or inflammation in the nasopharyngeal or otolaryngeal region. Clinically, a cock-robin wry position of the head is typical. This syndrome is a disease of childhood and is usually not seen after the age of 12. The treatment is conservative and includes the use of a cervical collar, analgesics, and antibiotics. Surgical intervention may rarely be required for patients who do not show that they benefit from conservative treatment. This can be a sequel of fibrosis that may develop in the atlantoaxial joint and that prevents the head from returning to its normal position. For this reason, the timing of the therapy is important. Once fibrosis has set in, the chances of a positive outcome after surgery decreases [22, 40].

Radiological examinations of our patient revealed persistent atlantoaxial rotatory dislocation after 2 weeks of conservative treatment. The rotatory misalignment can only temporarily be improved with traction, so we took the patient to surgery (under traction) and stabilized C1-C2 with wiring and bone grafting between the laminae of C1-C2.

Appendix

Anatomical Review

Upper Cervical Region Anatomy

This region consists of the flat occipital bone forming the posterior skull base, the clivus of the sphenoid bone anteriorly, and the C1 and C2 vertebrae. Instability at the craniocervical junction (CCJ) can arise from pathologies that develop in the C0-C1 and C1-C2 joints. The balance between stability and movement here is provided by strong ligaments. The craniocervical junction is stabilized anteriorly by five key ligaments: (1) the anterior atlantooccipital membrane (continues the anterior longitudinal ligament), (2) the tectorial membrane (continues the posterior longitudinal ligament), (3) the transverse ligament (provides attachment to the anterior arch of odontoid C1), (4) the alar ligament (connects the dense occipital condyles and axial rotation and adds resistance to lateral bending), and (5) the apical ligament (attaches the odontoid to the basion). The four structures that stabilize posteriorly are as follows: (1) the ligamentum nuchae, (2) the interspinous ligament, (3) the posterior atlantooccipital membrane, and (4) the ligamentum flavum and neck muscles (Fig. 15).

Neck muscles are multilayered and make serious contributions to stabilization. These muscles are divided into anterior, posterior, and lateral muscles. The posterior muscles are especially important when the cranium is to be firmly attached to the cervical region in some cases. These neck muscles and the muscles attached to the skull are stripped, and thus stabilization is performed. These muscles are then closed over the instrumentation area and sewn together. The better the muscles are preserved, the higher the chance of surgical success, as they will continue their stabilization duties.

The anterior neck muscles are a group of muscles that cover the front of the neck. They are further divided into the following subgroups: the superficial muscles, which are the most superficial in the anterior neck and include the platysma and sternocleidomastoid; the suprahyoid muscles, which as the name suggests, are located superior to the hyoid bone and include the digastric, mylohyoid, geniohyoid, and stylohyoid; and the infrahyoid muscles, which are located below the hyoid bone and consist of the sternohyoid, omohyoid, sternothyroid, and thyrohyoid.

The anterior vertebral muscles are a deep muscle group located just in front of the cervical vertebral column. These include the rectus capitis anterior, rectus capitis lateralis, longus capitis, and longus colli. These muscles are surrounded by the prevertebral fascia of the neck, so they are often referred to as the prevertebral muscles. The main function of these muscles is to provide varying degrees of flexion for the head.

The lateral neck muscles, also called the lateral vertebral muscles, are a group of muscles that run obliquely along the lateral sides of the neck. These include the anterior, middle, and posterior scalene muscles, which lie between the transverse processes of the cervical vertebrae and the upper two ribs. Because of their attachments, these muscles mainly produce ipsilateral flexion for the neck. They are related to neck movement rather than to the occipitocervical region.

The back of the neck is covered with the posterior group of muscles, which connect the skull to the spinal cord and pectoral girdle. These muscles can be divided into three layers: (1) the superficial layer, comprising the trapezius, splenius capitis, and splenius cervicis; (2) the deep layer, comprising the cervical transversospinalis

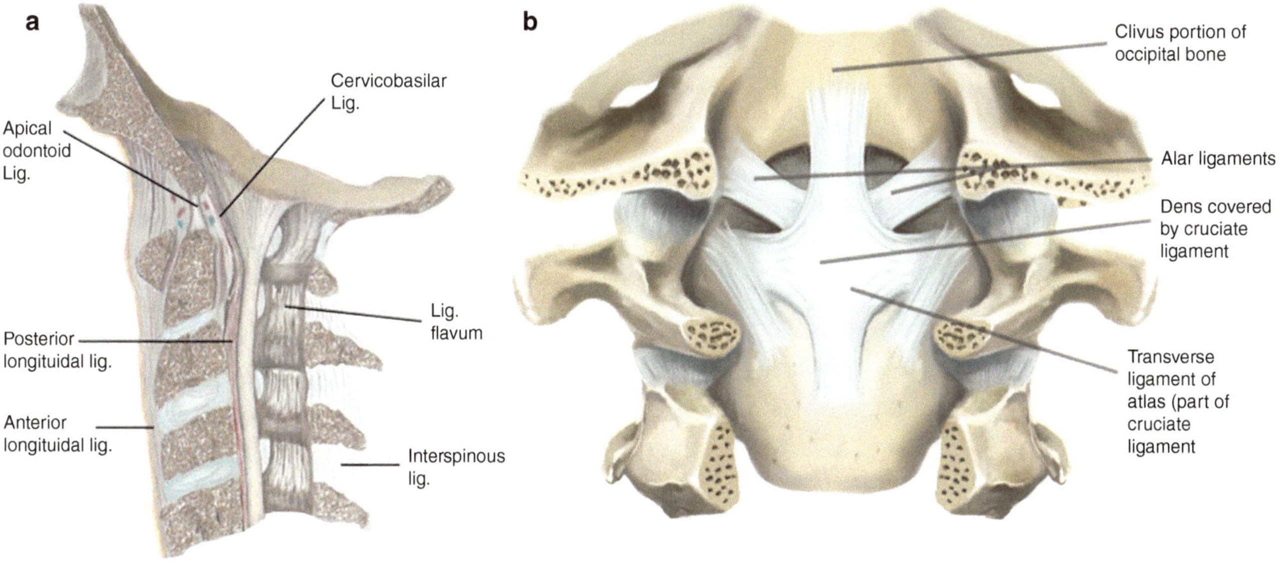

Fig. 15 (**a**) Occipitocervical region ligaments. (**b**) Cruciate ligament and alar ligaments connecting C1-C2-C3 are observed in the occipitocervical region. The accessory atlantoaxial ligament descends from both sides of the transverse ligament

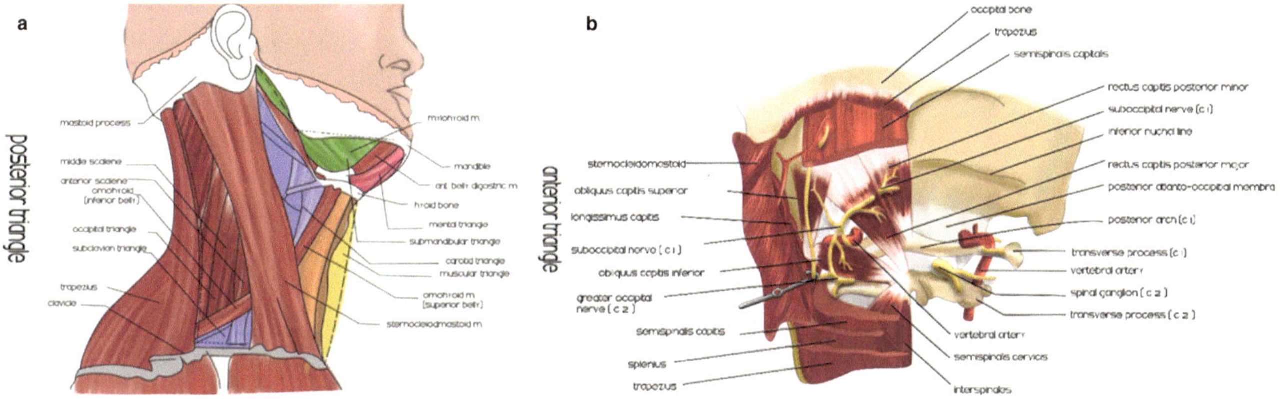

Fig. 16 (**a**) Deep and superficial neck muscles are seen. (**b**) Coronal section of deep and superficial muscles between cranium and cervical region

muscles (semispinalis capitis, semispinalis cervicis, and multifidus cervicis); and (3) the deepest layer, comprising the suboccipital muscles, interspinales cervicis muscles, and intertransversarii colli muscles (Fig. 16). Obviously, the overlapping layers effectively mix in stabilization while performing the flexion, extension, rotation, and bending movements of the neck.

Key Radiographic Metrics

Measurements of the Head in Neutral Position on the Cervical Spine

One fact to be pointed out is that cervical alignment is also affected by thoracic and lumbar pathologies, and as a result of pathologies occurring here, serious alignment disorders may occur. However, it especially causes the local deterioration of cervical alignment with cervical and occipitocervical pathologies. The alteration of normal cervical alignment as a result of pathology is the effort to keep the head level so that objects can continue to be seen in the horizontal plane. It is important in occipitocervical junction surgery in that if this alignment is not taken into account in a planned stabilization, any misalignment will end up as a permanent deformity that seriously disturbs forward gaze and that can seriously compromise the patient's gait (and thus mobility). Therefore, surgeons must ensure that the cervical alignment stays in the proper plane before any planned instrumentation (Fig. 17).

Important radiographic morphometric parameters are listed in the Appendix, which explains their relevance for the occipi-

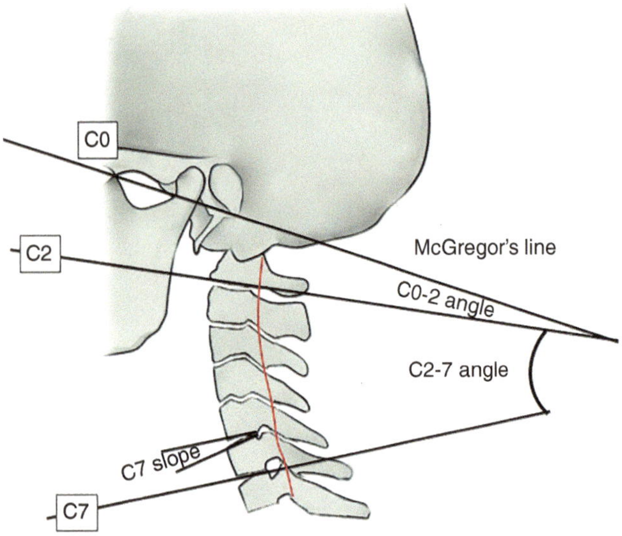

Fig. 17 C0-C2 angle and C7 slop angle measurements

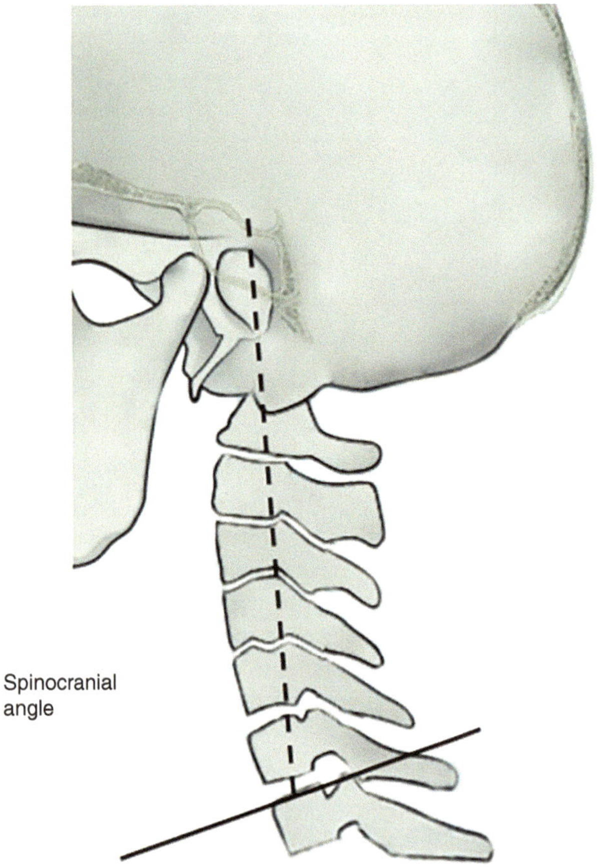

Fig. 18 Spinocranial angle. This is the angle between the line passing the upper border of the C7 vertebra body tangentially and the line drawn from the midpoint of C7 to the sella turcica. It gives the position of the head on C7-T1 and shows whether it is in sagittal balance

tocervical region. After any surgery, staying within the normative morphometric values is necessary to maintain the patient's visual perspective and to allow the head to have a healthy relationship with the remaining parameters of the spine (Fig. 18).

Measurements in the Occipitocervical Region

Anatomical markers constitute important parameters for occipitocervical craniometry. Such craniometry has been defined for conventional radiography, CT, and MRI. Measurements such as the Chamberlain, McGregor, McRae, and Wackenheim line formally describe the relationship between the cranium and the cervical region. While extremely helpful in diagnosis, knowing these measures and others (e.g., the atlantodental interval, ADI, power ratio, Harris rule, and clivoaxial angle) will also guide the planning of the surgery to be performed. Therefore, these basic measurements should be kept in mind.

Chamberlain Line: This measure is the line connecting the back of the hard palate with the opisthion, as seen in the lateral view of the craniocervical junction. Basilar invagination can be identified when the tip of the odontoid is >3 mm above this line (Fig. 19).

McGregor Line: This measure refers to a line connecting the posterior edge of the hard palate to the most caudal point of the occipital curve. An odontoid tip 4.5 mm above this line is indicative of basilar invagination.

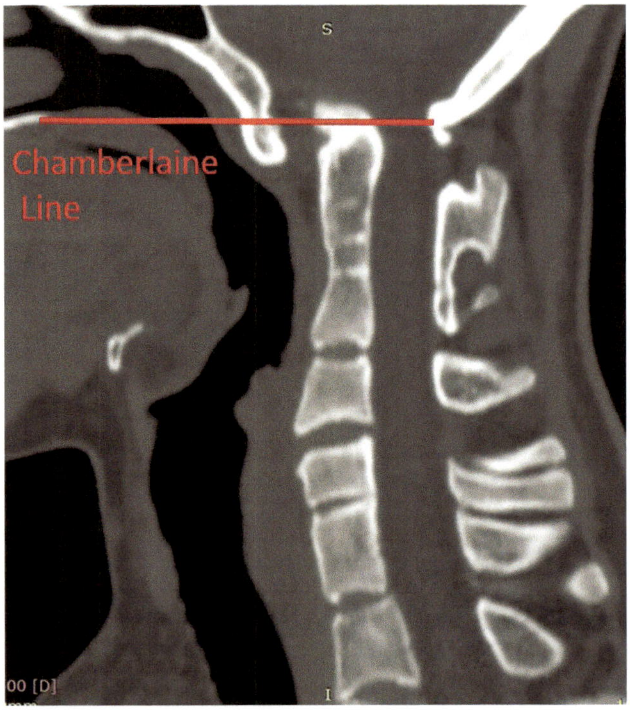

Fig. 19 Odontoid type I invagination appears above the Chamberlain line

McRae Line: A radiographic line drawn on a lateral skull radiograph or midsagittal section of CT or MRI connecting the anterior and posterior margins of the foramen magnum (basion to opisthion). It assesses the presence of basilar invagination (atlantoaxial impaction). The tip of the odontoid process is normally located about 5 mm below this line; basilar invagination is diagnosed when the odontoid tip crosses this line. The line also helps to measure the position and degree of cerebellar tonsillar descent since the cerebellar tonsils are normally found above this line, namely the foramen magnum. In cases of cerebellar ectopia with a caudal displacement of the tonsils >5 mm below the foramen magnum, a Chiari malformation may be diagnosed.

Wackenheim Line: This measure is also known as the clivus-canal line or the basilar line. It is created by drawing a line along the clivus and extending it below and into the upper cervical canal on a midsagittal view. Normally, the tip of the odontoid is ventral (anterior) to this line, and the tip of the odontoid is touching the line (tangential). In cases of basilar invagination, this line cuts through the odontoid. In posterior atlantooccipital dislocation, the line will extend behind the odontoid process.

Atlantodental Interval (ADI)

This measure is used to assess ligamentous stability at the C1/C2 junction, as seen on a lateral or axial view (plain X-ray or sagittal CT cut), and it aids in the diagnosis of atlantooccipital dissociation injuries and of isolated atlas and axis injuries, which can best be measured as the horizontal distance between the anterior arch of the atlas and the odontoid process of C2. It is the distance between the posterior cortex of the anterior arch of the atlas and the anterior cortex of the odontoid in the median (midsagittal) plane. On X-ray, its normal values are <3 mm in adults, <3 mm in men, < 2.5 mm in women, and <5 mm in children (regardless of sex). On CT, this distance is <2 mm in adults.

$$\textbf{Powers ratio} = C - D / A - B$$

C-D: Distance from the basion to the arch of posterior C1.

A-B: Distance from the anterior arch of C1 to the opisthion.

Importantly, if the ratio is ~1, it is considered normal. If the ratio is >1.0, there is a possibility of anterior dislocation. Conversely, if the ratio is <1.0, there is a probability of posterior atlantooccipital dislocation. With respect to the underlying pathology, there is a possibility of a fracture of the odontoid or a fracture of the atlas arch (Fig. 20).

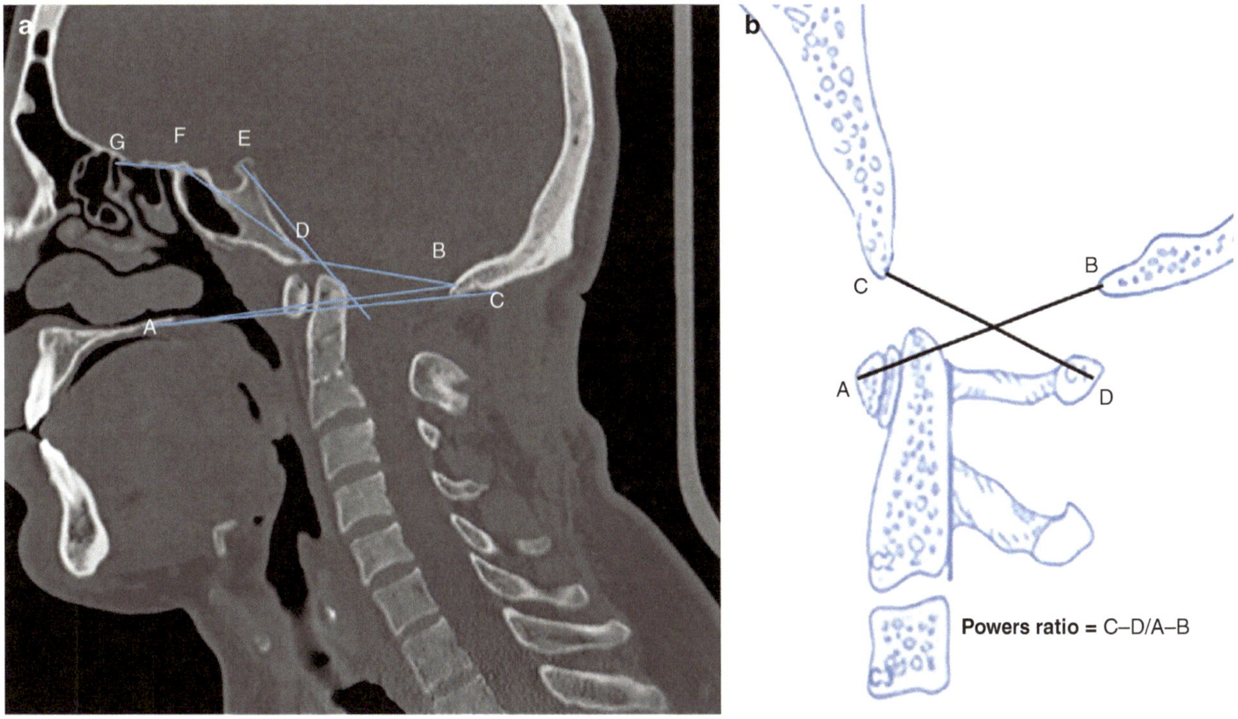

Fig. 20 (**a**) Parameters revealing the relationship between the cranium and occipitocervical region. AB Chamberlain line, AC McGregor line, DB McRae line, ED Wackenheim Clivus line. (**b**) Power's ratio is around 1. If it is >1, the dislocation is considered anterior; if <1, it is considered posterior

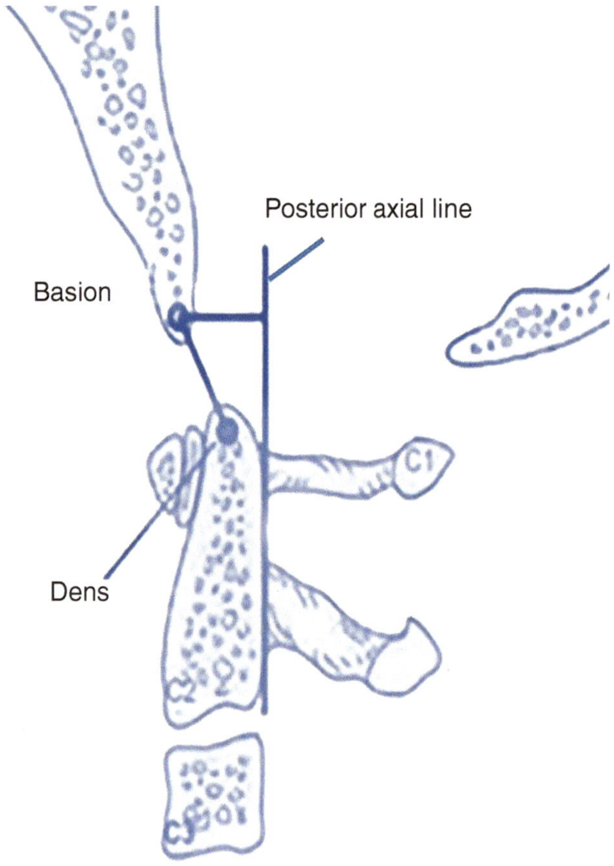

Fig. 21 Harris rule of 12: basion–dens interval or basion–posterior axial interval > 12 mm suggests occipitocervical dissociation

Harris Rule of 12

Occipitocervical dissociation is considered if the distance of the basion–dens measure (BDM) or the basion–axial measure (BAM) is >12 mm (Fig. 21). The clivoaxial angle is measured by drawing a line along the posterior (back—or, when lying more horizontally, the top) side of the lower clivus and intersecting that line with a line drawn on the posterior side of the axis. If the angle created is less than 135°, it is considered pathological. Like instability, a kyphotic clivoaxial angle is often seen in patients with connective tissue disorders and degenerative rheumatoid diseases (Fig. 22).

Further Important Parameters and their Relevance to the Occipitocervical Region

High C0-C2 Angle (High Cervical Angulation): This is the angle formed between the line starting from the end point of the bone projection of the upper palate and passing through the lowest part of the occipital bone (McGregor line) and a second line passing through the lower edge of C2. Its mean value is 15.8° (+7.15°), and it is always lordotic.

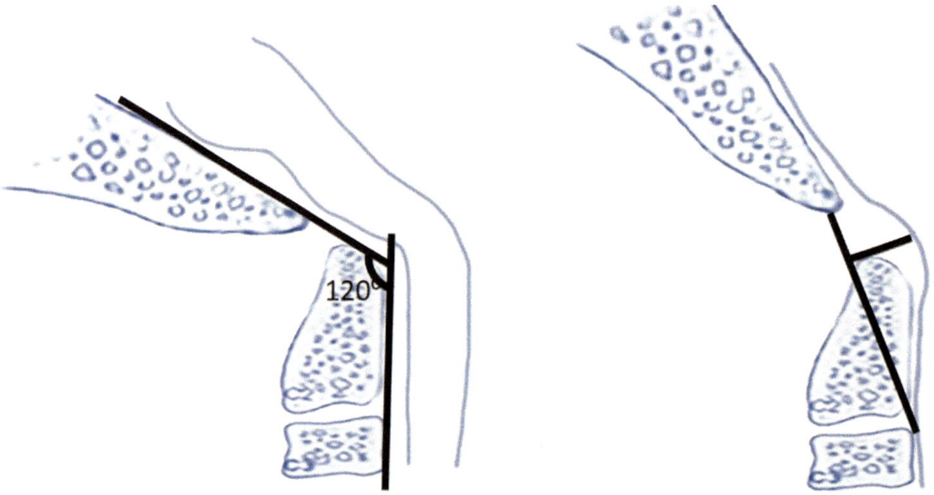

Fig. 22 The clivoaxial angle is formed by a line extrapolation at the posterior end of the lower clivus that intersects with a line drawn on the posterior side of the axis. If the enclosed angle created is less than 135°, it is considered pathological

Cervical Lordosis Angle: This is the angle between the tangential line passing through the lower face of the C2 vertebra and the perpendicular lines drawn to the tangential lines passing through the lower face of the C7 vertebra (the Cobb method). The average value is 30.73° ± 4.88°.

Spinocranial Angle (SCA): This is the angle between the tangential line passing through the upper edge of the C7 vertebral body and the line drawn from the midpoint of C7 to the sella turcica on this line. In asymptomatic people, the value of this angle is 83° ± 9°, on average. It is an important angle because it establishes the position of the head on C7-T1 and tells the observer whether the head is in good sagittal balance.

References

1. Ahmed R, Menezes AH. Management of operative complications related to occipitocervical instrumentation. Neurosurgery. 2013;72(2 Suppl Operative):ons214-28.
2. Bono CM, Vaccaro AR, Fehlings M, Fisher C, Dvorak M, Ludwig S, Harrop J. Spine trauma study group. Measurement techniques for upper cervical spine injuries: consensus statement of the spine trauma study group. Spine (Phila Pa 1976). 2007;32(5):593–600.
3. Harms J, Melcher RP. Posterior C1-C2 fusion with polyaxial screw and rod fixation. Spine (Phila Pa 1976). 2001;26(22):2467–71.
4. He B, Yan L, Xu Z, Chang Z, Hao D. The causes and treatment strategies for the postoperative complications of occipitocervical fusion: a 316 cases retrospective analysis. Eur Spine J. 2014;23(8):1720–4.
5. Hwang SW, Gressot LV, Chern JJ, Relyea K, Jea A. Complications of occipital screw placement for occipitocervical fusion in children. J Neurosurg Pediatr. 2012;9(6):586–93.
6. Le Huec JC, Thompson W, Mohsinaly Y, Barrey C, Faundez A. Sagittal balance of the spine. Eur Spine J. 2019;28(9):1889–905.
7. Mazur MD, Sivakumar W, Riva-Cambrin J, Jones J, Brockmeyer DL. Avoiding early complications and reoperation during occipitocervical fusion in pediatric patients. J Neurosurg Pediatr. 2014;14(5):465–75.
8. Yang D, Patel S, DiSilvestro K, Li N, Daniels A. Postoperative complication rates and hazards-model survival analysis of revision surgery following Occipitocervical and Atlanto-axial fusion. N Am Spine Soc J. 2020;3:100017.
9. Ankith NV, Avinash M, Srivijayanand KS, Shetty AP, Kanna RM, Rajasekaran S. Congenital osseous anomalies of the cervical spine: occurrence, morphological characteristics, embryological basis and clinical significance: a computed tomography based study. Asian Spine J. 2019;13(4):535–43.
10. Browd S, Healy LJ, Dobie G, Johnson JT 3rd, Jones GM, Rodriguez LF, Brockmeyer DL. Morphometric and qualitative analysis of congenital occipitocervical instability in children: implications for patients with Down syndrome. J Neurosurg. 2006;105(1 Suppl):50–4.
11. Dabaghi-Richerand A, Hensinger R, Farley F. Congenital disorders of the child's cervical spine. 2018 https://doi.org/10.1007/978-1-4939-7491-7-9.
12. Klimo P Jr, Rao G, Brockmeyer D. Congenital anomalies of the cervical spine. Neurosurg Clin N Am. 2007;18(3):463–78.
13. Rojas CA, Hayes A, Bertozzi JC, Guidi C, Martinez CR. Evaluation of the C1-C2 articulation on MDCT in healthy children and young adults. AJR Am J Roentgenol. 2009;193(5):1388–92.
14. Goel A, Laheri V. Plate and screw fixation for atlanto-axial subluxation. Acta Neurochir. 1994;129:47–53.
15. Guo J, Lu W, Ji X, Ren X, Tang X, Zhao Z, Hu H, Song T, Du Y, Li J, Shao C, Xu T, Xi Y. Surgical treatment of atlantoaxial subluxation by intraoperative skull traction and C1-C2 fixation. BMC Musculoskelet Disord. 2020;21(1):239.
16. Menezes AH, Ryken TC. Craniovertebral junction abnormalities. In: Weinstein SL, editor. The pediatric spine: principles and practice, 1st edn, vol. 1. New York: Raven Press; 1994. p. 307–21.
17. Menezes AH, VanGilder JC. Anomalies of the craniovertebral junction. In: Youmans J, editor. Neurological surgery, 3rd edn, vol. 2. Philadelphia: Saunders; 1990. p. 1359–420.
18. Salunke P, Sharma M, Sodhi HB, Mukherjee KK, Khandelwal NK. Congenital atlantoaxial dislocation: a dynamic process and role of facets in irreducibility. J Neurosurg Spine. 2011;15(6):678–85.
19. Yang SY, Boniello AJ, Poorman CE, Chang AL, Wang S, Passias PG. A review of the diagnosis and treatment of atlantoaxial dislocations. Global Spine J. 2014;4(3):197–210.
20. Goel A. Goel's classification of atlantoaxial "facetal" dislocation. J Craniovertebr Junction Spine. 2014;5(1):3–8.
21. Magerl F, Seemann P. Stable posterior fusion of the atlas and axis by transarticular screw fixation. In: Society CSR, editor. Cervical spine. New York: Springer-Verlag; 1986. p. 322–7.
22. Ozer AF, Marandi HJ, Sasani M, Oktenoglu T, Suzer T. Posttraumatic syringomyelia: a technical note. Turk Neurosurg. 2014;24(4):618–22.
23. Henderson FC. Cranio-cervical instability in patients with hypermobility connective disorders. J Spine. 2016;2016(5):2D.
24. Lustrin ES, Karakas SP, Ortiz AO, Cinnamon J, Castillo M, Vaheesan K, Brown JH, Diamond AS, Black K, Singh S. Pediatric cervical spine: normal anatomy, variants, and trauma. Radiographics. 2003;23(3):539–60.
25. Reynolds MD. Lateral subluxation of atlanto—axial joint. Ann Rheum Dis. 1979;38(5):499.
26. Fielding JW, Hawkins RJ. Atlanto-axial rotatory fixation. (fixed rotatory subluxation of the atlanto-axial joint). J Bone Joint Surg Am. 1977;59(1):37–44.
27. Riascos R, Bonfante E, Cotes C, Guirguis M, Hakimelahi R, West C. Imaging of Atlanto-occipital and atlantoaxial traumatic injuries: what the radiologist needs to know. Radiographics. 2015;35(7):2121–34.
28. Shin H, Barrenechea IJ, Lesser J, Sen C, Perin NI. Occipitocervical fusion after resection of craniovertebral junction tumors. J Neurosurg Spine. 2006;4(2):137–44.
29. Oh YG, Lee BJ, Jeon SR, Roh SW, Rhim SC, Park JH. Anterior odontoid screw fixation for the treatment of type 2 odontoid fracture with a kyphotic angulation or an anterior Down-slope: a technical note. Neurol Med Chir (Tokyo). 2019;59(8):321–5.
30. Fei Q, Li J, Lin J, Li D, Wang B, Meng H, Wang Q, Su N, Yang Y. Risk factors for surgical site infection after spinal surgery: a meta-analysis. World Neurosurg. 2016;95:507–15.
31. Ogihara S, Yamazaki T, Inanami H, Oka H, Maruyama T, Miyoshi K, Takano Y, Chikuda H, Azuma S, Kawamura N, Yamakawa K, Hara N, Oshima Y, Morii J, Okazaki R, Takeshita Y, Tanaka S, Saita K. Risk factors for surgical site infection after lumbar laminectomy and/or discectomy for degenerative diseases in adults: a prospective

multicenter surveillance study with registry of 4027 cases. PLoS One. 2018;13(10):e0205539.
32. Olsen MA, Mayfield J, Lauryssen C, Polish LB, Jones M, Vest J, Fraser VJ. Risk factors for surgical site infection in spinal surgery. J Neurosurg. 2003;98(2 Suppl):149–55.
33. Huckell CB, Buchowski JM, Richardson WJ, Williams D, Kostuik JP. Functional outcome of plate fusions for disorders of the occipitocervical junction. Clin Orthop Relat Res. 1999;359:136–45.
34. Lee CC, Liu YT. Occipitocervical fusion complicated with cerebellar abscess: a case report. BMC Musculoskelet Disord. 2020;21:129.
35. Nockels RP, Shaffrey CI, Kanter AS, Azeem S, York JE. Occipitocervical fusion with rigid internal fixation: long-term follow-up data in 69 patients. J Neurosurg Spine. 2007;7(2):117–23.
36. Ogihara S, Yamazaki T, Shiibashi M, Chikuda H, Maruyama T, Miyoshi K, Inanami H, Oshima Y, Azuma S, Kawamura N, Yamakawa K, Hara N, Morii J, Okazaki R, Takeshita Y, Nishimoto J, Tanaka S, Saita K. Risk factors for deep surgical site infection after posterior cervical spine surgery in adults: a multicentre observational cohort study. Sci Rep. 2021;11(1):7519.
37. Pharisa C, Lutz N, Roback MG, Gehri M. Neck complaints in the pediatric emergency department: a consecutive case series of 170 children. Pediatr Emerg Care. 2009;25:823–6.
38. Blankstein A, Pavlotsky F, Roizin H, Ganel A, Chechick A. Acquired torticollis in hospitalized children. Harefuah. 1997;133:616–9.
39. Iaccarino C, Francesca O, Piero S, Monica R, Armando R, de Bonis P, Ferdinando A, Trapella G, Mongardi L, Cavallo M, Giuseppe C, Franco S. Grisel's syndrome: non-traumatic atlantoaxial rotatory subluxation-report of five cases and review of the literature. Acta Neurochir Suppl. 2019;125:279–88.
40. Viscone A, Brembilla C, Gotti G. The importance and effectiveness of conservative treatment in Grisel's syndrome. J Pediatr Neurosci. 2014;9(2):200–1.

The Naked Neurosurgeon and the Anatomy of a Complication

Anil Pande, Siddhartha Ghosh, and G. Krishna Kumar

Abstract

Introduction

The neurosurgeon is always poised precariously between the operation and the abyss of a complication. As Wilder Penfield sagaciously wrote in 1961, "I will faithfully record and analyze my failures in the care of the sick, seeking the cause, so that those who follow may be warned of the danger."

Aim

This paper seeks to briefly overview the literature on complications in surgery, neurosurgery in particular.

Materials and Method

Progress in our specialty has been accomplished by the overcoming of complications via technique or technology. Dr. Samer Nashef commented sarcastically that surgeons are not, as a general rule, well known for their rapacious appetite for reading. But knowing the literature on complications from our field and others is essential for progress. We must know the anatomy of complications to avoid and manage them.

In 1992, Michael Apuzzo published his magnus opus, *Brain surgery: Complication avoidance and management*, which was admirably followed by Edward Benzel's edited work *Spine surgery: Techniques, complication avoidance and management*, setting standards in the science of complication avoidance and management in 1999 for years to come. In 2001, *Crossing the quality chasm: A new health system for the twenty-first century* was published in the United States by the Institute of Medicine. Lucian Leape (a pediatric and thoracic surgeon) published *Error in Medicine* in *JAMA* in December 1994, and in 1991, he published the *Harvard Medical Practice Study*, defining essential terms like *adverse event* and *negligence*. Atul Gawande, a general surgeon at Harvard University, wrote "The Bell Curve: What happens when patients find out how good their doctors really are," in the *New Yorker* on December 6, 2004; he went on to pen *Complications—A surgeon's notes on an imperfect science* in 2002 and *Better: A surgeon's notes on performance* in 2007; and he peaked with his classic *The Checklist Manifesto—How to get things right* in 2009. In 2015, *The Naked Surgeon—The power and peril of transparency in medicine* appeared. Written by a cardiothoracic surgeon, Samer Nashef, the book takes the study of complication avoidance to a different level and describes how cardiac surgery blazed the trail in quality monitoring and improvement, leaving no scope for other specialties but to follow. The era of the naked neurosurgeon may be beginning anytime.

Conclusion

Ever since E. C. Pearce delivered the 34th Rovenstine lecture, *40 years behind the mask—Safety revisited*, in 1996, the literature on complication avoidance and management has been growing exponentially. Cross-specialty discourse and the exchange of ideas are essential for neurosurgery to maintain its position as the emperor of all specialties.

Keywords

Neurosurgical complications · Anatomy of a complication · Era of the naked neurosurgeon · Complication avoidance · Management in neurosurgery

A. Pande (✉) · S. Ghosh · G. Krishna Kumar
Department of Neurosurgery, Institute of Neurosciences, Apollo Specialty Hospital, Chennai, Tamil Nadu, India

Introduction

The oldest myth in human civilization about the occurrence of a complication talks about when the devas and the asuras churned the ocean using a tortoise as a base, Mount Mandara as the churn, and the great snake Vasuki as the rope to try to

K. Turel, E. M. Kasper (eds.), *Complications in Neurosurgery II*, Acta Neurochirurgica Supplement 133,
https://doi.org/10.1007/978-3-031-61601-3_19

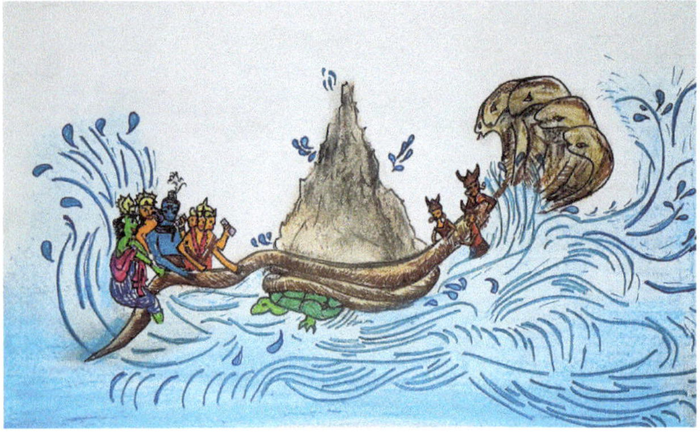

Fig. 1 The Samudra Manthan myth

obtain the elixir of immortality. The churn yielded not only the ultimate elixir of life (Amritha) but also the most powerful poison of all, called halahala (Fig. 1). As all existence was threatened, the gods called upon Shiva the Destroyer to deliver them from this dreaded complication, and he drank the poison, which turned his throat blue. The neurosurgeon is similarly always poised precariously between the operation and the abyss of a complication into which they and their patient may fall.

Nudges by Mentors

As Wilder Penfield sagaciously wrote in 1961, "I will faithfully record and analyze my failures in the care of the sick, seeking the cause, so that those who follow may be warned of the danger." Wilder Penfield was my teachers' mentor (Fig. 2). Prof Ramamurthi was once called by me to help out when I as a resident plunged in while doing a craniectomy for a young patient. He scrubbed, inspected the operative field, and then descrubbed, saying "go ahead; I've plunged 17 times." The mentor leading the novice by hand through the minefield of complications is played out every day in countless neurosurgical theaters (Fig. 3). Prof Ramamurthi had a photograph of a ropewalker high over the valley—under which was written the following legend: "The man who cannot afford to make a mistake—neurosurgeon." This frame hung behind his chair in his office and was pointed out to every resident that he trained (Fig. 4). Sir William Osler gave the following advice to young doctors: "Errors in judgment must occur in the practice which consists largely of balancing probabilities—you will draw from your errors the very lessons which may enable you to avoid their repetition," which holds good even today. Mentors like Ramamurthi, Yassargil, and Samii nudge not only their residents but the complete specialty to perform better, reduce errors, and improve the outcomes of our operative procedures.

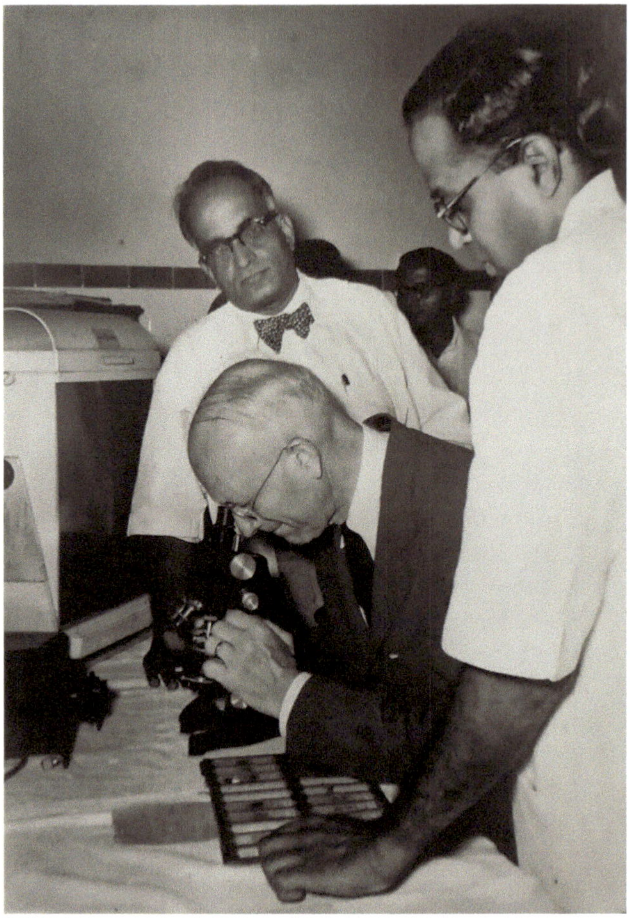

Fig. 2 S. T. Narasimhan, Wilder Penfield, B. Ramamurthi

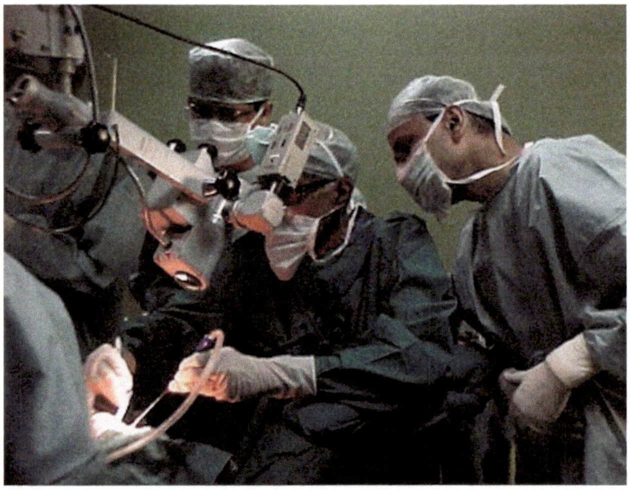

Fig. 3 Prof. Anil Pande, Prof. B. Ramamurthi and Dr. M. C. Vasudevan

Technique and Technology

Progress in our specialty has been seen in the overcoming of complications via technique or technology, and they occurred

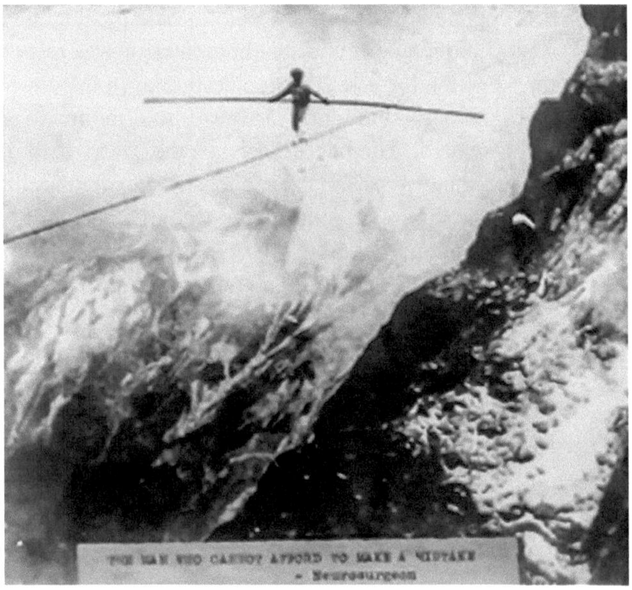

Fig. 4 "The man who cannot afford to make a mistake—neurosurgeon"

thanks to nudges by our mentors. The technology led innovations in current drills and craniotomes with safety features, which have made the Hudson brace and the plunging associated with it very rare indeed.

Anatomy of a Complication

In 1621, *The Anatomy of Melancholy* was published by Robert Burton, where he used the word *anatomy* to elaborate on "what it is: with all the kinds, causes, symptomes, prognostickes, and several cures of melancholy." The word is used in that context here. We must know the anatomy of complications to avoid and manage them. No neurosurgical complication anatomy is the same: The individual patient morphological characteristics, procedure variability, theater workspace, and personnel are different each time.

A complication is a problem of extreme complexity, says Atul Gawande. In the book *The Checklist Manifesto*, Gawande cites the classification of problems by Brenda Zimmerman and Sholom Glouberman, whose expertise is the science of complexity. They categorize problems as simple—e.g., baking a cake; in comparison, they categorize sending a rocket to the moon as a complicated problem and raising a child as a complex problem. With complexity increasing in neurosurgery, the possibility of a complication or mishap multiplies. Latent errors are lurking faults in the system, organization, management, training, technique, or equipment, and these cause a complication or an adverse event.

The new science of complications draws on wide and varied fields of human knowledge. Chaos theory, the science of heuristics, probability theory, Boolean logic, behavioral science, the dual process theory of cognition [1], and innumerable others are used to explain the etiology of why things go wrong.

The Swiss cheese model of accident causation is one such explanation proposed by James Reason. The human defense against complication is likened to slices of cheese with randomly and naturally placed holes arranged in parallel vertical arrays. The holes represent weaknesses, and rarely and randomly, they all align, creating a trajectory of accident causation. Measures that prevent such alignment need to be implemented, and leadership is extremely important in achieving and maintaining such quality measures in healthcare [2].

The neurosurgical practice—like all branches of surgery and medicine—is threatened by a pandemic of complications. A study in the United States attributed the frequent occurrence of these mishaps to having three fatal air crashes every day [3]. From the aviation industry, the medical profession learned various ways of documenting and eliminating the possibilities of critical events that can lead to mishaps. The new science of patient safety is central to the unraveling of this complexity, and if the neurosurgeon doesn't fail, the system might fail them and might also compromise the safety of the patient.

Learning About Complications from the Aviation Industry

Risk Analysis and the Management—The Preflight Checklist

The concept of checklists was born to manage the complexity of the Boeing B-17 bombers during World War II. The B-17 bomber was a great advance, with four engines and its resultant innumerable control panels and meters. However, the test flight was a disaster and led to the death of the pilots. The introduction of a preflight checklist made them flyable and safe. Detailed checklists were then used to fly these Flying Fortresses without mishaps by even relatively untrained pilots. The use of checklists was one of the main reasons for the victory of the allies in World War II, and they are now used to prevent error in medicine and surgery and many other complex human endeavors.

The sterile cockpit concept and rule is a safety rule that prohibits nonessential and distracting activity during the critical periods of the flight. Translated to the surgical theater, it heightens levels of awareness and prevents any distraction of attention for the surgeon, anesthetist, or theater personnel during critical parts of the operation. Fatigue and stress are important risks for failure and suboptimal performance. Recognizing the importance of teamwork, listening to juniors within a flexible hierarchy, and team-training techniques as developed in aviation are to be incorporated [4].

Critical Incident Analysis Technique

Critical incident investigation in the aviation industry dates back to the 1930–40 period and was responsible for improving the quality of pilots and military aircraft performance. In 1978, Cooper et al. used a modified version of adverse event analysis in anesthesia to reduce the occurrence of errors [5].

Checklists in Neurosurgery

As complexity increases, the need for a checklist becomes more relevant. Gawande et al. pointed out that the cognitive limitations of forgetting a surgical step and remembering but not carrying out or improperly executing a step are all common and happen to the most trained experienced surgeons. Memory is documented to be unreliable; we have many biases, and our cognition can become impaired. All this is to be understood and accepted from research, and checklists can help us to reduce mishaps. Checklists have thus reduced complications by 36%, deaths by 47%, and infections by 50% [6]. Kapur et al., in a review comparing the aviation industry with healthcare, advocated for specific training in cognitive bias avoidance [7]. Schelkun advocated the adoption of aviation's credo—"plan YOUR flight and fly your plan"—by surgeons and amended it accordingly: "plan your operation and operate your plan." [8].

The surgical career of most neurosurgeons can be informed by the insight that we all need to be observed by a mentor or a coach during all stages of our careers, and we can keep improving our patients care, outcomes, and satisfaction not only by adopting new innovations but also by continuously getting better at what we do.

Learning from Anesthesia

Beecher and Todd's study [9] *Deaths Associated with Anesthesia and Surgery* appeared in the annals of surgery in 1954, and this shook the foundations of both specialties (anesthesia and surgery) with its shocking revelations about mortality and morbidity and about system failures. Phillips and Capizzi [10] began their review of complications in anesthesia with a shocking but true statement: "You, the members of the medical profession, gentlemen, are in a favored position—the world acclaims your success and flowers cover your failures."

J. B. Cooper et al. [5] applied a modified critical incident analysis technique and found that human error was responsible for 82% of adverse events in anesthesia. In this much-criticized landmark study, only 14% of these failures were equipment related. Human error was the overwhelming cause of the majority of mishaps and critical events rather than equipment failure. A dedicated first conference on anesthetic complications was the *International Symposium on Preventable Anesthetic Morbidity and Mortality* held in Boston, Massachusetts, on October 8–10, 1984. Leroy Vandam assigned the subject "anesthesia accidents," to Ellison Pierce as a resident's talk. He was the one who later went on to deliver the famous and transformative 34th Rovenstine lecture, *40 years behind the mask –safety revisited*, in 1996. The science of complications is rapidly expanding, and terms like *near miss* [11] and *the stratification of risk* [12] continue to be defined.

The Literature on Complications

Samer Nashef commented sarcastically that surgeons are not, as a general rule, well known for their rapacious appetite for reading. Many of us practicing surgeons don't have the time or inclination to read about the new horizons in quality and outcome in surgery. But knowing the vast literature on complications from our field and others is essential for progress.

Landmarks in Neurosurgery

Horwitz and Rizzoli's *Postoperative Complications in Neurosurgical Practice: Recognition, Prevention and Management*, which appeared in 1967, was well received and well reviewed by authorities like Lawrence Pool and Charles B. Wilson [13, 14]. This continues to be a valuable resource and highlights the importance of building a collective consciousness of neurosurgical errors, mishaps, failings, and their recognition, prevention, and management.

Col. Ludwig G. Kemp's elaborately illustrated *Operative Neurosurgery*. The atlas was a brilliant individual work that set out to illustrate the simple steps of a procedure (comparable to a checklist of safety and reproducibility), which could be developed into complex and intricate operations. The book remains an important learning aid for neurosurgeons.

In 1992, Michael Apuzzo published his magnum opus, *Brain surgery: Complication avoidance and management*, and this classic made the avoidance of a complication central to the practice of cranial surgery. Neurosurgeons still partake in the distilled experience of senior surgeons who laid a secure foundation of safe neurosurgery. In 1999, Edward Benzel edited *Spine Surgery: Techniques, Complication*

Avoidance, and Management, which set the standards in the science of complication avoidance and management in spine neurosurgery.

The Prophets of the Quality Revolution in Medical Care

Ernest A. Codman and Florence Nightingale were among the early pioneers of the clinical audit and quality revolution in medicine. The work of luminaries like Deming [15], Donabedian [16], and others on quality and how it is accessed and measured was translated to medicine from the management and manufacturing industry. Donald M. Berwick [17] and others put the patient's experience as the benchmark of quality in healthcare. The patient was made king in a way akin to the marketing quality adage that the customer or consumer is king.

Dr. Lucian Leape, a pediatric cardiothoracic surgeon, published his *Error in Medicine* in *JAMA* in December 1994, and this sent shockwaves across the world, leading to a major revamp of the way that the quality of care and outcomes was perceived by doctors, healthcare workers, and public and private health providers [12, 18]. The *Harvard Medical Practice Study* was published in 1991, and terms like *adverse event* and *negligence* became common parlance. *The Bristol Report* [19] was published in 1998 and was an inquiry into what went wrong in pediatric cardiac surgery there between 1984 to 1995. This led to a revolution in quality improvement in cardiac surgery and the National Health Service (NHS).

Crossing the quality chasm: A new health system for the twenty-first century was published in the United States by the Institute of Medicine in 2001 [20]. This document set out to tackle the huge quality gap in healthcare.

Atul Gawande, a general surgeon at Harvard University, wrote *The Bell Curve: What happens when patients find out how good their doctors really are*, in the *New Yorker* on December 6, 2004; *Complications—A surgeon's notes on an imperfect science* 2002; and *Better: A surgeon's notes on performance* in 2007, and he peaked with his classic *The Checklist Manifesto—How to get things right* in 2009.

The Naked Neurosurgeon

In 2015, *The Naked Surgeon—The power and peril of transparency in medicine* appeared. Written by a cardiothoracic surgeon, Samer Nashef, the book takes the study of complication avoidance to a different level and describes how cardiac surgery blazed the trail in quality monitoring and improvement, leaving no scope for other specialties but to follow [21]. *The Hawthorne Effect* [22] explains how the simple close observation of one's surgical outcomes can improve the results and safety of the operations. In it, Nashef confidently predicts that all specialties will have to measure, document, and analyze their outcomes by using scores and risk adjustment. This unbiased and patient-reported outcome and feedback is essential in continuously informing and improving our interventions.

Complications and adverse events take a severe toll on the surgeon, and the stress due to this can be acute [23]. Henry Marsh, a renowned UK neurosurgeon, set out to record, as he put it, and "remember all my worst mistakes." The reluctance of the neurosurgical fraternity to mention any adverse event is a protective reflex. He, however, talks about the terrible failures and unexpected complications that cause severe stress and despair among neurosurgeons. He calls this a "defensive psychological armor" that leaves the surgeon as naked as the patient if it's removed. The era of the naked neurosurgeon may be beginning anytime.

The Neurosurgery Patient Safety Foundation of the World Federation of Neurosurgical Societies (WFNS) can be an international complication reporting and learning system. This could be modeled on the National Patient Safety Foundation Agenda for Research and Patient Safety [24]. This collective memory system, along with a promise to learn and act, will revolutionize neurosurgery in a way similar to its application in other fields [25]. For an online, continuously updated study of the *Deaths Associated with Neurosurgery* featuring the big killers, like infection, bleeding, surgeon recklessness, error in timing or judgment, unsafe anesthesia, and the great void, the unexpected has to be initiated. This big and ever-expanding database could be a downloadable cloud resource and later develop into a helpful learning tool during crisis management.

Cognitive Strategies for Neurosurgeons to Avoid Complications [26]

Training has to be in simulation, nonsimulation, and "surprise and startle" events. The nontechnical training of surgeons to survive instrument and technology failures during operations [27] is also essential.

The WFNS

A collective memory bank of complications is necessary. Complications usually may not strike the initial operations but as the Neurosurgeon's confidence grows, he takes on more difficult procedures and thus a high volume Neurosurgeon's complications can inform a Neurosurgeon with smaller volumes about complication avoidance. Guidelines, checklists, and timeout protocols developed in leading institutions around the globe could be made available worldwide through the World Federation of Neurological

Surgeons. In 2013, UCLA adopted a preoperative shunt checklist, a cerebrospinal fluid (CSF) shunt implementation protocol, and the CSF shunt supplementary timeout. These local initiatives could be standardized like the World Health Organization (WHO) Surgical Checklist and be implemented at other centers, thus improving safety and quality in all neurosurgical centers worldwide.

Conclusions

"Brain surgery is a terrible profession, and if I did not feel it will become different in my lifetime, I should hate it," remarked Wilder Penfield. Despite immense advances in technique, technology, and experience, the surgery of the nervous system continues to learn and grow from its complications, which are unlikely to go away completely.

Ever since E. C. Pearce delivered the 34th Rovenstine lecture, *40 years behind the mask—Safety revisited*, in 1996, the literature on complication avoidance and management has been growing exponentially. Cross-specialty discourse and the exchange of ideas are essential for neurosurgery to maintain its position as the emperor of all specialties.

Recommended Reading

1. *Complications: A young surgeon's notes on an imperfect science.* Atul Gawande Picador books. 2002
2. *Better: A surgeon's notes on performance.* Atul Gawande Penguin books 2007
3. *Checklist Manifesto: How to get things right.* Atul Gawande Penguin Viking 2009
4. *The Naked Surgeon: The power and peril of transparency in medicine.* Samer Naschef Scribe Publications 2015
5. *The Best Practice: How the new quality movement is transforming medicine.* Charles Kenney 2008. Public Affairs Books, Perseus Books Group.

Conflict of Interest Statement The authors have no conflicts of interest concerning the reported materials or methods.

References

1. Fargen K, Friedman W. The science of medical decision making: neurosurgery, errors, and personal cognitive strategies for improving quality of care. World Neurosurg. 2014;82:e21–9.
2. Eckenhoff JE. In: Lunn JN, editor. Leadership: a determining factor in quality care, quality of Care in Anesthetic Practice. London: Macmillan; 1984. p. 306–14.
3. Sullenberger C. In: Gordon S, Mendenhall P, O'Connor B, editors. Beyond the checklist. What else health care can learn from aviation teamwork and safety, Ithaca. Cornell University Press; 2013.
4. Sexton JB, Thomas EJ, Helmreich RL. Error, stress, and teamwork in medicine and aviation: cross-sectional surveys. Br Med J. 2000;320:754–9.
5. Cooper JB, Newbower RS, Long CD, McPeek B. Preventable anesthesia mishaps: a study of human factors. Anesthesiology. 1978;49:399–406.
6. Haynes AB, Berry WR, Gawande AA. What do we know about the safe surgery checklist now? Ann Surg. 2015;261(5):829–30.
7. Kapur N, Parand A, Soukup T, Reader T, Sevdalis N. Aviation and healthcare: a comparative review with implications for patient safety. JRSM Open; 2015.
8. Schelkun S. Lessons from aviation safety: 'plan your operation—operate your plan'. Patient Saf Surg. 2014;8:1–3.
9. Beecher HK, Todd DP. A study of the deaths associated with anesthesia and surgery. Ann Surg. 1954;140:2–34.
10. Philips OC, Capizzi LS. Anesthesia mortality, Public Health Aspects of Critical Care Medicine and Anesthesiology. Peter Safar. Philadelphia, FA Davis(eds) 1974 pp 220–39.
11. Nashef SA. What is a near miss? Lancet. 2001;361(9352):180–1.
12. Leape LL. Reporting of adverse events. N Engl J Med. 2002;347(20):1633–8.
13. Wilson CB. Postoperative complications in neurosurgical practice: recognition, prevention, and management. JAMA. 1967;200(12):1135.
14. Pool JL. Postoperative complications in neurosurgical practice. Arch Neurol. 1967;17(2):223.
15. Deming WE. Out of the crisis. Cambridge, MA: MIT Center for Advanced Engineering Study; 1986.
16. Donabedian A. The quality of care. How can it be assessed? JAMA. 1988;260:1743–8.
17. Berwick DM. Continuous improvement as an ideal in Health care. N Engl J Med. 1989;320(1):53–6.
18. Leape LL. Error in medicine. JAMA. 1994;272:1851–7.
19. The report of the public inquiry into children's heart surgery at the Bristol Royal Infirmatory 1984-1995:learning from Bristol (2001) Bristol Royal Infirmatory Inquiry, Department of health, London.
20. Crossing the quality chasm: a new health system for the 21st century (2001) Institute of Medicine (US) Committee on Quality of Health Care in America. National Academies Press Washington (DC): (US).
21. Nashef SA. European system for cardiac operative risk evaluation (EuroSCORE). Eur J Cardiothorac Surg. 1999;16(1):9–13.
22. Landsberger HA. Hawthorne revisited. Ithaca, New York: Cornell University Press; 1958.
23. Pinto A, Faiz O, Bicknell C, et al. Acute traumatic stress among surgeons after major surgical complications. Am J Surg. 2014;208:642–7.
24. Cooper JB, Gaba DM, Liang B. The National Patient Safety Foundation agenda for research and development in patient safety. Med Gen Med. 2000;2:E38.
25. Macrae C, Vincent C. Learning from failure: the need for independent safety investigation in healthcare. J R Soc Med. 2014;107:439–43.
26. Bhangu A, Bhangu S, Stevenson J, Bowley DM. Lessons for surgeons in the final moments of Air France Flight 447. World J Surg. 2013;37(6):1185–92.
27. Parsonnet V, Dean D, Bernstein AD. A method of uniform stratification of risk for evaluating the results of surgery in acquired adult heart disease. Circulation. 1989;79(6 Pt 2):I3–I12.

Effect of Staphylococcal Decolonization Regime on Post-Craniotomy Meningitis

Ankush Gupta and Vedantam Rajshekhar

Abstract

Post craniotomy meningitis (PCM), an uncommon complication following craniotomy can be categorized as either bacterial meningitis (BM) or aseptic meningitis (AM) based on the results of CSF culture. Staph. aureus is a common causative organism. Some patients who are nasal carriers of these organisms have been shown to be at a higher risk of acquiring surgical site infections (SSI) following general or gynecological surgeries. Staphylococcal decolonization regime (SDR), using chlorhexidine gluonate (CHG) showers and application of mupirocin ointment to the anterior nares, is an attempt to reduce the load of these bacteria in a patient prior to surgery. SDR targeted at those proven to be nasal carriers of staphylococcal bacteria, has shown to reduce SSI following general surgery, gynecological surgery and cardiothoracic surgery. However, its effectiveness in reducing PCM has been poorly investigated. In a review of the literature on the use of SDR in patients undergoing craniotomy, we found only one study where the authors used CHG showers but in a non-targeted fashion (all patients rather than only carriers). They showed a reduction in the incidence of both AM and BM following craniotomy compared to historical controls, but the study had a confounder in the form of a change of the prophylactic antibiotic used. While there is no high quality evidence that SDR is effective in reducing PCM, its relatively low cost, easy implementation and few and mild side effects, would make it attractive to adopt in patients undergoing craniotomy.

Keywords

Craniotomy · Meningitis · Staphylococcus · Decolonization · Efficacy

Introduction

Post-craniotomy meningitis (PCM), although a rare postoperative complication when compared to surgical site infections (SSIs) in neurosurgery, poses a formidable challenge to neurosurgeons in terms of both its identification and its treatment. Its incidence in the literature varies from 0.3% to 8.9% [1–9]. It results in severe morbidity and also significantly prolongs the duration of hospital stay for patients [2, 7]. The diagnosis of PCM remains more elusive than community-acquired meningitis because of its relatively indolent course and its masking of the classical signs of fever, neck rigidity, and altered sensorium following a recently concluded surgery. On the basis of the growth characteristics of microbiological cultures, PCM can be divided into bacterial meningitis (BM) and culture-negative "aseptic" meningitis (AM). A definitive distinction between the two can be made only by carrying out cerebrospinal fluid (CSF) cultures because other parameters, such as CSF glucose concentration and CSF white blood cell count, can be equivocally altered in either.

Commonly encountered bacteria that cause PCM are usually of staphylococcal origin, thought to be a contamination from microorganisms in the skin flora [10]. Patients who are nasal carriers of *Staph. aureus* tend to have a two to nine

A. Gupta · V. Rajshekhar (✉)
Department of Neurological Sciences, Christian Medical College, Vellore, India
e-mail: rajshekhar@cmcvellore.ac.in

K. Turel, E. M. Kasper (eds.), *Complications in Neurosurgery II*, Acta Neurochirurgica Supplement 133,
https://doi.org/10.1007/978-3-031-61601-3_20

times higher risk of acquiring SSI when compared to noncarriers [10]. Hence, in an attempt to reduce the incidence of PCM, a preoperative staphylococcal decolonization regimen (SDR) should logically reduce the incidence of SSI and PCM. However, only limited data are available in the neurosurgical literature on the impact of SDR on SSI and PCM. Hence, we aimed to review the existing literature on the effect of SDR on PCM to determine whether SDR should be routinely used prior to craniotomies.

Incidence of PCM

The incidence of PCM has been reported to vary from 0.3% to 8.9% [1–9]. A large multicenter prospective study assessing the incidence of neurosurgical site infections in 2944 patients concluded that the overall incidence of superficial surgical site infections (SSIs) was 4%, whereas that of deep infections, including meningitis, was 2.5% [11]. Korinek et al. [4] found the overall incidence of PCM to be 1.52% in their series of 6243 consecutive craniotomies. In another, very large Indian series of 18,092 patients, Srinivas et al. [8] found the incidence of PCM to be 2.1%. A previous study from our institution, including 1349 patients undergoing elective craniotomies, was coherent with this observation and found the incidence of PCM to be 3.2% and that of postoperative BM specifically to be 0.6% [12]. This incidence of BM had not changed much according to a comparison with another study from our institution, carried out 5 years earlier, which quoted the rate of postoperative BM to be 0.8% [13]. Reichert et al. [7] reported a relatively high incidence of PCM in their study (8.9%), of which only 32% grew out organisms on microbiological cultures for evaluation—the most common organism being *Acinetobacter baumanii*. Therefore, the majority of PCM in their patients might in fact have been AM. In a large study from China including 1162 neurosurgical patients, the incidence of PCM at 8.6% was also high, and the mean duration of hospital stay was significantly prolonged in those patients who developed PCM [2]. The relatively higher incidence of PCM in the series of these authors was attributed to the fact that their center was a large-volume referral center, translating into surgeries that were more challenging and time-consuming. The variability in the incidence of PCM in the literature is probably a result of the lack of standardized criteria for its diagnosis.

Risk Factors for PCM

Many studies have analyzed the risk factors for the development of PCM. Korinek et al. [11] found CSF leak and subsequent early reoperation to be the only independent risk factors associated with higher rates of infection, thereby emphasizing the need for meticulous surgical techniques and the prompt management of preoperative or postoperative hydrocephalus. In another study, they found CSF leakage, concomitant incisional infection, male gender, and surgical duration to be independent predictive risk factors for PCM [4]. Kourbeti et al. [5] concluded that the independent risk factors associated with PCM in their study were surgical entry into the paranasal sinuses, an increasing score on the American Society of Anesthesiology (ASA) scale, and the prolonged use of intracranial pressure (ICP) monitors or external ventricular drains (EVDs), especially when EVDs are in situ for >5 days. Reichert et al. [7] also found reoperation to be the only significant risk factor associated with PCM.

In our analysis of 1349 patients undergoing elective craniotomies, an infratentorial pathology and the presence of an intraventricular drain were the only significant risk factors for the development of postoperative AM [12]. Srinivas et al. [8] documented the presence of a pre-existing infection (such as post-pyogenic meningitis or tuberculosis with hydrocephalus) to be significant risk factors. In a study from China on 1162 neurosurgical patients, diabetes mellitus, EVDs, and lumbar drains were significant risk factors for the development of PCM [2].

Role of Prophylactic Antibiotics

The use of prophylactic perioperative antibiotics to reduce the incidence of PCM has long been a subject of debate. Barker et al. [14], in their meta-analysis of six randomized controlled trials, demonstrated a significant beneficial impact of prophylactic antibiotics on lowering the incidence of PCM as long as at least one preoperative antibiotic provided Gram-positive coverage. However, because the definitions of meningitis in those trials were variable and somewhat subjective, this result should be interpreted with caution. Another meta-analysis comprising 2365 patients concluded that prophylactic antibiotic use significantly reduced PCM [15]. On the other hand, Korinek et al. [4] concluded that although perioperative antibiotic prophylaxis did significantly reduce incision site infections, it did not provide any significant protection against PCM. On the downside, it resulted in selecting resistant microorganisms. Other studies have also corroborated these findings [2, 16]. The choice of prophylactic antibiotics also varies according to the regional microbiological flora and needs to be updated on a regular basis. Using multiple antibiotics should be avoided because this results in the selection of antibiotic-resistant microorganisms. We have provided evidence showing that a conservative prophylactic antibiotic policy does not result in an increase in the incidence of PCM [13].

Etiology of PCM

PCM can be either bacterial or aseptic, the latter accounting for up to 70% of all cases [17, 18]. Clinically, both AM and BM tend to present with signs of meningeal irritation, such as fever, worsening headache, and nuchal rigidity, but deterioration in the sensorium is generally associated with BM because these tend to have a more fulminant course. CSF white cell counts and CSF glucose are not very reliable markers in differentiating between the two in the immediate postoperative period. CSF lactate (upper normal cutoff value of 4 mmol/L) has shown promising results from its sensitivity to and specificity in predicting bacterial meningitis [19, 20]. However, the gold standard for diagnosing BM remains microbiological CSF culture data. A negative culture growth after 72 h points toward the diagnosis of AM, but occasionally, the lack of culture growth could be attributed to the administration of perioperative antibiotics. Some authors have argued that AM could be a form of low-grade BM, where bacterial DNA has been demonstrated in CSF samples after increasing the number of polymerase chain-reaction amplifications [21]. Broad-range 16S rRNA gene polymerase chain reaction (PCR) has also been proven to be useful in the identification of bacterial pathogens in culture-negative infections [22]. However, this finding has been challenged by Zarrouk et al. [23], who found no significant impact from the broad-range 16SrRNA PCR on the management of postoperative AM.

The reported culture-positivity rate in patients with suspected PCM ranges from 32% to nearly 100% [7, 9, 24]. In a large study from China, the culture-positivity rate was only 10.4%, which was possibly attributed to the usage of prophylactic antibiotics in almost all patients and to the lack of repeated CSF cultures. The most common organism in this study was *Acinetobacter baumanii* [2]. In another large study, comprising 2944 patients, *Staph. aureus* was the most common organism responsible for PCM [11]. Korinek et al. [4] found that the use of perioperative antibiotic prophylaxis probably resulted in patients' developing PCM caused by noncutaneous bacteria, especially *Enterobacteriaceae*. In the Indian population, the most common organisms responsible for PCM range from Gram-positive cocci (staphylococcal species) to Gram-negative bacilli (nonfermenting Gram-negative bacilli—i.e., *Pseudomonas* and *Acinetobacter*) [8, 12, 13]. Significant regional variability has been found in the bacterial organisms cultured in the CSF of patients with PCM, though no obvious geographic trend can be noted [16].

Morbidity and Mortality Associated with PCM

PCM results in significant postoperative morbidity and mortality, therefore mandating its prompt recognition and treatment. Many authors have found that PCM significantly prolongs hospital stay [2, 7]. Erdem et al. [3] reported a high mortality rate, that of 40.8%, in their patients who developed PCM. They concluded that mortality in these patients was significantly associated with the presence of a concomitant nosocomial infection, a GCS score <10, and a CSF glucose value <30 mg/dL. In another large study, comprising 3580 patients undergoing neurosurgical operations, the case fatality rate due to PCM was 8%, the predictors of mortality being low CSF glucose concentration (<1.66 mmol/L), increasing the value of the acute physiology and chronic health evaluation (APACHE) III score and Gram-negative etiology [25]. Kourbeti et al. [5] also reported a case fatality rate of 8% among their patients who developed postoperative meningitis (n = 25) in their series of 453 patients, although the authors reported that the deaths were not directly related to meningitis. Finally, Srinivas et al. [8] reported a mortality rate of 5% among patients who developed PCM in their cohort of 18,092 neurosurgical patients.

Staphylococcal Decolonization Protocols

As microorganisms from the skin flora are implicated in the majority of the SSIs and deeper infections, such as meningitis, interventions that help to reduce the skin microbes should theoretically reduce the incidence of SSIs. The most common organism responsible for hospital-acquired infections, especially in the intensive care unit (ICU), is *Staphylococcus aureus*. About 30% of healthy adults have been found to be colonized with *Staph. aureus*, most commonly in the anterior nares or in extra-nasal sites such as the throat, perineum, or skin [26]. Relatively higher rates of colonization have been detected in hospital inpatients, HIV-infected individuals, intravenous drug users, and insulin-dependent people with diabetes [27]. The risk of postoperative infection in nasal carriers is estimated to be two to 12 times higher than that of those not colonized with *Staph. aureus* [27].

Various interventions have been used for decontaminating the skin prior to surgery. However, only a very small percentage of these interventions have been used in neurosurgical patients. One such intervention uses a chlorhexidine gluconate (CHG) shower a minimum of three times prior to surgery. Instructions for the procedure are mentioned in a handout that can be given to patients [28]. Intranasal mupirocin ointment application has been quite extensively studied and has been shown to rapidly eradicate methicillin-resistant *Staphylococcus aureus* (MRSA) from the anterior nares. However, it does not offer long-term protection against colonization [26]. Harbarth et al. used real-time PCR testing to screen patients for MRSA colonization and used a combination of intranasal mupirocin ointment and chlorhexidine body wash for 5 days prior to surgery [29]. Chlorhexidine gluconate application to the nasopharynx and oropharynx has also been tried in patients undergoing cardiac surgery [30]. Multiple other topical agents and systemic agents have been tried for staphylococcal decolonization, but the most studied agents remain topical intranasal mupirocin ointment and chlorhexidine body wash [26].

There is some debate on whether SDR should be universally applied or applied only to those patients in whom colonization with staphylococcal organisms has been established through testing [12, 26, 29–31]. The former strategy is probably logistically easier to implement and more cost-effective, and it can be safely applied in all patients, except those who are allergic to the antiseptic agents used, because these agents have no known significant side effects [12, 31].

Impact of SDR

Very limited data are available on the impact of SDR on the incidence of PCM. This is due to two factors. First, SDR has been studied extensively in orthopedic and cardiovascular surgeries, but not in neurosurgery [27, 30, 32]. Second, the impact of SDR has been assessed for its impact on the incidence of SSI in neurosurgical patients, but not on PCM specifically.

In a large double-blind randomized control trial involving 6771 patients admitted to the departments of internal medicine, cardiothoracic surgery, vascular surgery, gastrointestinal surgery, orthopedics, or general surgery, the nasal carriage of *Staph. aureus* was determined by using real-time PCR, and those found to be carriers were then subjected to randomization to receive either SDR or the placebo. This study concluded that the implementation of an SDR in *Staph. aureus* carriers significantly reduces the risk of deep SSIs in surgical patients and reduces the average hospital stay by 2 days [33]. Lefebvre et al. [31] screened patients undergoing deep brain stimulation for the presence of *Staph. aureus* in the nasal passage and implemented an SDR in those who tested positive. They found a significant reduction in the incidence of SSI in those patients undergoing screening, from 10.9% to 1.6%. In a large cohort of 4266 patients undergoing spinal surgery, Chan et al. [34] found a significant reduction in the incidence of SSIs postoperatively, after an implementation of SDR involving CHG showers. On performing a subgroup analysis, they found a significant reduction in SSIs in the cohort of patients undergoing nonfusion surgeries, while the reduction in SSI in the cohort undergoing spinal fusion surgeries was not statistically significant.

In our study on the impact of SDR [12], we analyzed a total of 1349 patients undergoing elective craniotomies, who were subdivided into two groups: 622 patients before and 727 patients after the implementation of an SDR. The SDR included 4% chlorhexidine body bath once daily and a twice daily nasal application of a 10% betadine ointment, for at least 2 days prior to surgery, and it was implemented in all patients without performing screening for *Staph. aureus* nasal carriage. Along with this, the perioperative antibiotic prophylaxis was also changed for the latter group of patients from chloramphenicol to ceftriaxone. The overall incidence of PCM in our study was 3.2%. We found that the initiation of SDR in patients undergoing elective cranial surgery reduced the incidence of both BM (from 0.8% to 0.4%) and AM (from 3.7% to 1.7%), the reduction in incidence of AM being statistically significant. There was also no significant side effect of this decolonization regime. To our knowledge, this is the only study in the literature analyzing the incidence of PCM after the implementation of SDR.

Other conflicting reports in literature have failed to show any significant benefit of SDR on postoperative hospital-acquired infection. In one recent study including 3126 cranial procedures, the implementation of a preoperative CHG shower protocol did not significantly reduce the incidence of SSI [28]. The only factor that they found significant in reducing SSI was the insertion of surgical drains. They also found that the implementation of an SDR did not alter the causative microorganisms of SSIs in their cohort. Perl et al. [35] conducted a double-blind randomized control trial involving 4030 patients undergoing various general, gynecologic, neurologic, or cardiothoracic surgeries. They concluded that the intranasal application of mupirocin ointment did not reduce the incidence of *Staph. aureus* infections overall, but it did significantly reduce the SSIs in those patients who were confirmed to be nasal carriers of *Staph. aureus*. Another study involving patients undergoing cardiac surgery failed to show any significant benefit of prophylactic intranasal mupirocin application in reducing postoperative SSIs [36].

Conclusions

The implementation of SDR using a combination of nasal and extra-nasal agents probably provides protection against the development of hospital-acquired SSIs, especially in patients who are carriers of *Staph. aureus*. However, because no major adverse event is due to the SDR, it can prophylactically be used for all patients undergoing neurosurgical procedures. The most commonly used combination is that of intranasal mupirocin ointment application and chlorhexidine body wash. Although limited, some evidence has shown that SDR does reduce the incidence of PCM and SSIs in a neurosurgical setting.

References

1. Chen C-H, Chang C-Y, Lin L-J, Chen WL, Chang Y-J, Wang S-H, Cheng C-Y, Yen H-C. Risk factors associated with postcraniotomy meningitis: a retrospective study. Medicine (Baltimore). 2016;95:e4329.
2. Chen C, Zhang B, Yu S, Sun F, Ruan Q, Zhang W, Shao L, Chen S. The incidence and risk factors of meningitis after major craniotomy in China: a retrospective cohort study. PLoS One. 2014;9:e101961.
3. Erdem I, Hakan T, Ceran N, Metin F, Akcay SS, Kucukercan M, Berkman MZ, Goktas P. Clinical features, laboratory data, management and the risk factors that affect the mortality in patients with postoperative meningitis. Neurol India. 2008;56:433–7.
4. Korinek A-M, Baugnon T, Golmard J-L, van Effenterre R, Coriat P, Puybasset L. Risk factors for adult nosocomial meningitis after craniotomy role of antibiotic prophylaxis. Neurosurgery. 2006;59:126–33.
5. Kourbeti IS, Jacobs AV, Koslow M, Karabetsos D, Holzman RS. Risk factors associated with postcraniotomy meningitis. Neurosurgery. 2007;60:317–26.
6. McClelland S, Hall WA. Postoperative central nervous system infection: incidence and associated factors in 2111 neurosurgical procedures. Clin Infect Dis. 2007;45:55–9.
7. Reichert MCF, Medeiros EAS, Ferraz FAP. Hospital-acquired meningitis in patients undergoing craniotomy: incidence, evolution, and risk factors. Am J Infect Control. 2002;30:158–64.
8. Srinivas D, Kumari HV, Somanna S, Bhagavatula I, Anandappa CB. The incidence of postoperative meningitis in neurosurgery: an institutional experience. Neurol India. 2011;59:195.
9. Wang Y, Wang Y, Ma W. Etiology and risk factors for meningitis and/or bacteremia after craniotomy for patients with glioma. Zhong Nan Da Xue Xue Bao Yi Xue Ban. 2018;43:410–4.
10. Humphreys H, Becker K, Dohmen PM, Petrosillo N, Spencer M, van Rijen M, Wechsler-Fördös A, Pujol M, Dubouix A, Garau J. Staphylococcus aureus and surgical site infections: benefits of screening and decolonization before surgery. J Hosp Infect. 2016;94:295–304.
11. Korinek AM. Risk factors for neurosurgical site infections after craniotomy: a prospective multicenter study of 2944 patients. The French study Group of Neurosurgical Infections, the SEHP, and the C-CLIN Paris-Nord. Service Epidémiologie Hygiène et Prévention Neurosurgery. 1997;41:1073–9.
12. Gupta A, Nair RR, Moorthy RK, Rajshekhar V. Effect of staphylococcal decolonization regimen and change in antibiotic prophylaxis regimen on incidence of postcraniotomy aseptic meningitis. World Neurosurg. 2018;119:e534–40.
13. Moorthy RK, Sarkar H, Rajshekhar V. Conservative antibiotic policy in patients undergoing non-trauma cranial surgery does not result in higher rates of postoperative meningitis: an audit of nine years of narrow-spectrum prophylaxis. Br J Neurosurg. 2013;27:497–502.
14. Barker FG. Efficacy of prophylactic antibiotics against meningitis after craniotomy: a meta-analysis. Neurosurgery. 2007;60:887–94.
15. Alotaibi AF, Hulou MM, Vestal M, Alkholifi F, Asgarzadeh M, Cote DJ, Bi WL, Dunn IF, Mekary RA, Smith TR. The efficacy of antibacterial prophylaxis against the development of meningitis after craniotomy: a meta-analysis. World Neurosurg. 2016;90:597–603.
16. Hussein K, Bitterman R, Shofty B, Paul M, Neuberger A. Management of post-neurosurgical meningitis: narrative review. Clin Microbiol Infect. 2017;23:621–8.
17. Van de Beek D, Drake JM, Tunkel AR. Nosocomial bacterial meningitis. N Engl J Med. 2010;362:146–54.
18. Zarrouk V, Vassor I, Bert F, Bouccara D, Kalamarides M, Bendersky N, Redondo A, Sterkers O, Fantin B. Evaluation of the management of postoperative aseptic meningitis. Clin Infect Dis. 2007;44:1555–9.
19. Leib SL, Boscacci R, Gratzl O, Zimmerli W. Predictive value of cerebrospinal fluid (CSF) lactate level versus CSF/blood glucose ratio for the diagnosis of bacterial meningitis following neurosurgery. Clin Infect Dis. 1999;29:69–74.
20. Xiao X, Zhang Y, Zhang L, Kang P, Ji N. The diagnostic value of cerebrospinal fluid lactate for post-neurosurgical bacterial meningitis: a meta-analysis. BMC Infect Dis. 2016;16:1–9.
21. Druel B, Vandenesch F, Greenland T, Verneau V, Grando J, Salord F, Christen R, Etienne J. Aseptic meningitis after neurosurgery: a demonstration of bacterial involvement. Clin Microbiol Infect. 1996;1:230–4.
22. Rampini SK, Bloemberg GV, Keller PM, Büchler AC, Dollenmaier G, Speck RF, Böttger EC. Broad-range 16S rRNA gene polymerase chain reaction for diagnosis of culture-negative bacterial infections. Clin Infect Dis. 2011;53:1245–51.
23. Zarrouk V, Leflon-Guibout V, Robineaux S, Kalamarides M, Nicolas-Chanoine M-H, Sterkers O, Fantin B. Broad-range 16S rRNA PCR with cerebrospinal fluid may be unreliable for management of postoperative aseptic meningitis. J Clin Microbiol. 2010;48:3331–3.
24. Kourbeti IS, Vakis AF, Ziakas P, Karabetsos D, Potolidis E, Christou S, Samonis G. Infections in patients undergoing craniotomy: risk factors associated with post-craniotomy meningitis. J Neurosurg. 2015;122:1113–9.
25. Federico G, Tumbarello M, Spanu T, Rosell R, Iacoangeli M, Scerrati M, Tacconelli E. Risk factors and prognostic indicators of bacterial meningitis in a cohort of 3580 postneurosurgical patients. Scand J Infect Dis. 2001;33:533–7.
26. Simor AE. Staphylococcal decolonisation: an effective strategy for prevention of infection? Lancet Infect Dis. 2011;11:952–62.
27. Kluytmans J, van Belkum A, Verbrugh H. Nasal carriage of Staphylococcus aureus: epidemiology, underlying mechanisms, and associated risks. Clin Microbiol Rev. 1997;10:505–20.
28. Ammanuel SG, Edwards CS, Chan AK, Mummaneni PV, Kidane J, Vargas E, D'Souza S, Nichols AD, Sankaran S, Abla AA. Are preoperative chlorhexidine gluconate showers associated with a reduction in surgical site infection following craniotomy? A retrospective cohort analysis of 3126 surgical procedures. J Neurosurg. 2021;1:1–9.
29. Harbarth S, Fankhauser C, Schrenzel J, Christenson J, Gervaz P, Bandiera-Clerc C, Renzi G, Vernaz N, Sax H, Pittet D. Universal screening for methicillin-resistant Staphylococcus aureus at hospital admission and nosocomial infection in surgical patients. JAMA. 2008;299:1149–57.
30. Segers P, Speekenbrink RGH, Ubbink DT, van Ogtrop ML, de Mol BA. Prevention of nosocomial infection in cardiac surgery by decontamination of the nasopharynx and oropharynx with chlorhexidine gluconate: a randomized controlled trial. JAMA. 2006;296:2460–6.
31. Lefebvre J, Buffet-Bataillon S, Henaux PL, Riffaud L, Morandi X, Haegelen C. Staphylococcus aureus screening and decolonization reduces the risk of surgical site infections in patients undergoing deep brain stimulation surgery. J Hosp Infect. 2017;95:144–7.
32. Rao N, Cannella B, Crossett LS, Yates AJJ, McGough RI. A preoperative decolonization protocol for Staphylococcus aureus prevents orthopaedic infections. Clin Orthop Relat Res. 2008;466:1343–8.

33. Bode LGM, Kluytmans JAJW, Wertheim HFL, et al. Preventing surgical-site infections in nasal carriers of Staphylococcus aureus. N Engl J Med. 2010;362:9–17.
34. Chan AK, Ammanuel SG, Chan AY, et al. Chlorhexidine showers are associated with a reduction in surgical site infection following spine surgery: an analysis of 4266 consecutive surgeries. Neurosurgery. 2019;85:817–26.
35. Perl TM, Cullen JJ, Wenzel RP, Zimmerman MB, Pfaller MA, Sheppard D, Twombley J, French PP, Herwaldt LA, Mupirocin and the Risk of Staphylococcus aureus Study Team. Intranasal mupirocin to prevent postoperative Staphylococcus aureus infections. N Engl J Med. 2002;346:1871–7.
36. Konvalinka A, Errett L, Fong IW. Impact of treating Staphylococcus aureus nasal carriers on wound infections in cardiac surgery. J Hosp Infect. 2006;64:162–8.

Cerebral Vasospasm Following the Endoscopic Endonasal Resection of Craniopharyngioma

Shejoy P. Joshua, Dilip Panikar, and Vineeth Viswam

Abstract

Cerebral vasospasm following an endoscopic endonasal resection of a craniopharyngioma is a rare, devastating occurrence that can lead to delayed cerebral ischemia and a poor neurological outcome if not diagnosed and treated in a timely manner. The etiology of this condition is not well understood. In this chapter, we present a case of cerebral vasospasm following transsphenoidal surgery (TSS) for craniopharyngioma, review the literature, and identify common presenting symptoms, probable predisposing factors, and essential management strategies to treat this condition.

Keywords

Vasospasm · Endoscopic surgery · Craniopharyngioma

Introduction

Craniopharyngiomas are rare epithelial tumors arising from the remnants of the embryonic epithelial cells of the craniopharyngeal duct. They account for 1.2–4% of all primary intracranial neoplasms and up to 5–10% of intracranial tumors in children in a tertiary referral center [1]. Considerable morbidity and mortality are associated with the surgical treatment of these tumors because of their proximity to critical neurovascular structures, particularly the visual pathway and hypothalamus. Advances in open and endoscopic skull base techniques have made safe resection possible in many patients; however, little is known about vasospasm, leading to delayed cerebral ischemia following endoscopic surgery on these lesions.

Cerebral vasospasm is a complication best known in the setting of aneurysmal subarachnoid hemorrhage with its associated morbidity and mortality. However, encountering vasospasm following endoscopic endonasal surgery for lesions extending into the suprasellar cisterns is uncommon. This condition can lead to delayed cerebral ischemia and a poor neurologic outcome if not diagnosed and treated in a timely manner [2]. Its pathophysiology is related to the structural and biochemical changes in the vascular endothelium and smooth muscle [3, 4].

The common management strategy is based on the treatment of vasospasm in aneurysmal subarachnoid hemorrhages. In this report, the need for high vigilance over this potentially devastating, delayed complication of transsphenoidal surgery; its probable causes; and its management are discussed.

Case Report

A 47-year-old nonsmoker presented with visual deterioration for about 2 months. On evaluation, he showed bitemporal hemianopia and panhypopituitarism. His MRI showed a solid cystic lesion in the sellar region with suprasellar extension suggestive of craniopharyngioma (Fig. 1). The lesion was excised via an endoscopic endonasal approach. He underwent an uneventful postoperative course. Postoperative MRI showed the complete resection of the lesion with minimal subarachnoid hemorrhage (SAH) in the surgical bed and left Sylvian fissure (Fig. 2a, b). However, on the tenth postoperative day, he developed right-sided hemiplegia and aphasia. MRI showed multiple acute infarcts in both cerebral hemispheres, the left side being more affected than the right with middle cerebral artery (MCA) and anterior cerebral artery (ACA) territory

S. P. Joshua (✉) · D. Panikar · V. Viswam
Department of Neurosurgery and Otorhinolaryngology, Aster Medcity, Kochi, Kerala, India
e-mail: drshejoy.joshua@asterhospital.com; drdilip.panikar@asterhospital.com; drvineeth.viswam@asterhospital.com

K. Turel, E. M. Kasper (eds.), *Complications in Neurosurgery II*, Acta Neurochirurgica Supplement 133,
https://doi.org/10.1007/978-3-031-61601-3_21

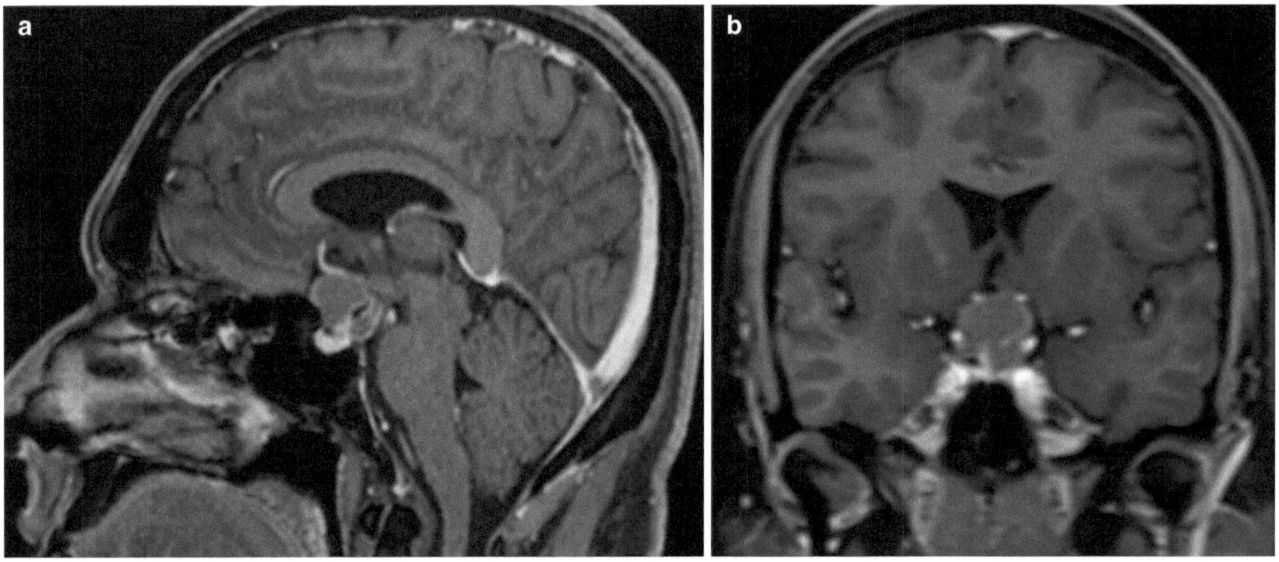

Fig. 1 (**a**) Preoperative MRI T1 post-gadolinium contrast sagittal images and (**b**) coronal images showing suprasellar extension of the lesion abutting the ICA and splaying the ACA superiorly

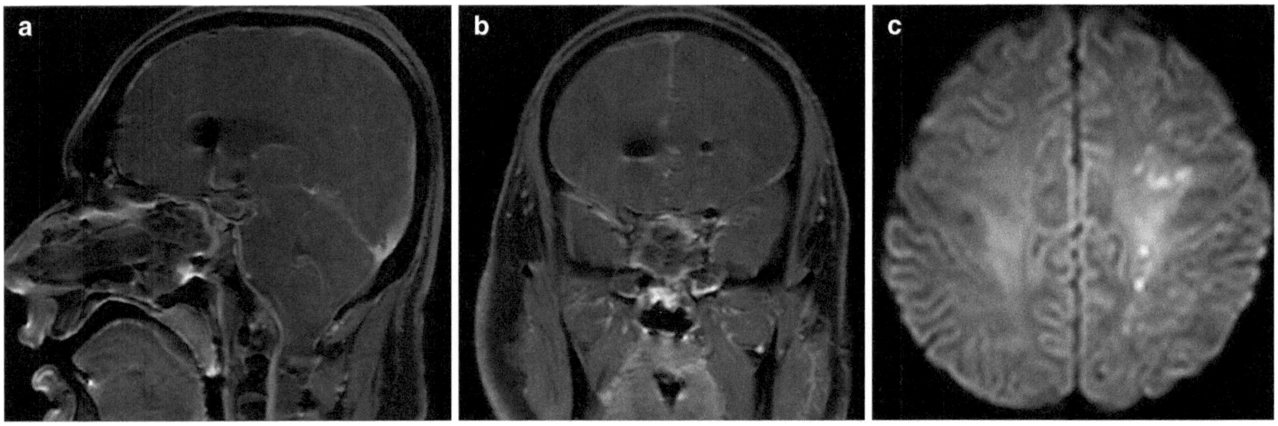

Fig. 2 (**a**) Postoperative MRI T1 post-gadolinium contrast sagittal images and (**b**) coronal images showing complete excision of the lesion; (**c**) diffusion-weighted MRI brain on tenth postoperative day showing bilateral cerebral ischemic changes (left > right)

infarcts (Fig. 2c). A transcranial doppler (TCD) evaluation showed characteristic features suggestive of bilateral middle cerebral artery vasospasm. This was confirmed on digital subtraction angiogram (DSA), which showed a significant spasm involving the bilateral middle (M1 segment) and anterior cerebral arteries (Fig. 3a, c). An intra-arterial bolus infusion of 2 mg of nifedipine was given bilaterally. The post-infusion angiogram showed an improvement in the spasm bilaterally (right side > left side) (Fig. 3b, d). He was then maintained on hypertensive therapy and euvolemia. After 48 hours, however, he was found to have persistent vasospasm on TCD assessments. A repeat catheter angiography showed 70% stenosis of the bilateral distal internal cerebral artery (ICA), M1, and M2 segments of the MCA with post-spasm vasodilatation. A microwire and Sceptre C 4 × 10 mm balloon catheter (Microvention—Terumo, California) was used to perform angioplasty by dilating the bilateral ICA, M1, and M2 segments with a 50% balloon diameter. After the angioplasty, he showed good flow across the ICA and resolution of the vasospasm (Fig. 4). He was maintained on hypertensive therapy. Repeat TCD assessments showed improvements in vascular velocities, and physical rehabilitation and speech therapy were initiated.

His hemiplegia and speech improved in 10 days, and he was ambulant with support at the time of discharge. A repeat MRI brain with magnetic resosnance angiogram (MRA), prior to discharge, showed no further extension of the areas affected by the infarcts and no vasospasm. Sequential MRI at 3-month, 1-year, and 2-year follow-ups showed no recurrence of the lesion and small patchy gliotic areas at the previous infarcts (Fig. 5).

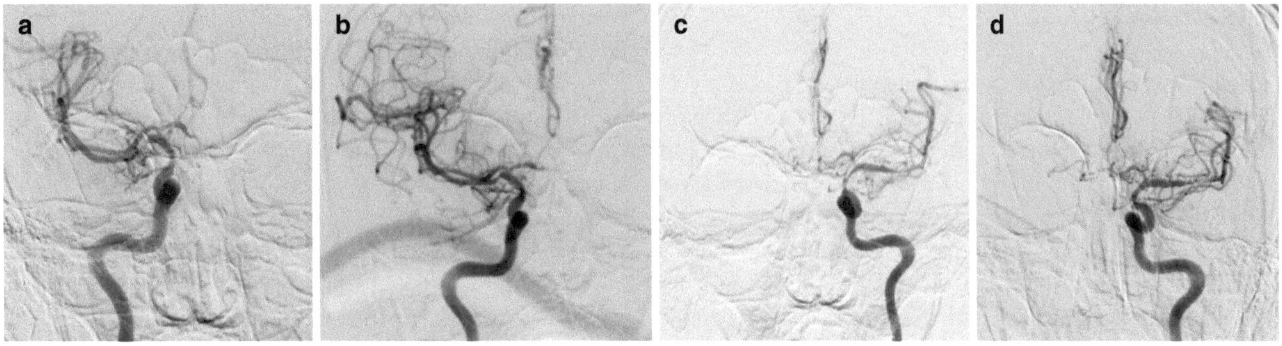

Fig. 3 DSA images: (**a**) right ICA injection, prior to nifedipine infusion, showing vessel in spasm; (**b**) post-nifedipine right ICA injection showing dilatation of vessels; (**c**) left ICA injection, prior to nifedipine infusion, showing vessel in spasm; (**d**) post-nifedipine left ICA injection showing dilatation of vessels. Post-infusion angiogram showed improvement in spasm bilaterally (right side > left side)

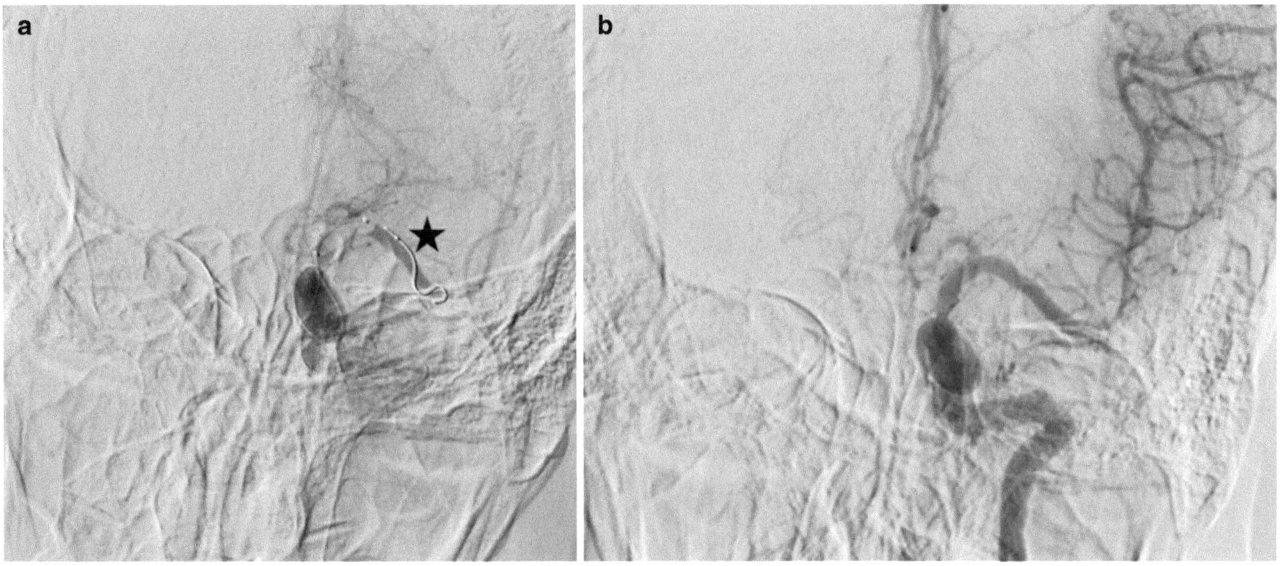

Fig. 4 DSA image showing (**a**) Sceptre C balloon catheter (*) at the MCA and (**b**) post–balloon angioplasty of left ICA injection showing dilatation of vessel with good flow in the MCA

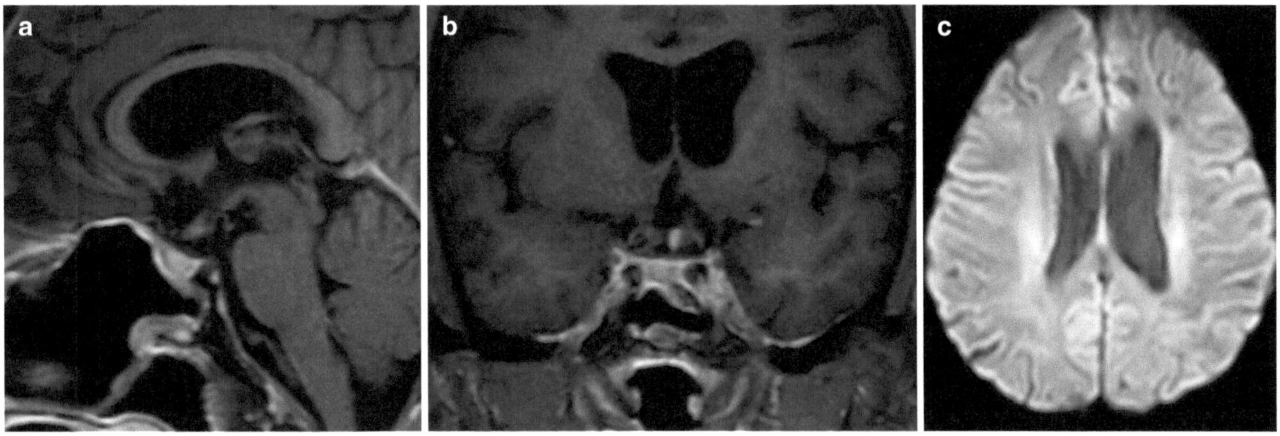

Fig. 5 (**a**) 2-year follow-up MRI T1 post-gadolinium contrast sagittal images and (**b**) coronal images showing no recurrence of the lesion. (**c**) Diffusion weighted images showing complete resolution of restriction

Discussion

Cerebral vasospasm following transsphenoidal surgery for craniopharyngioma is a rare complication, where only a few cases have been reported in literature. Because of the little awareness of this complication, it is poorly understood and often recognized late. This delay can cause serious and permanent neurological deficits. No clear protocol of management has been described in the literature, so the treatment is based on the lessons learned from the management of vasospasm in aneurysmal subarachnoid hemorrhage.

Eseonu et al. reviewed 12 reported cases of vasospasm following transsphenoidal surgery for pituitary adenoma and found that intraoperative subarachnoid hemorrhage occurred in 84% of cases. Hemoglobin degradation products (oxyhemoglobin and methemoglobin) and synthetic hemostatic material factors activate proinflammatory cytokines, which lead to oxidative stress and reduce endothelium nitric oxide, which in turn cause arterial vasospasm [5]. The postoperative MRI in our own case showed minimal blood in the surgical bed and left Sylvian fissure. The presence of subarachnoid hemorrhage on the postoperative imaging should warn the surgeon of the possibility of delayed cerebral ischemia (DCI) from vasospasm.

The onset of vasospasm after transsphenoidal surgery for suprasellar lesions appears to follow the same time course as that seen in aneurysmal subarachnoid hemorrhage, ranging from 3 to 14 days and peaking at 8–9 days postoperatively [5]. Hyponatremia serves as an early sign of DCI [6].

Causes of vasospasm other than SAH include the rupture of the cyst contents into the cisternal spaces, which causes chemical meningitis and the inflammation of vessel walls. Arterial spasm in the femoral arteries of rats following the direct instillation of craniopharyngioma cyst fluid has been reported [7]. Hence, avoiding the rupture of the cyst contents into the cisterns and proper irrigation can aid in avoiding DCI. Fat can cause aseptic meningitis, and the products of lipid metabolism have also been shown to cause vasospasm in a model studying canine basilar arteries. Hence, fat should be judiciously used for reconstruction [8]. The other rare causes of vasospasm are hypothalamic injury, especially of the median eminence [9], and the manipulation of the vessels of the circle of Willis [10].

Multiple treatment modalities have been proposed for postoperative TSS vasospasm, including hemodynamic augmentation therapy using hypertension and euvolemia, thromboxane A2 antagonists, calcium channel blockers, endovascular angioplasty or intra-arterial vasodilators, and intrathecal thrombolytics [11, 12].

Medical therapy may be sufficient in many cases. However, the early identification of this complication is the key to obtaining a good outcome, as it was in our case. A very low threshold for diagnostic DSA and endovascular therapy ensures the ability to re-establish the adequate perfusion of the brain and avoids progressive infarction. We also observed that transcranial doppler data (TCD) correlated well with the catheter angiogram findings. The diligent use of TCD can be used to monitor responses to therapy. Follow-up DSA also has a role to play in ensuring that the treatment strategies are effective, especially in cases featuring persistent vasospasm on TCD assessments.

Because most studies have suggested that blood in the cisterns predisposes the development of DCI, proper hemostasis and ample irrigation during surgery may minimize the occurrence of vasospasm. One could postulate that utilizing prophylactic nimodipine after TSS might reduce the incidence of neurological deficits once SAH has been observed. However, as a next step, additional comprehensive prospective multicenter studies are needed to determine this and more-standardized management approaches to TSS vasospasm.

Conclusion

Cerebral vasospasm following endonasal endoscopic surgery, even though a rare entity, can cause significant morbidity if not identified and treated early. Intraoperative cerebrospinal fluid (CSF) leak, the rupture of a craniopharyngioma cyst, the handling of major vessels, and postoperative peritumoral subarachnoid hemorrhage are the predisposing factors. Close observation for new-onset neurological deficits with a high index of suspicion will pick up this condition early. Effective treatment options to obtain complete neurologic recovery are hypertensive therapy, maintaining euvolemia, intra-arterial nimodipine or milrinone, and balloon angioplasty.

Conflict of Interest The authors declare that they have no conflicts of interest.

References

1. Samii M, Tatagiba M. Surgical management of craniopharyngiomas: a review. Neurol Med Chir (Tokyo). 1997;37:141–9.
2. PuriAS ZG, Zarzour H, Laws E, Frerichs K. Cerebral vasospasm after transsphenoidal resection of pituitary macroadenomas: report of 3 cases and review of the literature. Neurosurgery. 2012;71:173–80.
3. Calabrese LH, Dodick DW, Schwedt TJ, Singhal AB. Narrative review: reversible cerebral vasoconstriction syndromes. Ann Intern Med. 2007;146(1):34–44.
4. Keyrouz SG, Diringer MN. Clinical review: prevention and therapy of vasospasm in subarachnoid hemorrhage. Crit Care. 2007;11(4):220.
5. Eseonu CI, ReFaey K, Geocadin RG, Quinones-Hinojosa A. Postoperative cerebral vasospasm following transsphenoidal pituitary adenoma surgery. World Neurosurg. 2016;92:7–14.

6. Kim EH, Oh MC, Kim SH. Angiographically documented cerebral vasospasm following transsphenoidal surgery for pituitary tumors. Pituitary. 2013;16(2):260–9. https://doi.org/10.1007/s11102-012-0415-7.
7. Kamal R, Jindal A, Suri A, Mahapatra AK. Effect of craniopharyngioma fluid on femoral vessels of rat. Neurol Res. 1999;21:796–8.
8. Sasaki T, Wakai S, Asano T. The effect of a lipid hydroperoxide of arachidonic acid on the canine basilar artery. J Neurosurg. 1981;54:357–65.
9. Wilkins RH. Cerebral vasospasm in conditions other than subarachnoid hemorrhage. Neurosurg Clin N Am. 1990;1(2):329–34.
10. Gupta R, Sharma A, Vaishya R, Tandon M. Ischemic complications after pituitary surgery: a report of two cases. J Neurol Surg A Cent Eur Neurosurg. 2013;74(Suppl 1):e119–e23.
11. Kasliwal MK, Srivastava R, Sinha S, et al. Vasospasm after transsphenoidal pituitary surgery: a case report and review of the literature. Neurol India. 2008;56(1):81–3.
12. Nishioka H, Ito H, Haraoka J. Cerebral vasospasm following transsphenoidal removal of a pituitary adenoma. Br J Neurosurg. 2001;15(1):44–7.

Complications Following Decompressive Craniectomy

Dhaval P. Shukla

Abstract

Decompressive craniectomy (DC) is performed to treat refractory intracranial hypertension following traumatic brain injury and stroke. Though technically not demanding, DC is still associated with several early and delayed complications. Early complications can be fatal, whereas delayed complications may result in regression of recovery. Adequately sized DC along with aggressive medical management mitigates most of the acute complications whereas early cranioplasty prevents delayed complications.

Keywords

Decompressive craniectomy · Subdural hygroma · Cranioplasty · Syndrome of the trephined · Hinge craniotomy

Through the decades of using decompressive craniectomy (DC) in the management of refractory intracranial hypertension, it has found its place as a life-saving procedure capable of a radical reduction in intracranial pressure (ICP). Clinical results and the rate of survival after decompressive craniectomy vary according to the underlying primary diagnosis. Though technically sounding as simple as opening the lid of a pressure cooker, DC may be among the most frustrating procedures performed by neurosurgeons. These surgeries are often performed by less-experienced or more-junior surgeons. Moreover, these operations frequently occur at night. Surgery is also complicated by more-frequent adverse intraoperative events such as heavy bleeding and massive brain swelling. The decision to remove additional brain tissue (temporal lobectomy or frontal lobectomy) or cut the tent and open up any of the basilar cisterns may be difficult during surgery [1, 2].

Given the unfavorable circumstances during which DCs are mostly performed, attention also needs to be focused on complications associated with DC. One in ten patients who undergo DC develops a complication for which additional medical intervention or neurosurgical intervention, or both, are required. These complications are based not only on the procedures themselves but also on the pathophysiological changes associated with a conversion of the closed intracranial compartment to an open one. The complications may further disturb the postoperative care and convalescence in the survivors, and therefore, in salvageable patients, the indication of DC should be based on information about the expected outcome and complication rate.

At the same time, anyone undertaking DC should address key aspects such as the prevention, early recognition, and adequate therapy of complications. This review discusses the causes and consequences of and the measures to avoid or treat complications following a DC [1, 2].

Early Complications

All the following listed complications are encountered either immediately after surgery or during acute care while the patient is still in the hospital:

- Hemorrhage (hematoma expansion)
- External cerebral herniation
- Wound complications
- Cerebrospinal spinal fluid (CSF) leak/fistulae
- Postoperative infection
- Seizures

D. P. Shukla (✉)
Department of Neurosurgery, National Institute of Mental health and Neurosciences, Bangalore, Karnataka, India
e-mail: dhavalshukla@nimhans.ac.in

K. Turel, E. M. Kasper (eds.), *Complications in Neurosurgery II*, Acta Neurochirurgica Supplement 133,
https://doi.org/10.1007/978-3-031-61601-3_22

Late or Delayed Complications

The following complications are encountered after discharge from acute care, during rehabilitation, or at follow-up in the outpatient department:

- Subdural hygroma
- Hydrocephalus
- Syndrome of the trephined

Hemorrhage (Hematoma Expansion)

A new hemorrhage or expansion of pre-existing small hematoma/cerebral contusion occurs from a sudden decompression or can be due to coagulopathy. Sometimes inadvertent brain injury during craniotomy or when applying dural hitching stitches can cause a hematoma as well. These hematomas can be in any plane and are named accordingly: extradural hematoma (EDH), subdural hematoma (SDH), or intraparenchymal hematoma. Extradural and subdural hematomas can occur after any craniotomy, but the progression or expansion of brain parenchymal contusion or hematoma is unique to DC (Fig. 1).

This type of hemorrhagic expansion typically presents with a tense scalp flap bulge, with or without deterioration in the sensorium of the patient (which may not be easily picked up if the patient remains intubated and sedated after a traumatic brain injury (TBI)). Such a hematoma can be detected with bedside ultrasonography, which may be sufficient for deciding whether urgent re-exploration and evacuation are needed. If the patient is medically and neurologically stable, then a computerized tomography (CT) scan can be performed before taking any patient back for surgery. Before taking patients back to the theater for re-exploration, an in-depth review of the antithrombotic/anticoagulant medication should be carried out, and a reversal of coagulopathy should be performed. Small hematomas may not require re-exploration; however, big hematomas causing the worsening or persistence of midline shift require evacuation. The final size of an expansion of hematoma cannot be predicted. Therefore, early and more-frequent scans—such as bedside ultrasonography (USG) or CT—after DC, especially in patients with contusions and contralateral calvarial fractures, should be conducted to detect such hemorrhagic expansion early [1].

External Cerebral Herniation

The commonest cause of external brain herniation is the inadequate size of DC (Fig. 2). The inadequate medical man-

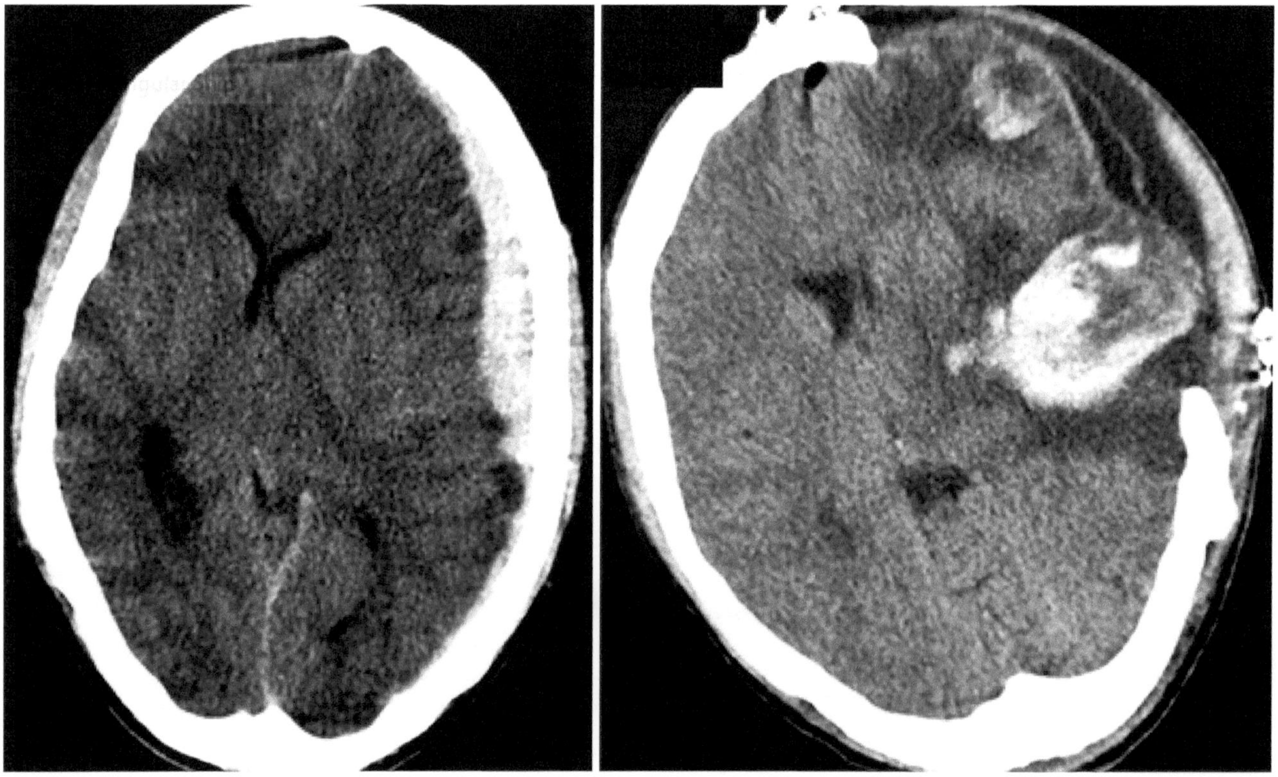

Fig. 1 CT scan (left) showing left hemispheric acute SDH. Postoperative CT scan (right) shows intraparenchymal hematoma after DC

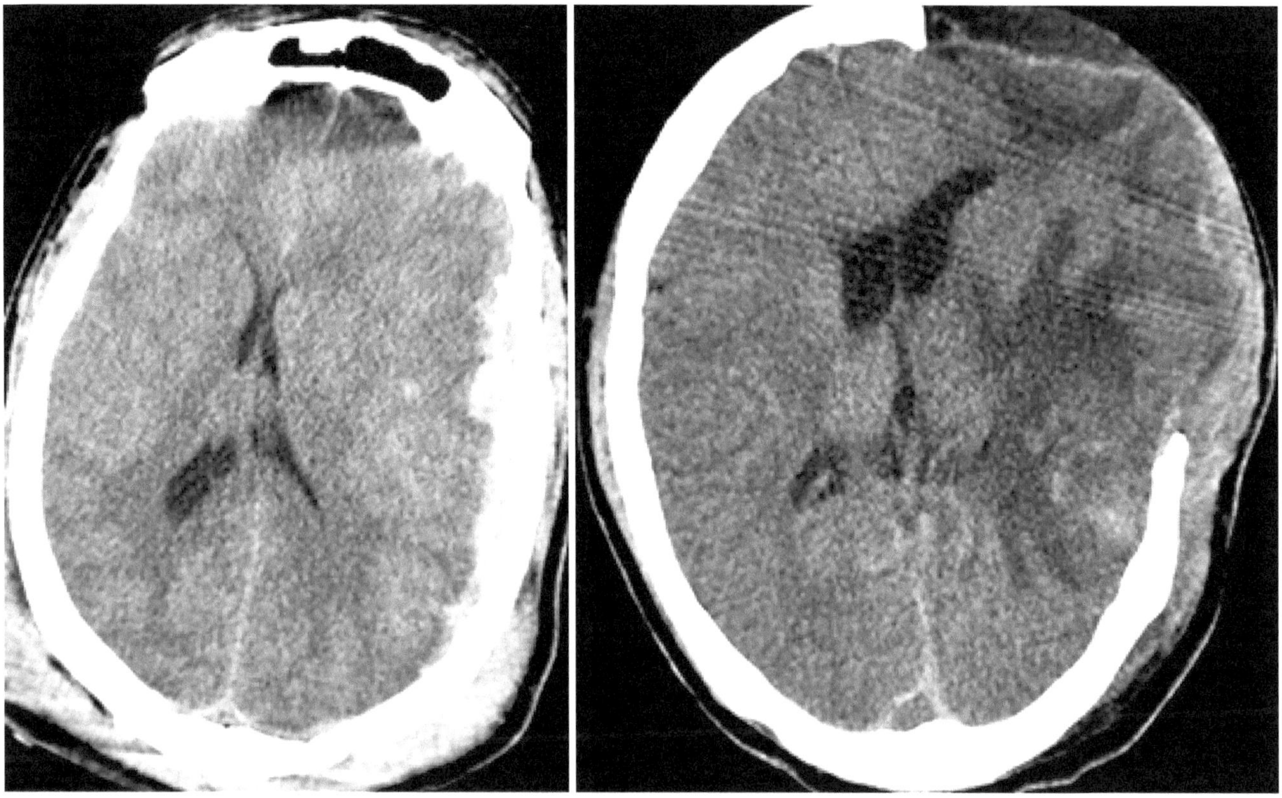

Fig. 2 CT scan following DC (right) for acute SDH (left) showing external brain herniation due to small craniectomy

agement of brain edema can also lead to external brain herniation. The bone flap should be large, at least 12 cm × 15 cm [3]. The veins over a herniating brain get compressed against the skull bone and can thrombose or get blocked, leading to the further worsening of the cerebral edema or hemorrhagic infarct. Gelfoam pledgets placed on either side of the veins between the skull bone and the brain can prevent venous occlusion. At times, the herniated brain will necrose and start oozing from the scalp wound. This can also be a cause of wound infection. In such cases, re-exploration, widening the craniectomy, and necrosectomy are required [1].

Wound Complications

Wound gaping, cerebrospinal spinal fluid (CSF) leak, and surgical site infection are not uncommon after a DC. The main causes of wound complications are brain bulge, an inability to perform watertight dural closure, and single-layer scalp closure. Though surgeons have reached consensus on expansile dural graft—e.g., sutured duraplasty or onlay—they still disagree about the optimal materials for duraplasty and the necessity of suturing expansile duraplasty [3]. We recommend a pericranial graft and watertight dura closure for the prevention of wound complications whenever possible. This can be time-consuming and difficult in the presence of a bulging brain. However, harvesting a pericranial graft does not significantly add to the duration of surgery. Because most DCs are sequential treatments after adequate medical treatment, rushing is not needed to finish the craniotomy, as in the case of an EDH, and sometimes, it can be spared to harvest the pericranial graft even before the osteotomy. The two-surgeon technique can be used for dural closure. One surgeon opens the dura, and at the same time, another surgeon starts stitching the pericranial graft to the dura to prevent brain bulge. Dural closure alone is not enough, though, and the scalp flap should be closed in two layers—galea and skin—to prevent wound disruption. At times, because of massive brain bulge, a single-layer rescue closure can be performed. Patients who require such rescue closure may not survive, and the relatives of the patients should be counseled after surgery.

Scalp flap necrosis is an extreme form of a wound complication after DC (Fig. 3). Conventionally, a reverse question mark trauma flap is raised for DC. When performed in

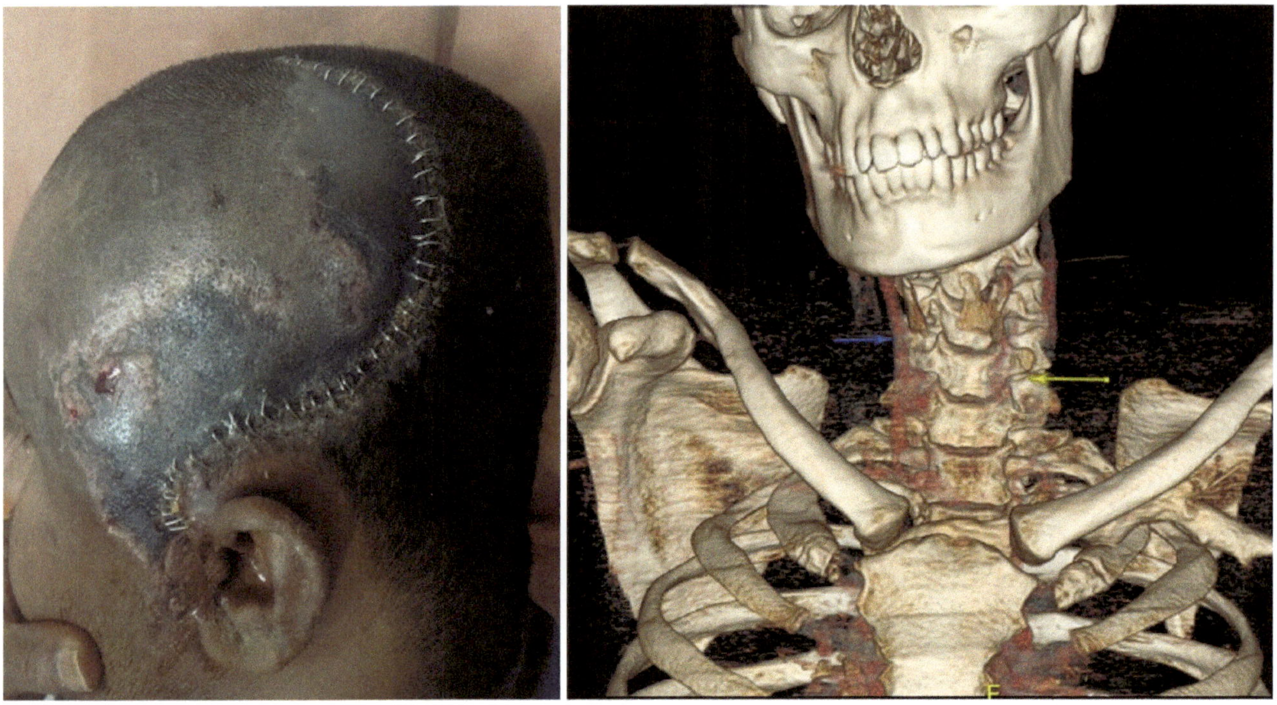

Fig. 3 A case of scalp flap necrosis (left) following DC for hemispheric malignant infarction. CT angiogram (right) showing complete occlusion of the left common carotid artery. The complete occlusion of the common carotid artery may be the reason for the devascularization of the scalp flap

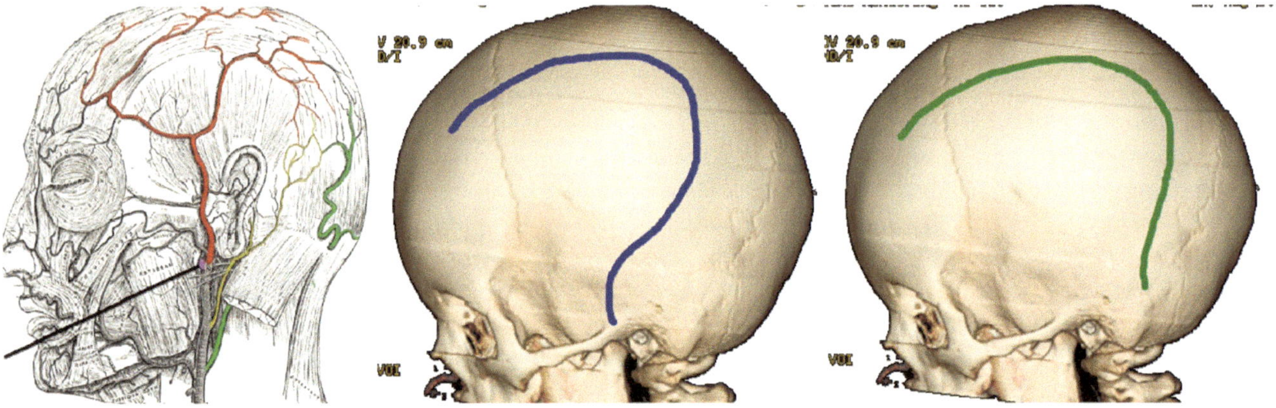

Fig. 4 Blood supply of scalp (left) showing three main arteries: the superficial temporal artery (STA), posterior auricular artery (PAA), and occipital artery. A conventional reverse question mark flap (middle) will disrupt the blood supply from STA and PAA. A retroauricular incision (right) will preserve the blood supply from STA and PAA

a hurry, the superficial temporal artery may get cut, and when the flap extends more posteriorly to the pinna, even the postauricular artery can get cut, leading to a reduction in the blood supply of the flap itself (Fig. 4). Alternative incisions have been proposed in the literature to mitigate postoperative wound complications [4, 5]. The retroauricular (RA) incision is an alternative incision that increases calvarium exposure to maximize the removal of the hemicranium and decreases wound-related complications when compared to a standard preauricular incision [5]. The Kempe incision (T shaped, one limb on midline vertex from the frontal hairline to the inion, and another perpendicular limb from mid vertex to mid zygoma) has been proposed for DC for TBI patients and stroke patients

(Fig. 5). The outcomes were comparable, with a trend toward a larger decompression with the Kempe incision. This incision can also be easily converted to bilateral or bifrontal [4].

A significant brain bulge can cause wound-healing problems. If possible, an external ventricular drain (EVD) should be inserted to monitor and reduce ICP by draining CSF.

The main dreaded consequence of wound problems is meningitis. In extreme cases, even a brain abscess can occur below the scalp flap (Fig. 6). The intracranial infection leads to greater mortality, an increase in the duration of hospital stay, and a delay in cranioplasty.

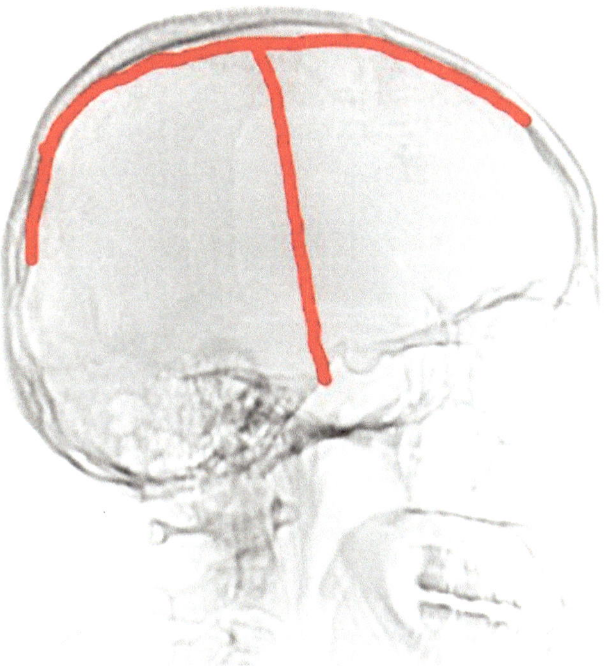

Fig. 5 Kempe incision

These wound complications cannot be ignored. They require early detection and prompt management. At times, a plastic surgeon consultation may help improve and accelerate wound healing.

Subdural Effusion and Hydrocephalus

The DC results in a loss of pressure gradient between CSF spaces and venous sinuses. This results in a dampening of the pulsatility of CSF, likely resulting in an impaired absorption of CSF. The altered CSF flow abnormality can cause subdural effusions, which may be ipsilateral, interhemispheric, and contralateral (Fig. 7) [6]. Hydrocephalus is also a consequence of altered CSF flow abnormalities (Fig. 8) [7]. Most of the time, the CSF flow abnormality resolves on its own. Any persistent subdural effusion or hydrocephalus results in worse neurological outcomes. The presence of any of them should be suspected if the scalp bulge reappears after a flat postoperative period, if the patient fails to hold the gains of initial improvement, or if the deterioration is delayed.

Restricting the superior and medial margins of the craniotomy to 2.5 cm from the midline helps to prevent CSF flow abnormalities. The Pacchionian granulations and arachnoidal villi are present in the paramedian dura. The presence of a strip of bone over the midline retains the pressure gradient between the CSF and the venous sinus, allowing for better CSF absorption. Moreover, avoiding craniotomy too close to the midline also results in less blood loss.

We have observed a relatively low incidence of subdural effusions in our cases of DC. We routinely close the dura by using pericranium as our duraplasty material of choice. We hypothe-

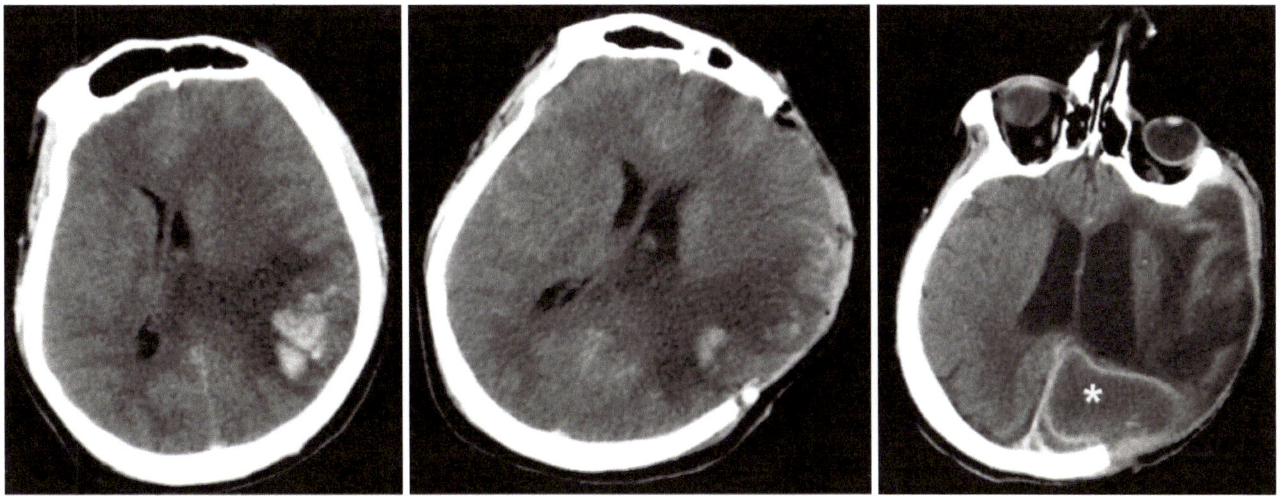

Fig. 6 A case of malignant cerebral edema due to cerebral venous infarct (left). The CT scan after DC (middle) showed adequate decompression. The patient developed a surgical site infection, which led to the development of the brain abscess (right)

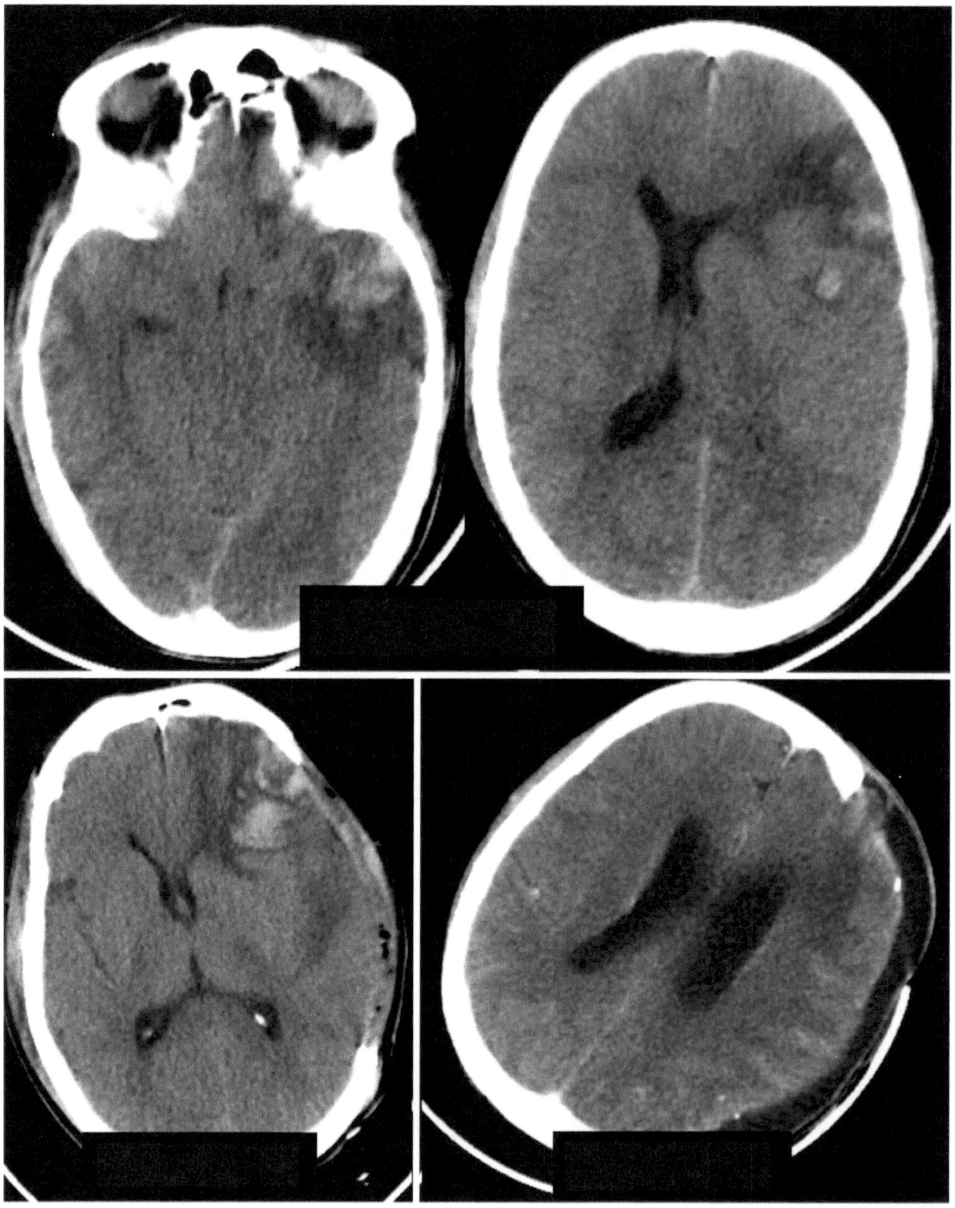

Fig. 7 Serial CT scans showing the development of subdural hygroma following DC

size that the pericranium acts as a semipermeable membrane allowing the absorption of CSF in the subcutaneous tissue.

Early cranioplasty also helps in the prevention of subdural hygromas and hydrocephalus. Cranioplasty often results in the resolution of subdural effusions [6].

The management of hydrocephalus following DC is controversial. No consensus has been reached on the timing of any shunt and cranioplasty. We prefer to place an EVD in the perioperative period during cranioplasty. If the symptomatic hydrocephalus persists after cranioplasty, then a ventriculoperitoneal (VP) shunt is inserted. A programmable VP shunt with an antisiphon device is preferred for hydrocephalus secondary to DC.

Sunken Scalp Flap Syndrome

Syndrome of the trephined, also known as sinking skin flap syndrome, results from a lack of structural support and subatmospheric intracranial pressure (Fig. 9). Changes in blood flow and fluid shifts cause the symptoms of this syndrome. The consequences of this syndrome can be diverse and include multiple new neurological symptoms, failure to hold the gains of initial improvement, delayed deterioration, and delayed community integration despite good neurological recovery. Early cranioplasty is indicated to prevent and treat the syndrome of the trephined [1].

Paradoxical Herniation

When a lumbar puncture is performed in a patient who has undergone a DC, a rapid fluid collection is seen in the subdural space causing midline shift, resulting in paradoxical herniation (Fig. 10). Paradoxical herniation can also result from dehydration, mannitol therapy, CSF leak, or hyperventila-

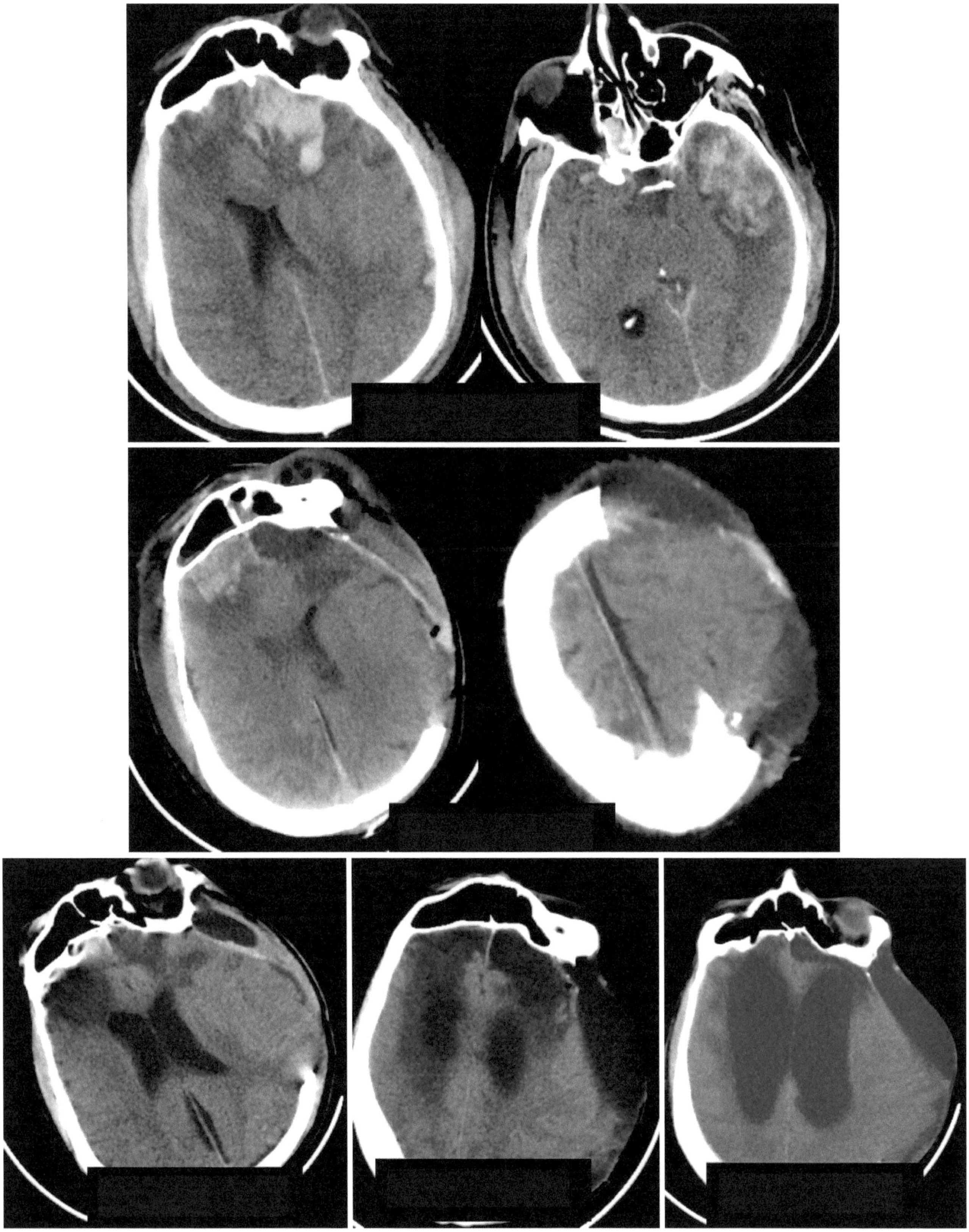

Fig. 8 Serial CT scans showing the development of hydrocephalus following DC

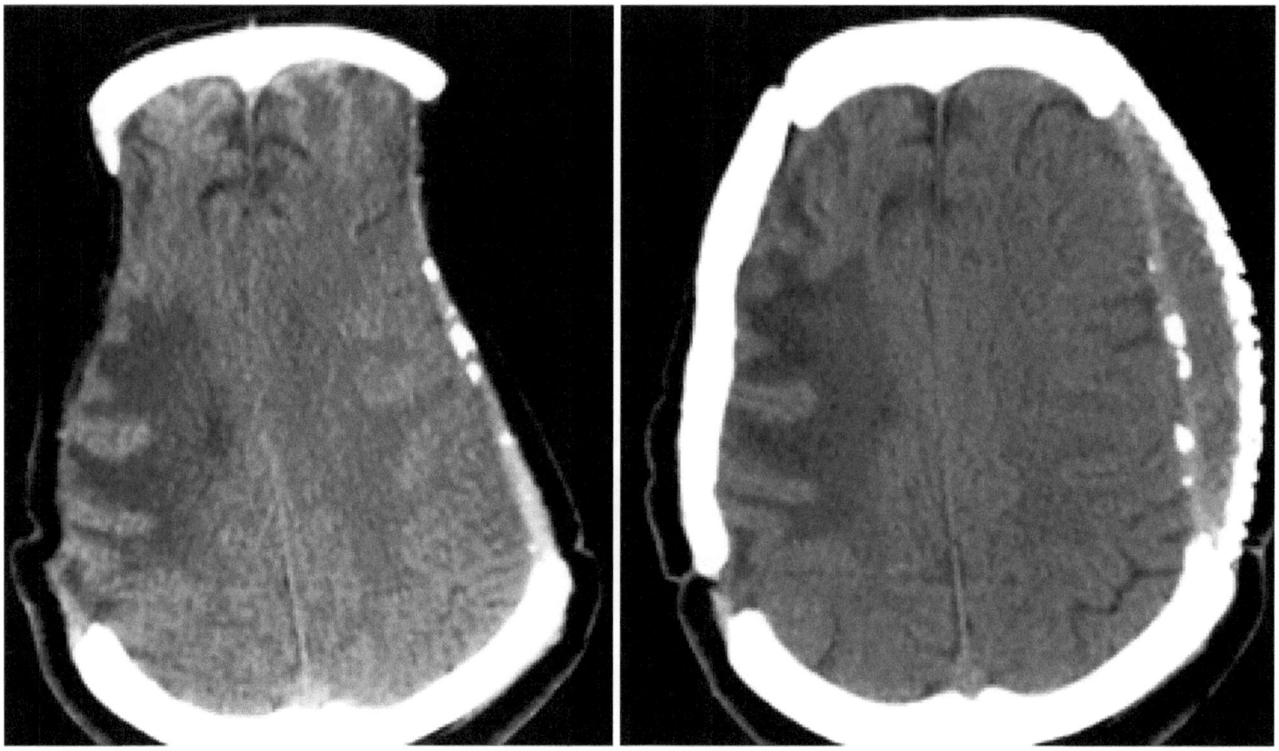

Fig. 9 A case of sunken flap syndrome following bilateral DC, which resolved following cranioplasty (right)

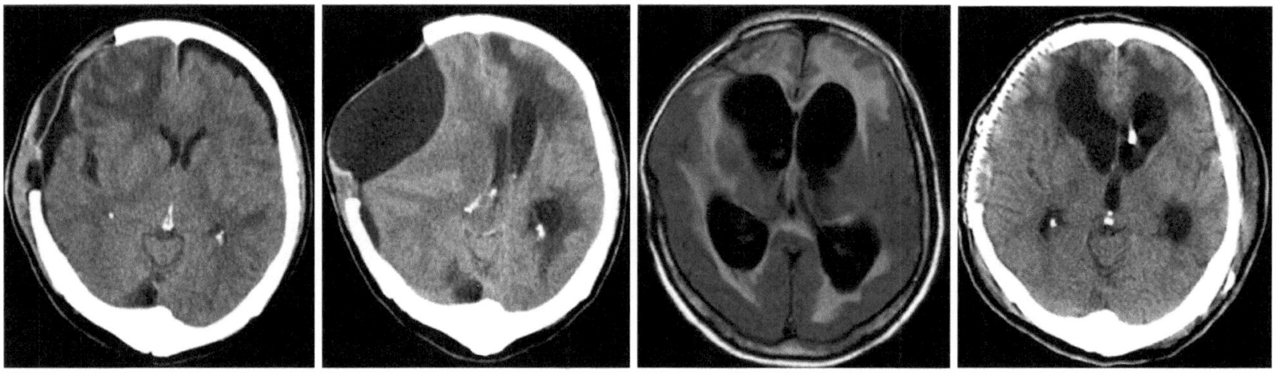

Fig. 10 Serial CT scans showing the development of subdural hygroma (second from left) following drainage lumbar puncture, leading to paradoxical herniation

tion. Among the consequences of paradoxical herniation are new neurological deficits and deterioration in the sensorium. The treatments for paradoxical herniation are intravenous hydration, the Trendelenburg position, and a blood patch. An early cranioplasty can mitigate this complication [1].

Paradoxical Neurological Deterioration

The causes of paradoxical neurological deterioration from DC are paradoxical brain swelling and distortions in the white matter tracts. A pre-emptive DC before the development of midline shift in cases of stroke leads to an increase in edema, which we term *paradoxical brain swelling*. Such patients are usually conscious before surgery but become unconscious after surgery. The treatment is the aggressive management of raised ICP with medical therapy and ventilation [1].

Alternatives to DC

DC not only results in complications but also necessitates an additional neurosurgical procedure, cranioplasty, in the survivors. Cranioplasty itself is associated with its own complications. The alternative to DC is hinged craniotomy or expansile craniotomy (Figs. 11, 12 and 13). The expansile craniotomy leads to a comparable brain volume expansion and ICP reduction in DC, precluding the need for cranioplasty after index surgery [8].

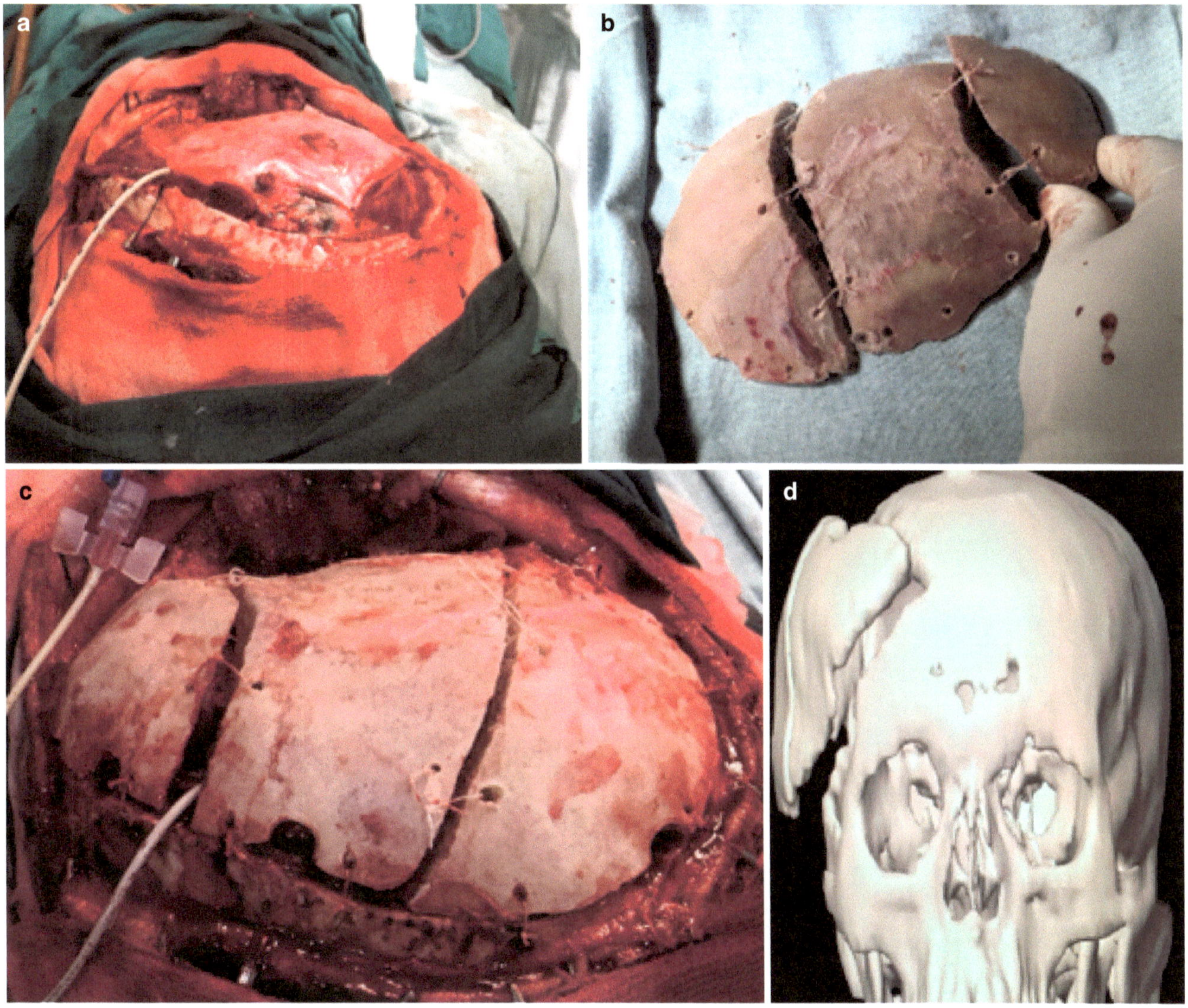

Fig. 11. A case of expansile craniotomy: (**a**) Brain bulge after craniotomy. (**b**) Bone flap divided into three pieces. (**c**) Bone fragments placed back and tied loosely to the skull. (**d**) Postoperative CT showing bulging bone fragments

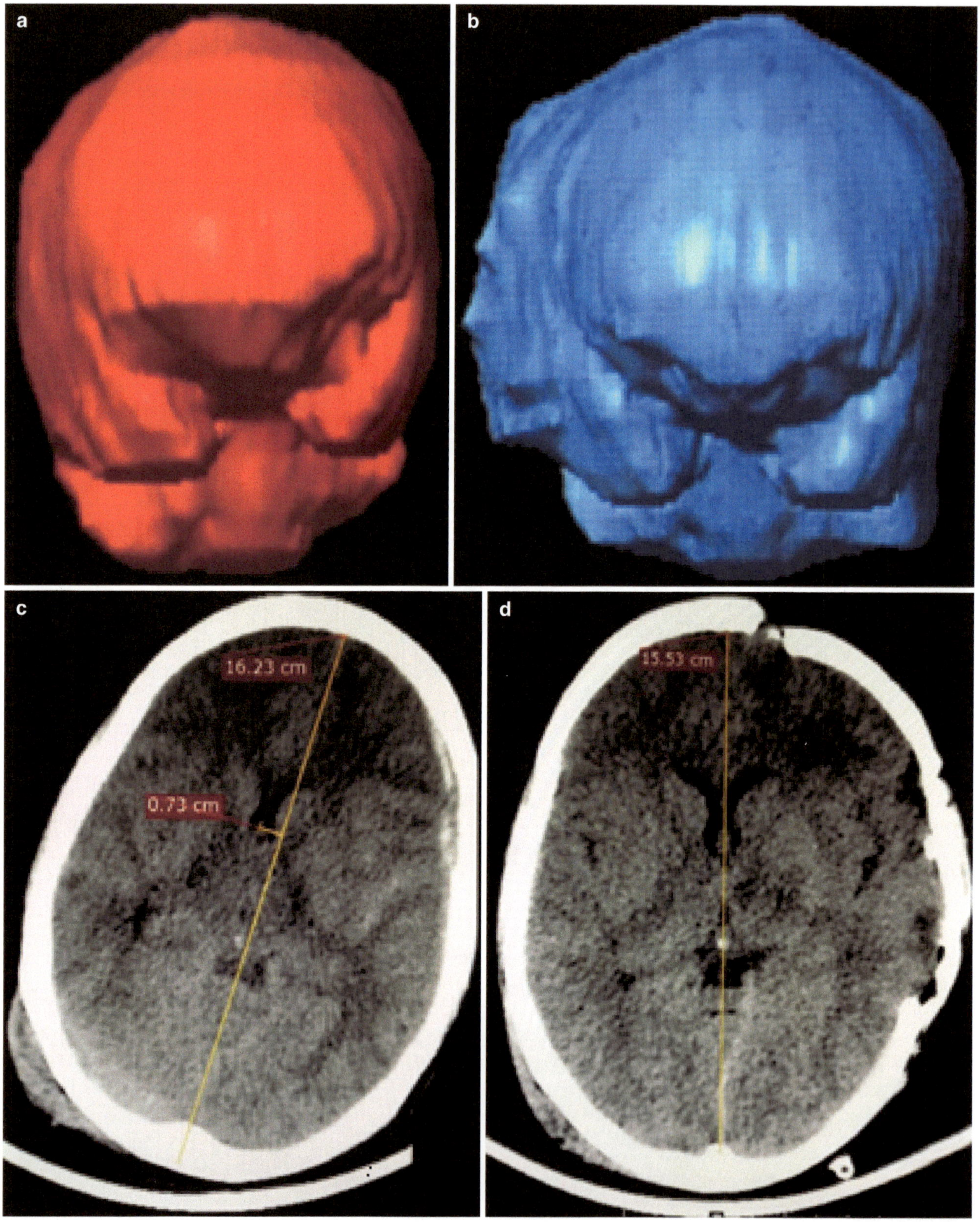

Fig. 12 Volume expansion and subsidence of midline shift following expansile craniotomy: (**a**) Preoperative intracranial volume. (**b**) Postoperative intracranial volume. (**c**) Preoperative CT scan showing midline shift. (**d**) Postoperative CT scan showing subsidence of midline shift

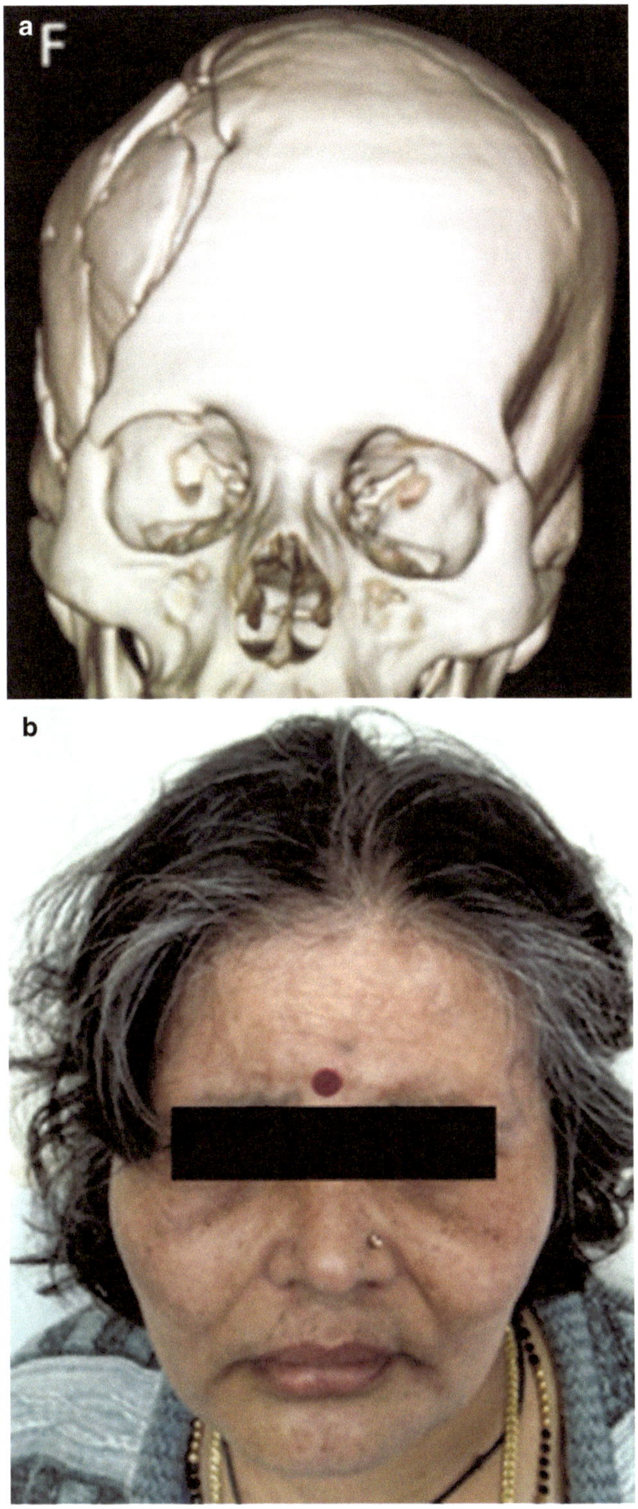

Fig. 13 (**a**) CT scan at follow-up showing settling of bone fragments of expansile craniotomy on the skull. (**b**) Clinical photograph showing a good cosmetic outcome

Conclusion

DC should be the last resort for the treatment of raised ICP. One in ten patients develops a complication for which additional medical or neurosurgical intervention is required. One should consider EVD or the removal of ICH/contusion for the further reduction of ICP before proceeding with DC. The commonest error is to make the craniectomy too small, which results in the inadequate relief of intracranial hypertension and results in brain herniation out of the defect and further secondary brain injury. Cranioplasty should be performed as soon as brain swelling has subsided, to prevent delayed complications following DC.

Declaration Author B.I.D. is a member of the National Institute of Health Research and its Global Health Research Group on Neurotrauma. The latter is supported by the National Institute of Health Research using Official Development Assistance (ODA) funding (16/137/105). The views expressed in this publication are those of the author(s) and not necessarily those of the National Health Service (NHS), the National Institute for Health Research, or the Department of Health.

References

1. Gopalakrishnan MS, Shanbhag NC, Shukla DP, Konar SK, Bhat DI, Devi BI. Complications of decompressive craniectomy. Front Neurol. 2018; https://doi.org/10.3389/fneur.2018.00977.
2. Kurland DB, Khaladj-Ghom A, Stokum JA, Carusillo B, Karimy JK, Gerzanich V, Sahuquillo J, Simard JM. Complications associated with decompressive craniectomy: a systematic review. Neurocrit Care. 2015;23(2):292–304.
3. Hutchinson PJ, Kolias AG, Tajsic T, et al. Consensus statement from the international consensus meeting on the role of decompressive craniectomy in the management of traumatic brain injury: consensus statement. Acta Neurochir. 2019;161(7):1261–74.
4. Abecassis IJ, Young CC, Caldwell DJ, Feroze AH, Williams JR, Meyer RM, Kellogg RT, Bonow RH, Chesnut RM. The Kempe incision for decompressive craniectomy, craniotomy, and cranioplasty in traumatic brain injury and stroke. J Neurosurg. 2021:1–10.
5. Dowlati E, Mortazavi A, Keating G, et al. The retroauricular incision as an effective and safe alternative incision for decompressive hemicraniectomy. Oper Neurosurg (Hagerstown, Md). 2021;20(6):549–58.
6. Wang H, Chen F, Wen L, Zhu Y, Chen Z, Yang X. Cranioplasty as the treatment for contralateral subdural effusion secondary to decompressive craniectomy: a case report and review of the relevant literature. J Int Med Res. 2020;48(11):300060520966890.
7. Ding J, Guo Y, Tian H. The influence of decompressive craniectomy on the development of hydrocephalus: a review. Arq Neuropsiquiatr. 2014;72(9):715–20.
8. Kishore K, Mishra T, Taploo D, Bhat D, Shukla D, Devi BI. A novel technique of expansile craniotomy as an alternative for decompressive craniectomy in traumatic brain injury (abstract). The 3rd Joint Symposium of the International and National Neurotrauma Societies and AANS/CNS Section on Neurotrauma and Critica. J Neurotrauma. 2018;35(16):A197.

A Clinical Learning Curve Should Be Avoided in Neurosurgery

Allan Taylor, David Le Feuvre, and Bettina Taylor

Abstract

Achieving competence in performing complex neurosurgical operations and learning new techniques after qualification take time. The improvement in skill over time (or as more procedures are performed) can be represented graphically as a learning curve. While surgeons are operating on patients to acquire the required skills, patients might be harmed. This is often referred to colloquially but incorrectly as "a steep learning curve." Although this may be an accepted learning practice for surgeons, it is unlikely to be acceptable to patients. Surgeons need to find ways of reaching a competent level of practice before operating on patients. To this end, the need for new techniques, what skills they require, and how they can be learned in a nonclinical environment should be defined. This can help surgeons determine where they start on a learning curve and what skills they need to achieve competence.

Keywords

Learning curve · Surgical training · Mentorship · Apprenticeship · Complications

A. Taylor (✉)
University of Cape Town and Groote Schuur Hospital, Cape Town, South Africa

Division of Neurosurgery, Neuroscience Building, Groote Schuur Hospital, Observatory, Cape Town, South Africa
e-mail: allan.taylor@uct.ac.za

D. Le Feuvre
University of Cape Town and Groote Schuur Hospital, Cape Town, South Africa

B. Taylor
EthiQal Medical Professional Indemnity, Cape Town, South Africa
e-mail: bettinat@ethiqal.co.za

Learning Curve Theory

A learning curve is a graphic representation of a learner's performance of a task (Y-axis) over time or the number of times the task is performed (X-axis). A learner's performance is expected to improve over time as the task is learned. If the task is easily learned, the graph will show a steep rise. The learner will rapidly improve performance, but then a plateau will be reached where further improvement is unlikely. If the task is difficult, the graph will show a gradual rise. Initial learning is slow but increases until proficiency has been reached. In most real-world situations, like learning a surgical technique, a sigmoid curve would be expected. Initial learning is difficult, and slow progress is made as the basic steps are learned. As the surgeon repeats the technique, proficiency accelerates, but once it has been mastered, their capacity to improve decreases and the curve flattens (Fig. 1). Some have also proposed that the skill required to reach the plateau phase may not be retained [1]. Dexterity may be lost with aging, or sufficient cases may not be performed to retain the required skill.

A learning curve requires a variable that is measurable and repeatable. In a production line, this may be the number of working units manufactured within a certain time or the time taken to produce a unit. Surgical operations have similarities to manufacturing in that they often involve repetitive steps. Doing the operation over and over makes it "automatic" for the surgeon, and thus, the procedure is often performed in less time with greater success. One difficulty is measuring this "success." The outcome measure may be time, blood loss, the extent of tumor resection, or the number of encountered complications. Only one such measure at a time may be plotted, and determining what reflects mastery of a particular procedure can be difficult.

Assuming that a group of surgeons need to learn a new operation, all of them will likely not be starting at the same skill level. Their starting point on the learning curve would then be different. Their progress may also differ in that some

K. Turel, E. M. Kasper (eds.), *Complications in Neurosurgery II*, Acta Neurochirurgica Supplement 133,
https://doi.org/10.1007/978-3-031-61601-3_23

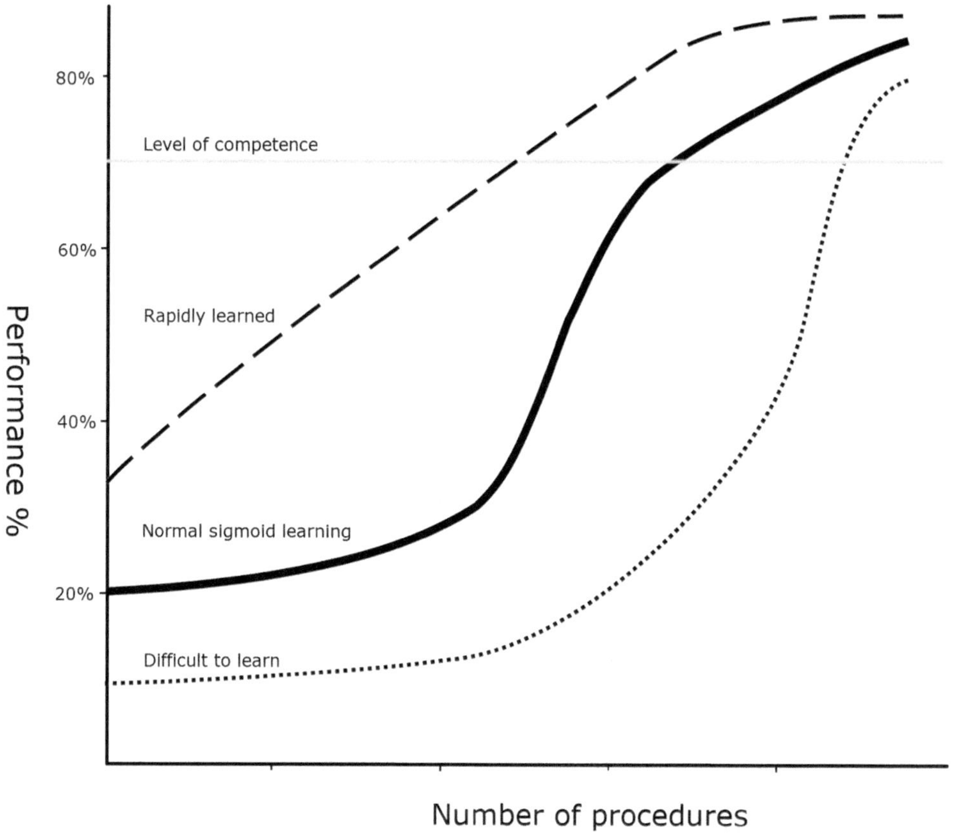

Fig. 1 Theoretical learning curve plots: Simple procedures may be rapidly learned, and surgeons may start close to a competent level (dashed line). Complex procedures take many repetitions to master, and surgeons may start with a low skill level (dotted line). Complex procedure learning may also be represented by a sigmoid curve where the initial learning is slow but as skills are acquired proficiency increases to reach a plateau (solid line)

may learn faster, in which case each surgeon will have a different slope on the graph. Their proficiency may also plateau at a different level. This is acceptable as long as all surgeons are operating at a point on the graph that is above the status defined as "competent." Competency is the skill level required to complete the surgery with acceptable morbidity and mortality. We rarely define or audit these levels in clinical practice, but this is sometimes a requirement for operating in a clinical trial. While surgeons are acquiring skill between the starting and competency points, patient morbidity and perhaps mortality can be assumed to increase. In colloquial speech, surgeons often refer to a "steep learning curve" when talking about starting a new operation. This is the wrong description for the graph curve. What they mean is that learning the procedure is challenging and that mistakes are made in the beginning. Hiding behind this term is the reality that patients are harmed while surgeons are training or learning new operations.

Surgical Training and Innovation

Training programs in neurosurgery are usually a combination of didactic and practical teaching. The practical skill acquisition occurs in a step-wise way. Junior trainees start with simple operations and laboratory training and as they advance are allowed to perform more-difficult operations. Often this happens as part of an apprenticeship where trainees first observe and assist before being allowed to operate while a senior person observes. It is a slow process. Quality control and patient safety are ensured through immediate supervision and tools like morbidity and mortality (M&M) meetings or adverse-event reporting.

Because the apprenticeship process is slow, all neurosurgery graduates are unlikely to be at a competent level for all neurosurgery procedures. This implies that they are still on a learning curve for a variety of these, including some for which a competent point has not yet been reached. In addition, surgical innovation continues during a surgeon's career, and they are pressured to adopt new techniques, particularly minimally invasive ones that are often rather technical and difficult to learn. This additional learning at the level of an independent and licensed specialist is often done without supervision or limited proctor supervision. It may be industry driven through observation or participation in workshops, but rarely is it associated with the rigor applied when compared to the step-by-step learning in a formal training program. This leads to the colloquial "steep learning curve," which has become an accepted part of surgical practice but would not be acceptable if patients could determine that surgeons were below the point of competence. Airline pilots require training and certification before flying passengers.

Their learning curve takes place in a simulator, and for this reason, travel by flight is safe. This does not occur in surgery, primarily because this type of professional training is time-intensive and expensive. Of course, advances have been made in surgical training. "See one, do one, teach one" may have been where training started, but skills, laboratories, logbooks, and competency-based rather than time-based learning have been incorporated into many programs [2]. These are more likely to be implemented in established training programs and applied to a catalog of simpler operations performed by junior trainees. Complex, high-risk surgeries remain a challenge to teach, and qualified surgeons are not required to submit to competency accreditation when undertaking a new operation. Surgeons wanting to learn a new operation have the options of self-teaching through reading and watching videos or observing operations in workshops, and if they are fortunate, they can perform the surgery with a proctor or mentor. Although these strategies may reduce unnecessary complications, they are unlikely to avoid the excess morbidity associated with a learning curve.

Avoiding the Clinical Learning Curve

Certifying the technical expertise of surgeons who are already advanced in their career (and board certified) is difficult, controversial, and unlikely to be widely applied. Continuing medical education programs are widely implemented but do not address practical technical competence. Recertification is not a requirement for most surgeons around the globe, and although it examines knowledge and decision-making, it does not address operative competence [3]. Ultimately, this leaves the responsibility of ensuring competence with the individual surgeon. Most surgeons believe that they are ethical and ascribe to the Hippocratic principle of "first do no harm," but many conflicts hamper our ability to do this properly. Surgeons must undertake difficult procedures that carry a significant risk of causing harm to patients. To do this, they must have the self-belief (reassurance) that they are competent, creating a potential bias toward exaggeration. Surgery is competitive in that surgeons aim not just to reap the financial rewards that come with performing operations but also to earn recognition. In a nonregulated healthcare market, surgeons naturally need to advertise their ability in order to get referrals and be noticed. The pressures are not all from within, though. Industry may well be an external force pushing surgeons to use new tools and implant more devices. This may be through flattery ("Dr. X, we have chosen you to implant the first 20 of device Y."), pressure ("All the other surgeons use device Y. Why not you?"), or financial incentives like consultancy fees. The disclosure of any conflict of interest is seen as a solution, but it assumes that the physician is aware of the conflict and fully discloses and that this added step has the desired effect [4]. How then do we avoid making learning errors at the expense of patients?

Reduce the Pressure to Perform New Procedures

Innovation must take place, but it should happen as part of research trials. Once confirmed as having benefit there, consideration should be given to how the new technique can be taught safely. Statements like "anyone can do this" or "it's easy" should be avoided during presentations at congresses and workshops.

Is the New Approach Essential?

The advantages of new techniques should not be overemphasized. Although minimally invasive operations have theoretical advantages, these have seldom been proven in head-to-head randomized trials with conventional techniques. Surgeons are concerned about being left behind or not competitive with their colleagues, so new approaches are rapidly adopted—sometimes too rapidly. Even if a new technique offers advantages, the extra morbidity created while learning should be taken into account. In a study looking at learning curves and their associated morbidity during minimally invasive esophagectomy by van Workum, the researcher determined that 119 cases of surgery are required for a surgical team to reach anastomosis competence. However, during the learning period under assessment, 357 patients had surgery by three teams, and the pooled anastomosis leak was 18.8% compared to a leak incidence of 4.5% after the learning curve plateau had been reached [5]. This means that 36 patients (or 10.1% of the "learning curve" patients) had a complication that could have been avoided by not starting the technique. If a learning curve is unavoidable, this extra morbidity needs to be taken into account when assessing the appropriateness of adopting a new technique. To be acceptable from a public health point of view, the new procedure would have to offer significant and relevant advantages. Even if the plateau offers a clear advantage, such that many patients will benefit in the future, how can this be justified to those patients who have surgery during the learning phase and potentially suffer a complication?

Determine the Starting Level on a Learning Curve

Surgeons have different levels of technical skill, training, and experience, and this should be taken into account when starting to learn a new procedure. Some basic skills might be required before learning a new technique. A vascular neurosurgeon cannot learn to coil an aneurysm without learning the basics of catheterization. A spinal surgeon cannot undertake endoscopic microdiscectomy without first learning how to use an endoscope. Surgeons should consider the skills required for a particular technique rather than how many of a similar procedure have been done in the past.

Define a Competent Level of Practice

Because surgical innovation aims to build on existing techniques, the outcome and complication incidence of established operations can be used to benchmark new operations. This data may come from published trials, but using real-world data to define acceptable outcome and complication rates may be more suitable. While all surgeons should aspire to the best possible outcomes, we need to be honest and transparent about our own abilities. Whereas trial-level outcomes may not be possible immediately, this is acceptable as long as competence is achieved and informed consent was obtained (see below).

Safe Learning from Start to Competence

Performing new surgery on patients is not an acceptable way to learn, and fortunately, we have other ways to attain the required skills. Real and virtual simulation models are now available for many procedures [6]. Preserved cadaver dissection may be criticized for not offering a real tissue feeling or ability to simulate bleeding, but fresh specimen dissection can offer a lifelike experience [7]. Just as pilots use simulation to train for routine flights and emergencies, surgeons should do the same. The most valuable way to learn is with a more experienced surgeon who acts as a mentor or proctor. Not only can they offer advice, but they can step in should the need arise.

Informing Patients

This may be the hardest step in learning. How can we inform patients about our level of skill and training without having the patient lose faith in the surgeon's ability? Informed consent is considered a standard of care in modern bioethics, and it implies that we inform patients not only about their disease and the treatment options but also about our ability to manage their care. This becomes much easier if the surgeon is confident that they are at a competent level. Surgeons should be able to say, "this is a new procedure for me, but I have done the required training, and I am competent." We are able to offer even more security to patients if we can say, "this is the experienced surgeon who will be operating with me today."

Conclusion

Surgical innovation and the need for surgeons to learn new techniques will continue. New techniques may be difficult to learn, and many repetitions are required to achieve a competent level of practice. This learning curve and its associated patient morbidity and mortality should not be acceptable in neurosurgery. As much as possible, learning should take place in a nonclinical and carefully supervised environment.

Conflict of Interest Statement The authors have no conflicts of interest to declare. No funding was received for this paper.

References

1. Hopper A, Jamison M, Lewis W. Learning curves in surgical practice. Postgrad Med J. 2007;83:777–9.
2. Kotsis S, Chung K. Application of see one, do one, teach one concept in surgical training. Plast Reconstr Surg. 2016;131(5):1194–201.
3. Cruft G, Humphreys J Jr, Hermann R, Meskauskas J. Recertification in surgery, 1980. Arch Surg. 1981;116(8):1093–6.
4. DiRisio A, Muskens I, Cote D, et al. Oversight and ethical regulation of conflict of interest in neurosurgery in the United States. Neurosurgery. 2019;84(2):305–12.
5. Workum F, Stenstra M, Berkelmans G, et al. Learning curve and associated morbidity of minimally invasive Esophagectomy, a retrospective multicenter study. Ann Surg. 2019;269(1):88–94.
6. Bernardo A. Virtual reality and simulation in neurosurgical training. World Neurosurg. 2017;106:1015–29.
7. Grabo D, Bardes J, Sharon M, Borgstrom D. Initial report on the impact of a perfused fresh cadaver training program in general surgery resident trauma education. Am J Surg. 2020;220:109–13.

Recurrent Symptomatic Cage Migration After Minimally Invasive L4-5 TLIF

Mazda K. Turel and Bhushan Meshram

Abstract

A 70-year-old man presented with severe lower-back pain and left L5 radiculopathy that was resistant to all forms of conservative treatment. Imaging showed a grade 1 unstable degenerative listhesis at L4/5 that resulted in severe left lateral recess stenosis. To this end, he underwent an uneventful minimally invasive L4/5 unilateral transforaminal lumbar interbody fusion (TLIF), and he was discharged 3 days later with complete relief of leg pain. But 2 weeks later, he presented to the emergency room with a recurrence of severe left leg pain. A plain X-ray obtained in the ER showed a displaced interbody cage (backout). The patient underwent revision surgery, where the cage was removed. A larger cage was reinserted, and right-sided pedicle screw and rod fixation was performed. This resulted in complete pain relief until 2 weeks later, when the patient experienced yet another recurrence of cage migration. This time, the cage was removed, and the interbody space was successfully impacted with a bone graft. Since then, he has been pain-free over a 6-month period. The possible reasons for cage backout and strategies to prevent it are discussed.

Keywords

Transforaminal lumbar interbody fusion · Cage migration · Cage retropulsion

Introduction

Transforaminal lumbar interbody fusion (TLIF) with pedicle screw and rod fixation is a well-established surgical procedure for the stabilization of vertebral segments with excellent short- and long-term results. Nonetheless, perioperative and postoperative complications are still encountered in significant numbers. Implant failure can result in debilitating pain and even neurological deficits. While posterior cage migration has been previously reported, the repeated retropulsion of an implanted cage is extremely rare. We discuss such a case in an elderly male patient who required three operations—two for recurrent cage migration (backout) within a span of around 1 month.

Case Report

History and Examination

A 70-year-old man presented with a 1-year history of progressively worsening lower-back pain and left lower-limb pain radiating to the lateral aspect of the thigh and the calf. He experienced lower-limb paresthesia and a claudication time of 5 min. His pain was so severe that he had begun to limp. A trial of medication, physiotherapy, and an epidural injection failed to provide any substantial relief.

Upon presentation, his physical examination was found to be unremarkable for any motor or sensory deficit. The MRI (Fig. 1) showed severe left lateral recess stenosis at L4/5 in combination with bilateral facet arthropathy. Dynamic X-rays (Fig. 2) showed a grade 1 listhesis with significant motion. We discussed the options of performing only a left lateral recess decompression versus performing a transforaminal lumbar interbody fusion (TLIF) possibly in combination with a unilateral L4/5 pedicle screw and rod fixation. The later option was considered because the entire medial facet needed to be resected for a thorough decompression. The patient wished to proceed with this surgery, and informed consent was obtained.

M. K. Turel (✉) · B. Meshram
Wockhardt Hospitals, Mumbai Central, Mumbai, India

K. Turel, E. M. Kasper (eds.), *Complications in Neurosurgery II*, Acta Neurochirurgica Supplement 133,
https://doi.org/10.1007/978-3-031-61601-3_24

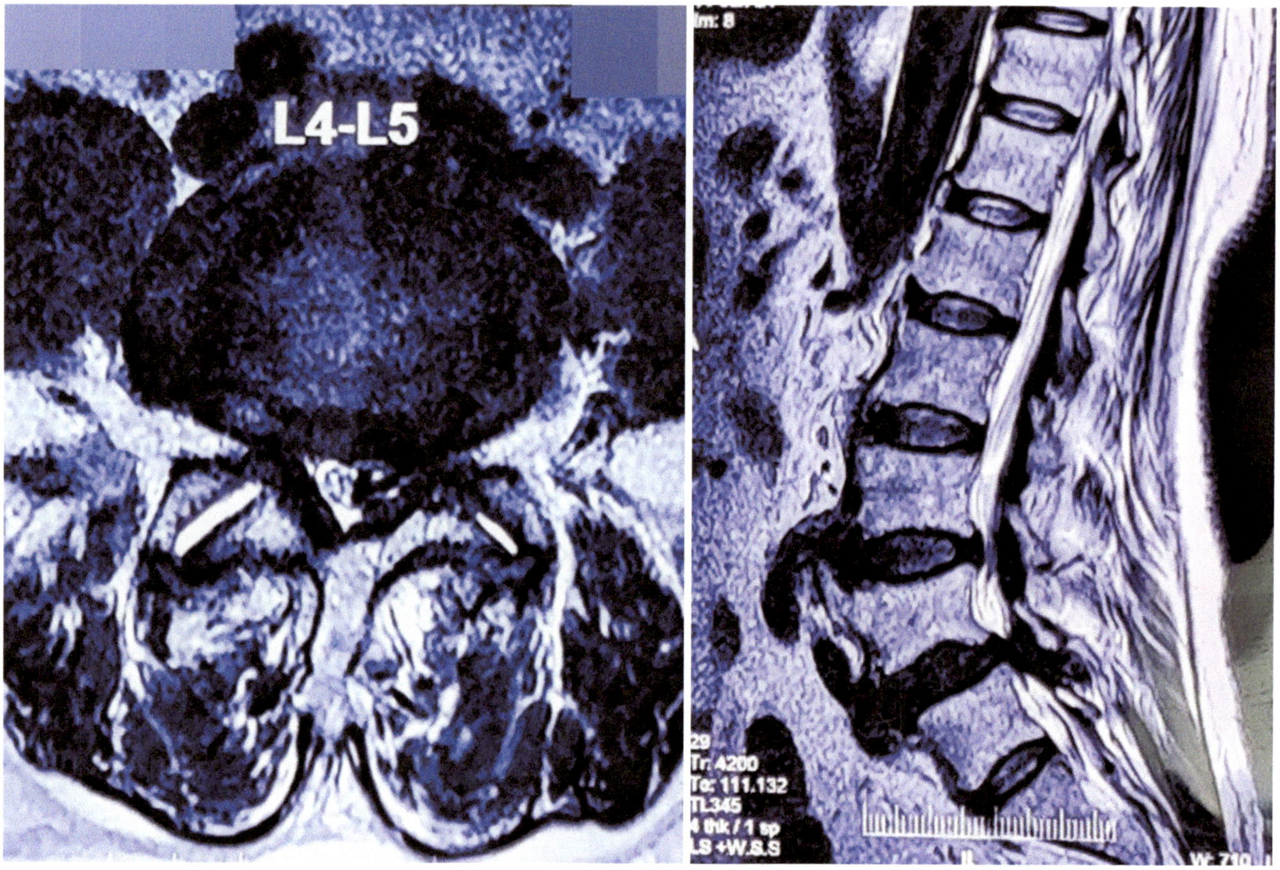

Fig. 1 T2-weighted sagittal and axial MRI of the lumbar spine showed stenosis at L45, more on the left due to facetal hypertrophy and ligamentum flavum thickening; there were significant facet effusions bilaterally

Surgery

A minimally invasive tubular TLIF was undertaken via a paramedian incision. A 22 × 60 mm Medtronic quadrant tube was docked at the L4/5 facet joint, and the medial facet was removed in a standard fashion. The thickened ligamentum flavum was removed, and the thecal sac and the nerve root were completely decompressed. Using a series of instruments and shavers, a L4/5 discectomy was performed, including endplate preparation. We then inserted a 11 × 24 mm polyetheretherketone (PEEK) cage into the prepared disc space, which was filled with bone graft. This was followed by a unilateral L4/5 pedicle screw and rod fixation. The wound was closed in layers without the need of a drain. Postoperatively, the patient showed complete relief from his leg pain, and the X-ray at discharge 3 days later showed the optimal positioning of the cage and instrumentation (Fig. 3).

Postoperative Course

But 2 weeks later, after a period of being completely pain-free, his left leg pain suddenly recurred on waking up one morning, and he was barely able to walk. A repeat X-ray (Fig. 4) was obtained, which showed the posterior migration of the cage. He was advised to undergo a redo operation, which he reluctantly agreed to. We opened the previous incision and upon exploration found the cage severely indenting the L5 root. We engaged the cage, removed it, inserted a larger cage (12 × 24 mm), compressed the existing screws during the final tightening, and inserted pedicle screws on the opposite side via another paramedian incision. Once again, he had complete relief from his leg pain, and the X-ray at discharge 3 days later showed the optimal positioning of the instrumentation (Fig. 5).

Once again, 2 weeks later, after being pain-free and fully mobilized for this period, his left leg pain recurred upon awakening. To our surprise, the X-ray (Fig. 6) once again showed the posterior migration of the recently inserted larger cage. After extensive consultation, we took him back to surgery the next day, removed the cage, packed the disc space with bone graft, and impacted it firmly. The postoperative X-ray performed at discharge showed optimal positioning once more (Fig. 7), and the patient remains pain-free at his 6-month follow-up for back and leg pain with no focal neurological deficit.

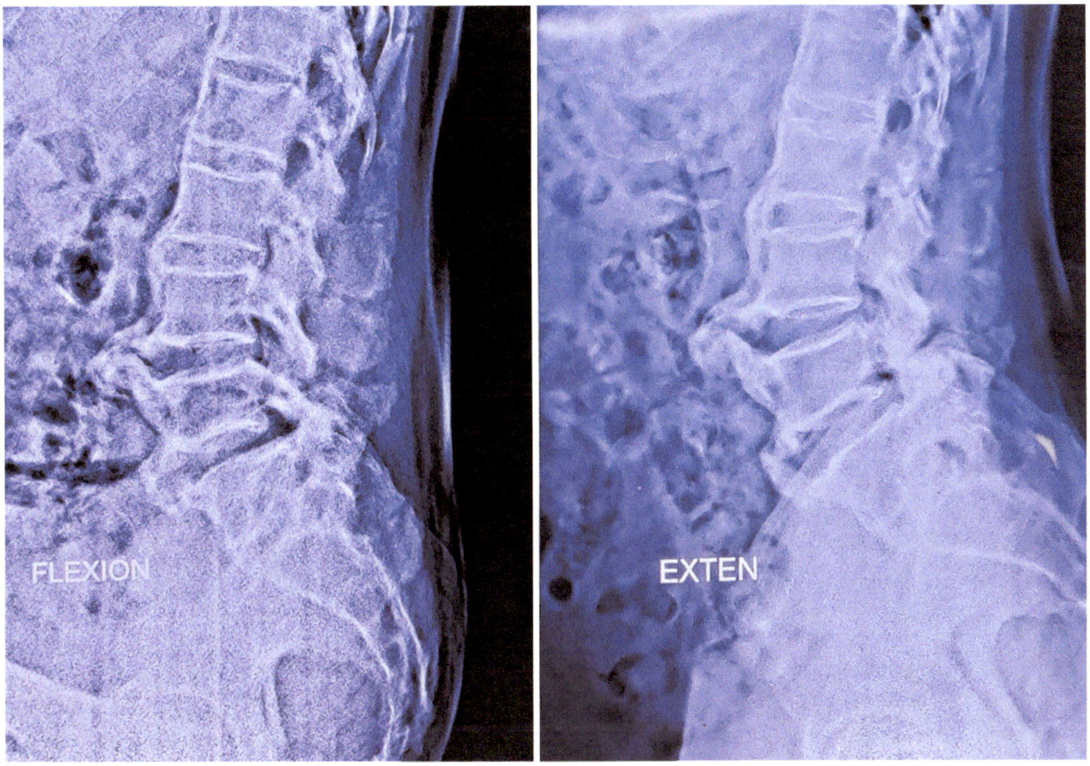

Fig. 2 Lateral X-rays of the lumbar sacral (LS) spine showed a grade 1 mobile listhesis with foraminal compromise

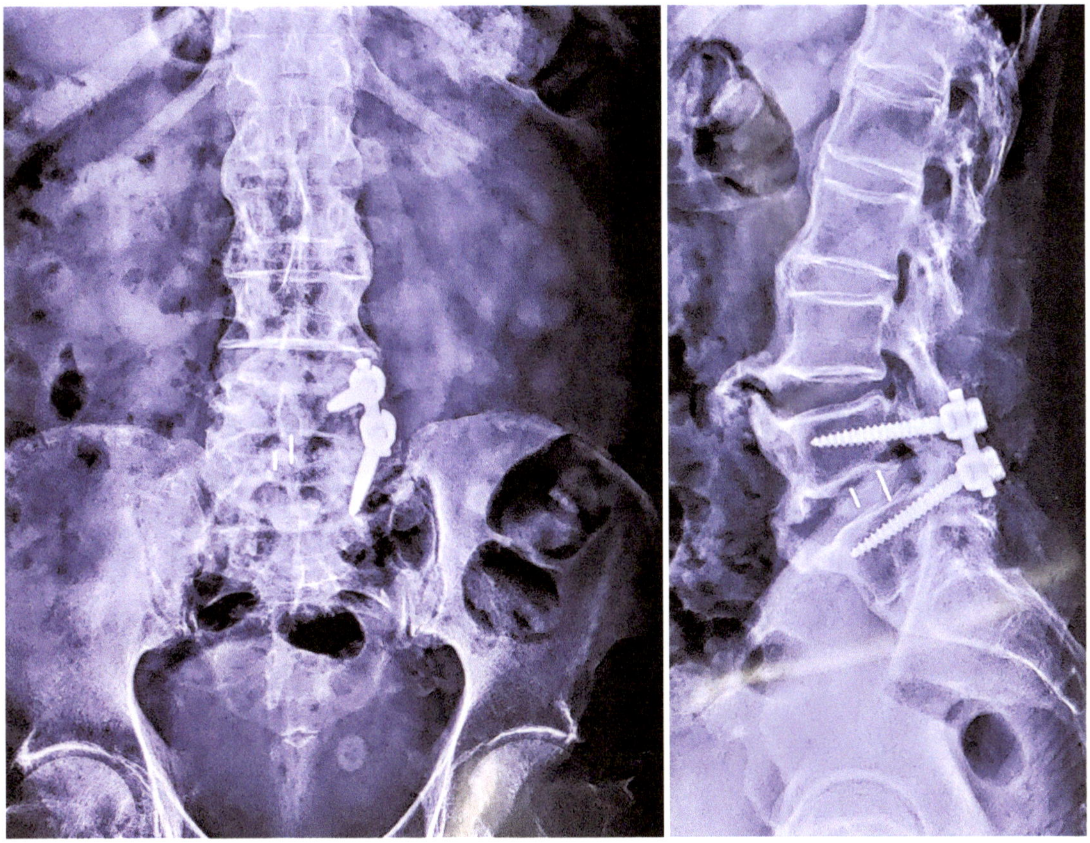

Fig. 3 Postoperative antero-posterior (AP) and lateral X-ray performed after the first surgery showed the optimal positioning of the instrumentation

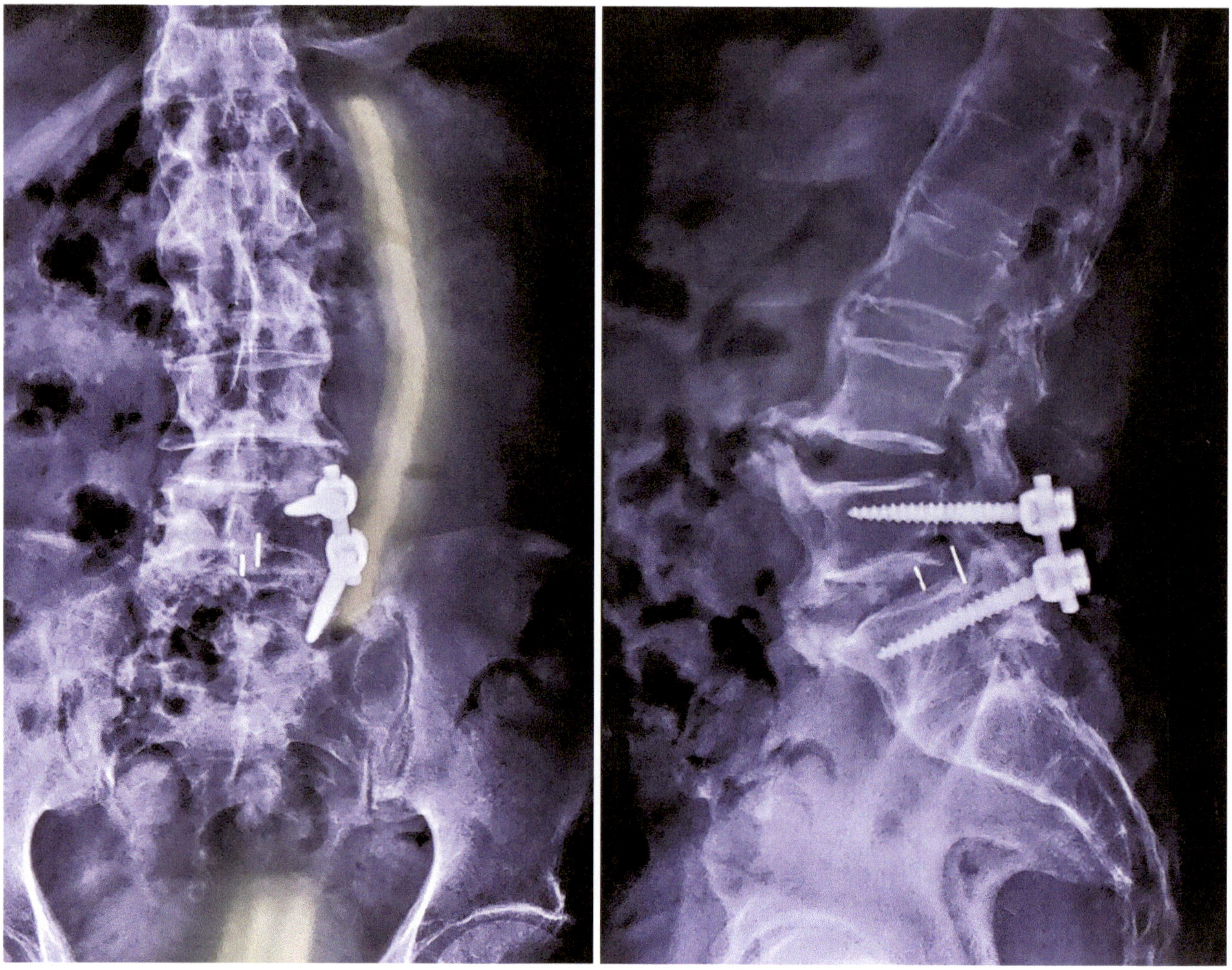

Fig. 4 Postoperative AP and lateral X-ray performed 2 weeks later showed the posterior migration of the cage

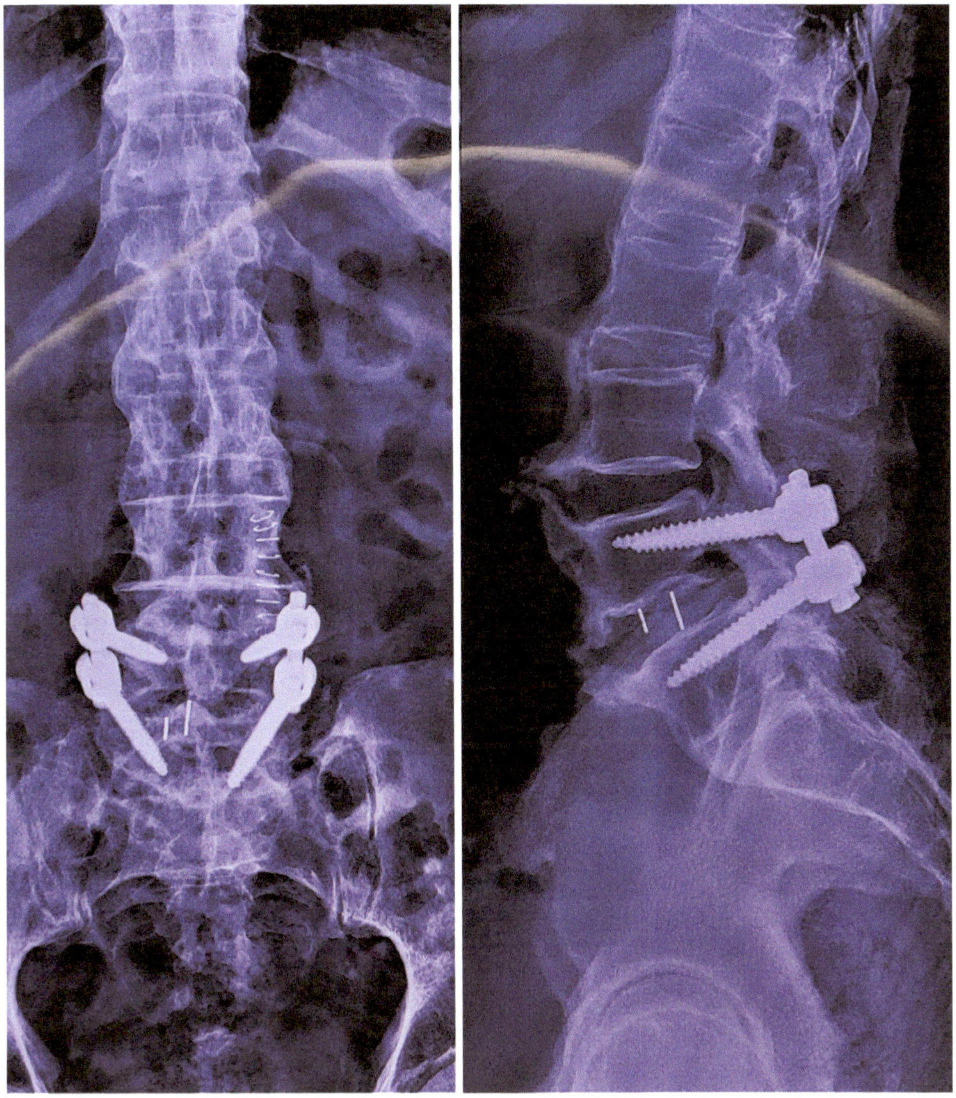

Fig. 5 AP and lateral X-ray performed at discharge after the second surgery showed the optimal positioning of the instrumentation

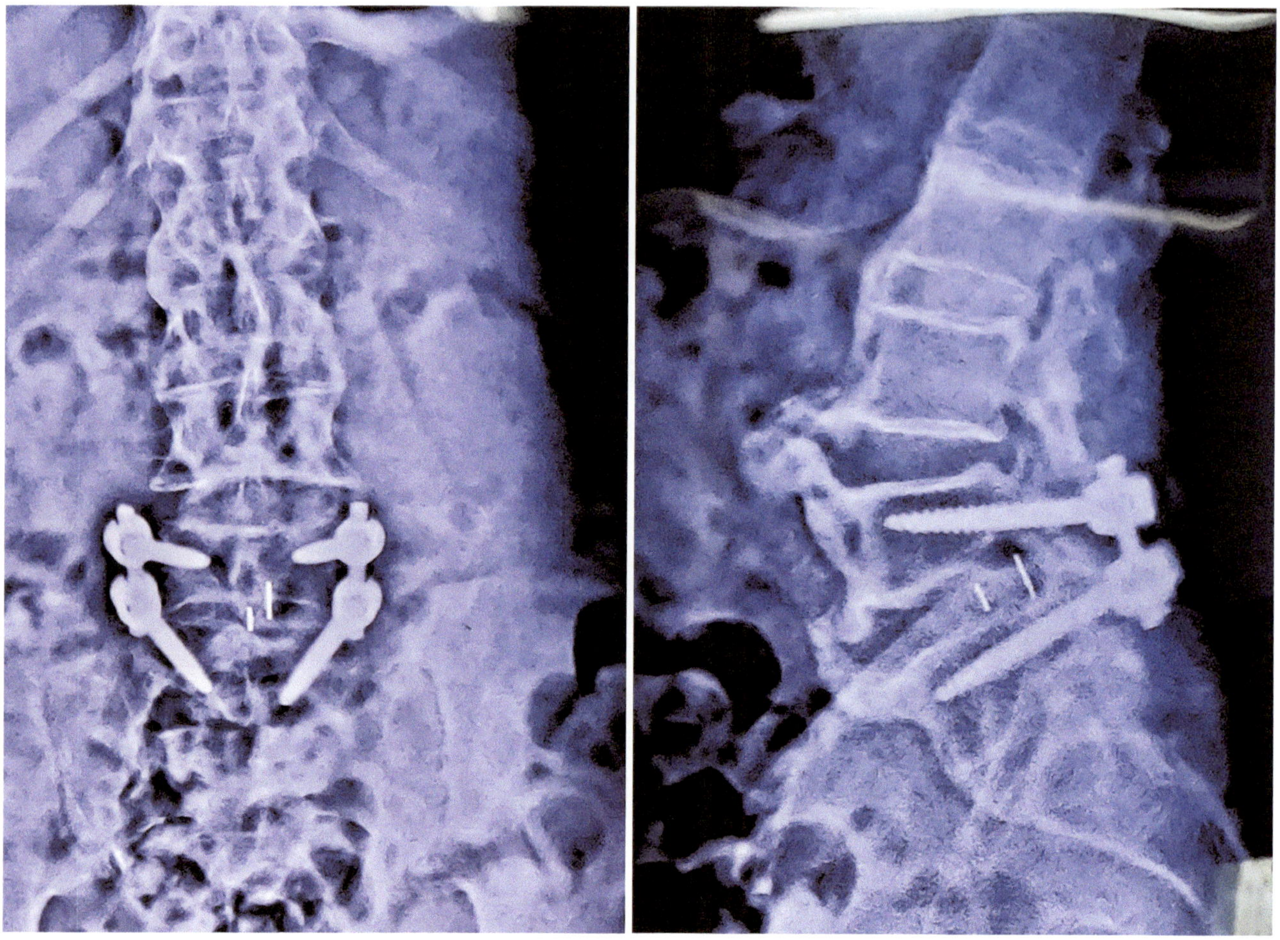

Fig. 6 AP and lateral X-ray 2 weeks after the second surgery once again showed the posterior migration of the cage

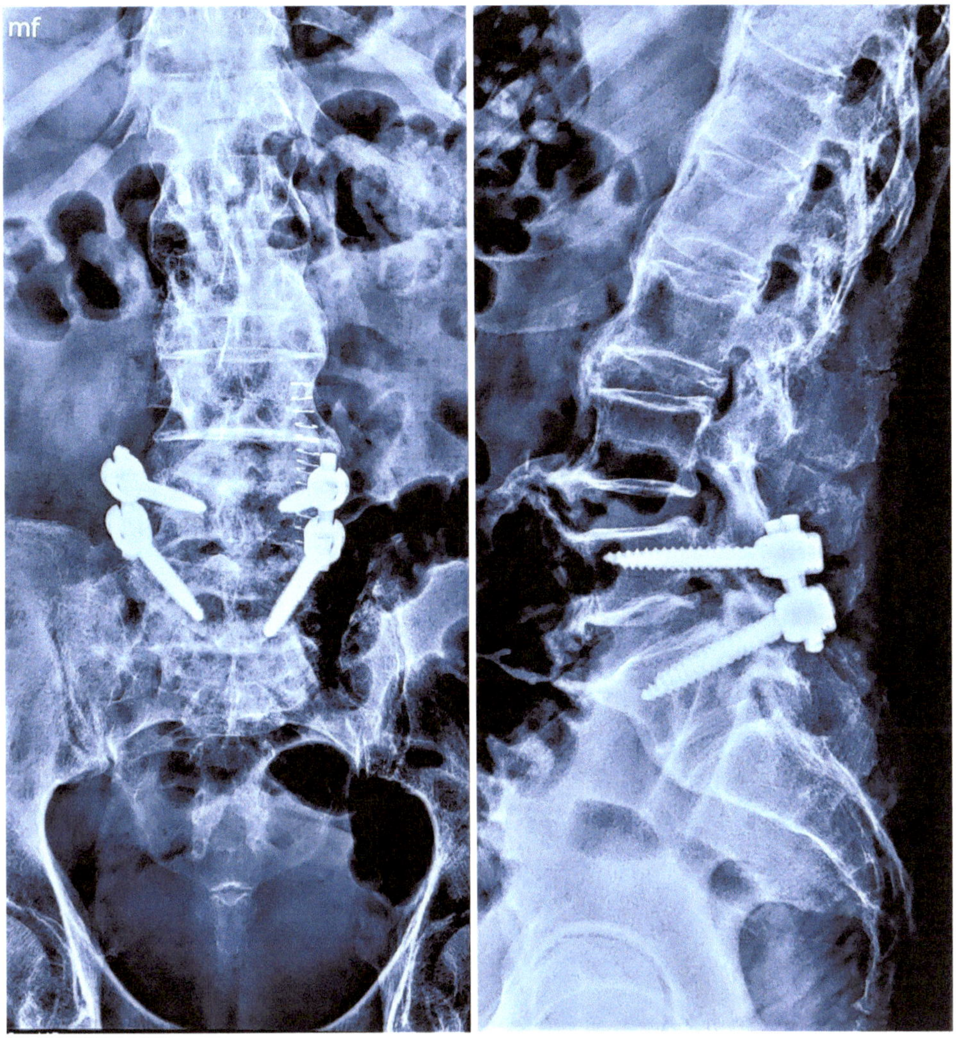

Fig. 7 The postoperative AP and lateral X-ray performed at discharge after the third surgery showed the optimal positioning of the screws with no cage

Discussion

Given the need of three surgeries to accomplish our goal of a rather standard decompression and instrumented fusion for degenerative spondylolisthesis, we reviewed the case in detail to analyze the causes of this complication. The cage might not have been inserted anterior enough the first time. Ideally, it should cross the midline and be positioned over the anterior third of the body. The alignment might not have been suboptimal, where the lordosis was overcorrected. According to previous reports on such a complication, some authors have argued that the posterior migration of the cage may occur because of constitutional factors such as osteoporosis or a pear-shaped disc or may occur iatrogenically from the posterior positing of the cage and endplate injury. Studying the constitutional factors preoperatively and a diligent surgical technique would help to avoid this complication [1].

Kimura et al. [2] reported that the risk factors of cage retropulsion after an interbody fusion are (1) a multilevel fusion procedure, (2) the involvement of the L5/S1 level, (3) a greater range of motion (ROM) of the disc space (>10° on lateral radiographs), and (4) taller discs (>10 mm at the midpoint of endplates on computed tomography scans). In such cases, more compressive force should probably be applied during pedicle screw insertion to prevent repeated cage migration.

To the best of our knowledge, only one other report of repeated cage migration has appeared in the literature [3].

References

1. Lee DY, Park YJ, Song SY, Jeong ST, Kim DH. Risk factors for posterior cage migration after lumbar interbody fusion surgery. Asian Spine J. 2018;12:59–68.
2. Kimura H, Shikata J, Odate S, Soeda T, Yamamura S. Risk factors for cage retropulsion after posterior lumbar interbody fusion: analysis of 1,070 cases. Spine. 2012;37:1164–9.
3. Lee JG, Lee SM, Kim SW, Shin H. Repeated migration of a fusion cage after posterior lumbar interbody fusion. Korean. J Spine. 2013;10:25–7.

Complications Following Microvascular Decompression (MVD) for Trigeminal Neuralgia (TN)

Keki Turel

Abstract

This article descibes the surgical management of classic trigeminal neuralgia via microvascular decompression of the neuro-vascular conflict zone. This treatment has been proven to be higly effective with an immediate relief of debilitating symptoms and a durable response. The article reports on cases with associated complications and their avoidance.

Keywords

Trigeminal neuralgia · Microvascular decompression · Complications

Patients with classical or idiopathic neuralgia that has an MRI-proven neurovascular conflict (NVC) and that is not amenable to conservative treatment are subjected to microvascular decompression (MVD). This is an excellent, proven procedure that gives relief to most patients immediately after surgery and in the long run. In every way, it has been found to be superior to other, less-invasive procedures. However, no surgical or medical treatment is exempt from complications.

Though the surgery of MVD appears elegant and straightforward in an area that is familiar to all neurosurgeons (cerebellopontine angle) and given that there is no significant distortion of neuraxsis or the cranial nerves, such as by a tumour, MVD is not free of complications and is liable to occur in several such surgeries. They may be minor or major, transient or permanent. Complications should not be surprising given that several important neurovascular structures are lodged in the cerebellopontine angle (CPA). Complications may be related to the pathology or variations in the anatomy of the posterior fossa and CPA in particular. But just as most airline disasters are due to pilot error, most complications while performing MVD are related to surgical error. They may pertain to one of the following:

1. Brain or blood vessel injury (petrosal venous injuries are more common than arterial injuries), resulting in infarction or a haemorrhage in the cerebellum or brain stem
2. Cranial nerve disturbances

Trigeminal nerve disorder (hypaesthesia or keratitis) is due to direct handling is more frequently than the neighbouring seventh (facial palsy) or eighth cranial neuropathies (tinnitus, dizziness, hearing impairment), occurring because of over-retraction and stretch injury, and the sixth (diplopia) occurs because of cranial nerves.

Cerebrospinal fluid (CSF) leak is the most common complication of posterior fossa surgery, and though well known to occur and hence ought to be avoidable, it still occurs as a major postoperative event in over 5% of patients and is liable to result in meningitis.

Wound infection can occur, as it can with any surgery, but headache is another disturbing postoperative complication, managing which can sometimes be a quite a headache for the surgeon. Mercifully, the dreaded complication of anaesthesia dolorosa is extremely uncommon following MVD. the following is a compilation of various complications in the literature [1]:

- Minor complications include dizziness, tinnitus, tiredness, wound infection, headache, scar tissue pain, permanent mild hypaesthesia, transient ataxia, diplopia, hypaesthesia (mild to severe), trigeminal motor weakness, facial nerve palsy, hearing impairment, and an altered sense of taste. (*Transient* was defined as lasting less than 12 months.)

K. Turel (✉)
Department of Neurosurgery, Bombay Hospital Institute of Medical Sciences, Mumbai, Maharashtra, India

K. Turel, E. M. Kasper (eds.), *Complications in Neurosurgery II*, Acta Neurochirurgica Supplement 133,
https://doi.org/10.1007/978-3-031-61601-3_25

- Major complications include death, stroke, meningitis, cerebrospinal fluid leak, hydrocephalus, anaesthesia dolorosa, permanent ataxia, diplopia, keratitis, severe hypaesthesia, facial weakness/nerve palsy, and hearing impairment or loss. (Permanent ones are those lasting longer than 12 months.)

Factors associated with complications are age, surgical difficulties, and surgical mishaps. Complications should be assessed/evaluated by appropriate specialists, preferably those not involved with the surgery.

Although MVD carries a risk of potentially serious complications, our study shows that almost all operated patients would recommend the procedure to other patients—even the operated patients who suffered major complications. This may reflect the high chance of a clinically significant outcome and the high degree of disability caused by the intense pain. According to our findings and clinical experience, we argue that while a risk of surgical complications after MVD has been documented, this risk should be weighed against the high chance of a clinically relevant surgical outcome combined with the weight of excruciating and intense pain and debilitating medical side effects.

Significantly, more women than men tend to have a failed outcome. The most frequent major complications were permanent hearing impairment, permanent severe hypaesthesia, permanent ataxia, and stroke.

The recurrence of pain falls under the category of treatment outcomes, not complications, although some recurrences could be the direct result of insufficient decompression or inadequate surgery/exploration.

Case Study

A 40-year-old female patient (Mrs SSG), was first seen by us in December 2018, for classic trigeminal neuralgia (TN) in her right cheek for 15 months, which later radiated to her right lower jaw. It was precipitated by all facial movements. Her pain was not controlled by the full range of conventional medications used for TN.

MRI Findings

The presence of a small vessel (probably a vein) a few millimetres lateral to the root entry zone (REZ) on heavily T2-weighted three-dimensional (3D) imaging (3D CISS/FIESTA) and time of flight (TOF) magnetic resonance angiography (MRA). Retrospectively, we can see the enlarged suprameatal tubercle (SMT) on that side in contrast to the opposite side (Fig. 1). Audiometry (Fig. 2) was 25–30 dB loss at 2.0 k.

Operation Details

A right retrosigmoid craniotomy was performed in the left lateral park-bench position. A 2.5 cm craniotomy was performed to expose the borders of the right transverse and sigmoid sinuses. The dura was opened with a curvilinear incision running along the sinuses. The posterior fossa was unduly small, and time was taken to drain CSF from the basal cisterns, permitting reasonable cerebellar retraction to visualise the trigeminal nerve and neighbouring structures (tentorium, petrosal vein anterior inferior cerebellar artery (AICA), and the REZ of vagal nerve (VN) and VII-VIII cranial nerve (CN) complex). The brainstem appeared anterior to the medial part of VN, appearing very close to the petrous bone because of a very narrow CPA. The unusually enlarged suprameatal tubercle (SMT) was seen encroaching into much of the limited space in the rostral part of the CPA, resulting in a suboptimal working space and very limited visualisation of VN and NVC, caused by the petrosal vein, which was submerged beneath the SMT and was to be later uncovered, which was made possible only after drilling the SMT.

Postoperatively, she had transient dizziness and vertigo for 2–3 days, mild (20%) persistent numbness on the right side of her face, and significant hearing impairment in her right ear (Fig. 3).

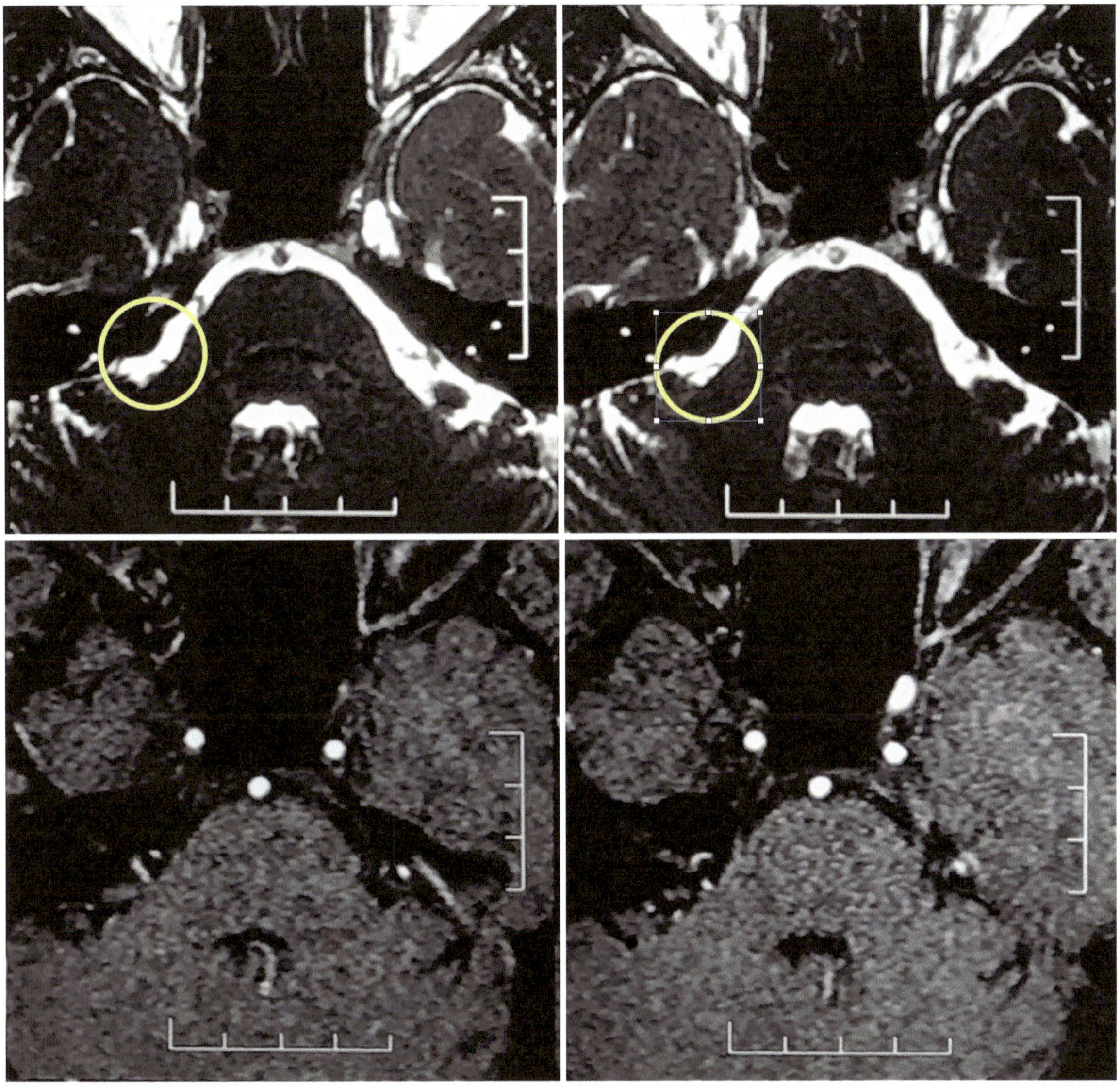

Fig. 1 Preoperative audiometry (25 December 2018)

Operation Findings

- A loop of AICA and a small vein crossing the REZ of VN
- Prominent suprameatal tubercle overhanging a very foreshortened, stoutish VN, narrowing the CP angle space even further, thus restricting the full view of VN and any other structure causing NVC
- Suprameatal tubercle drilled away, thus revealing a significant petrosal vein abutting against VN laterally, caudally, and rostrally (Figs. 4, 5, 6, 7, 8, 9, 10, 11 and 12)
- Lateral placement of Teflon between VN and vein and both VN and AICA at REZ (Figs. 13 and 14)
- Early postoperative audiometry (18 days after MVD, on 19 January) showed severe sensorineural deafness (Fig. 3)

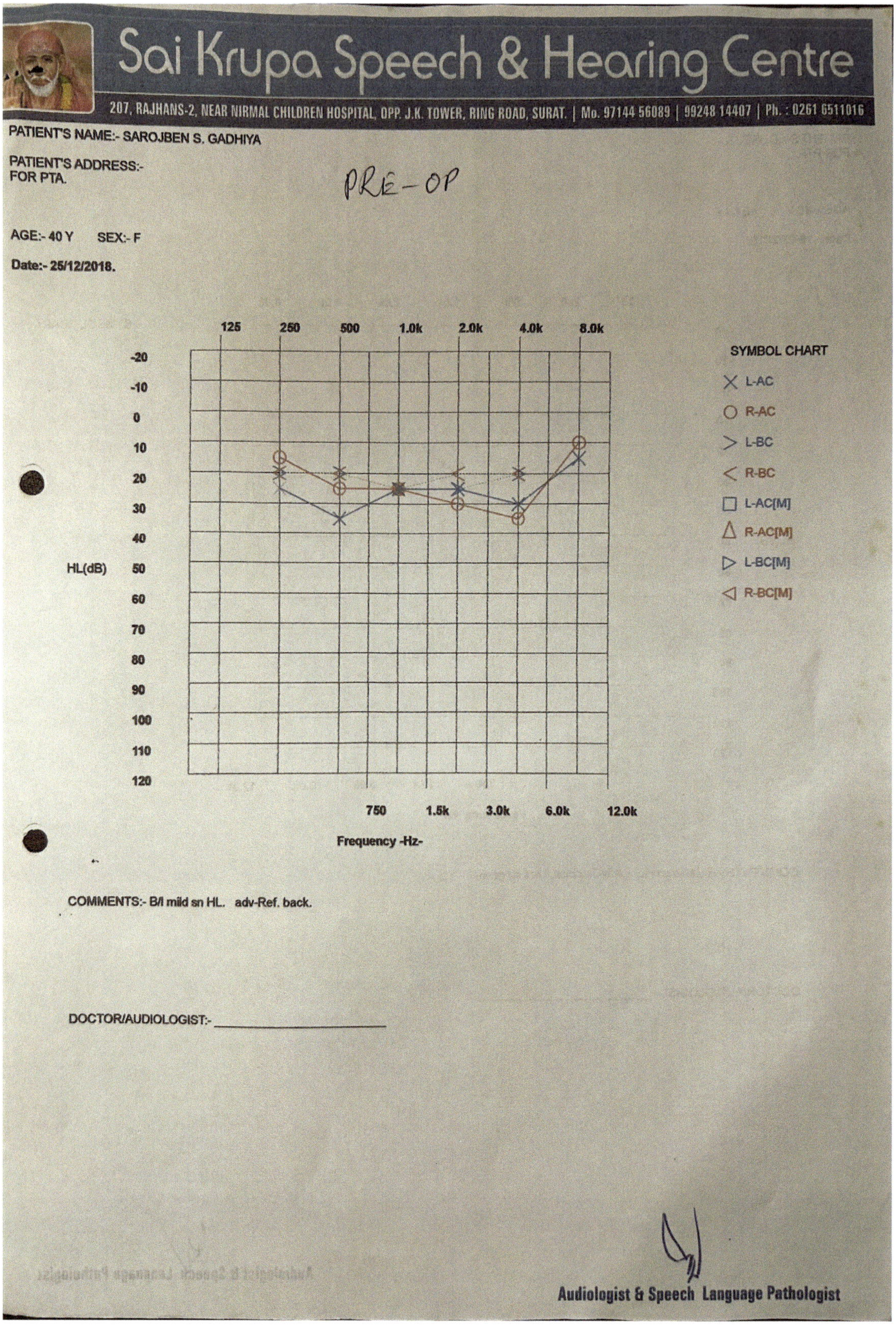
Sai Krupa Speech & Hearing Centre

207, RAJHANS-2, NEAR NIRMAL CHILDREN HOSPITAL, OPP. J.K. TOWER, RING ROAD, SURAT. | Mo. 97144 56089 | 99248 14407 | Ph. : 0261 6511016

PATIENT'S NAME:- SAROJBEN S. GADHIYA

PATIENT'S ADDRESS:-
FOR PTA.

PRE-OP

AGE:- 40 Y SEX:- F

Date:- 25/12/2018.

COMMENTS:- B/l mild sn HL. adv-Ref. back.

DOCTOR/AUDIOLOGIST:- ______________________

Audiologist & Speech Language Pathologist

Fig. 2 19-day postoperative audiometry (19 January 2019)

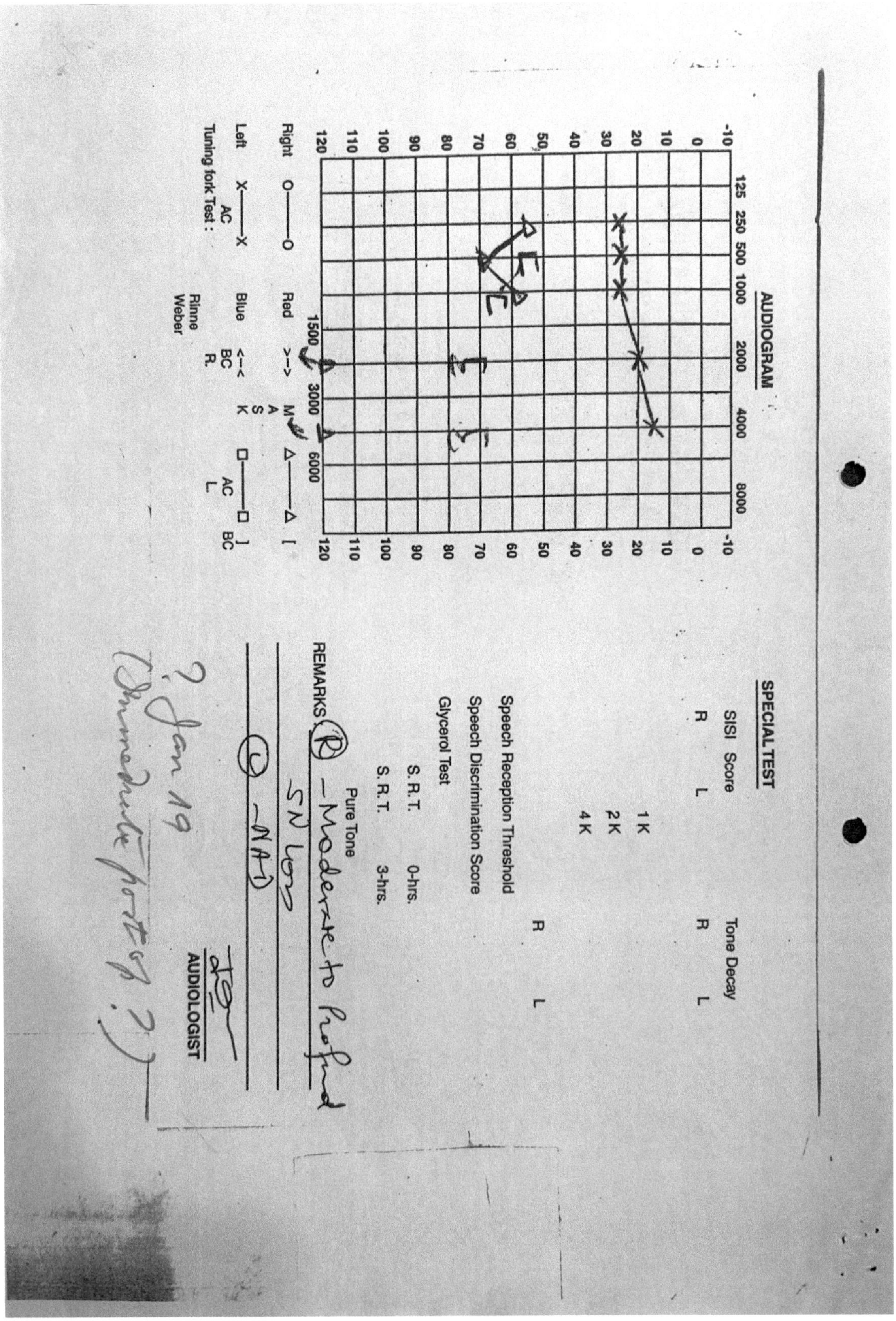

Fig. 3 Overpowering presence of a large suprameatal tubercle in CPA

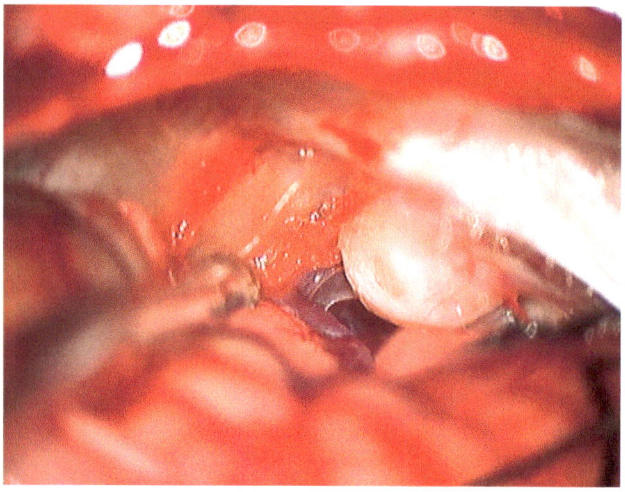

Fig. 4 Very restricted CPA, with brainstem almost reaching the petrous bone, the REZ of VN "sitting" atop it; petrosal vein seen on either side of SMT, its continuity concealed by the enlarged SMT

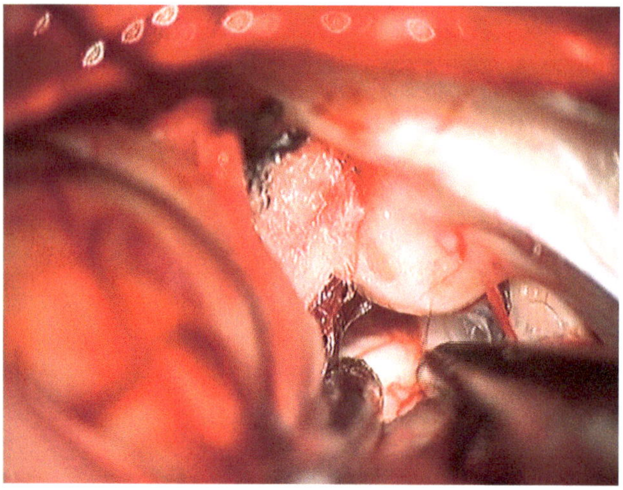

Fig. 5 Overview of anatomy upon further brain relaxation, after release of CSF

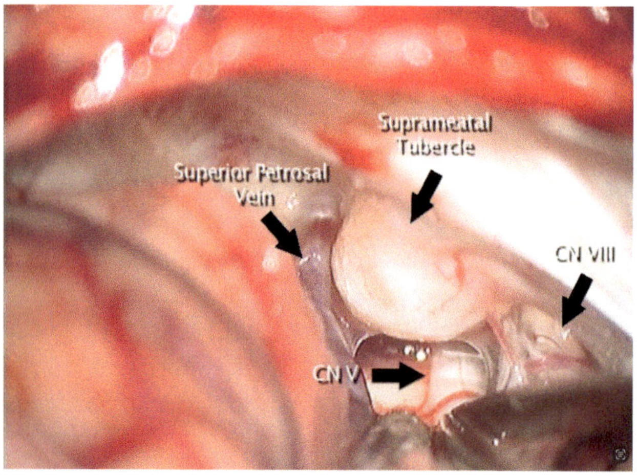

Fig. 6 Beneath SMT, the erstwhile hidden transverse pontine vein crosses VN to join petrosal vein, causing NVC

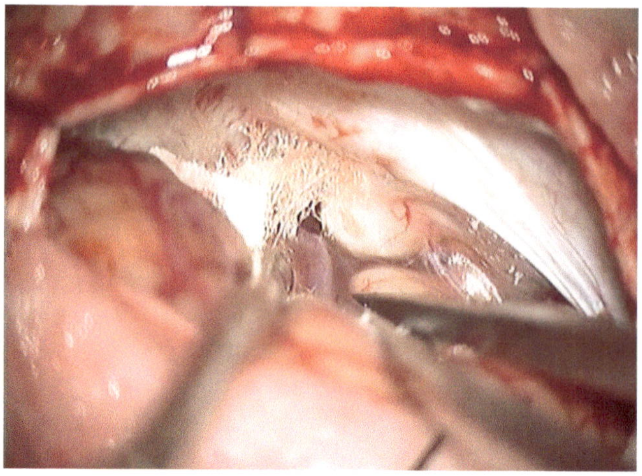

Fig. 7 Transverse pontine vein at the caudal end of VN

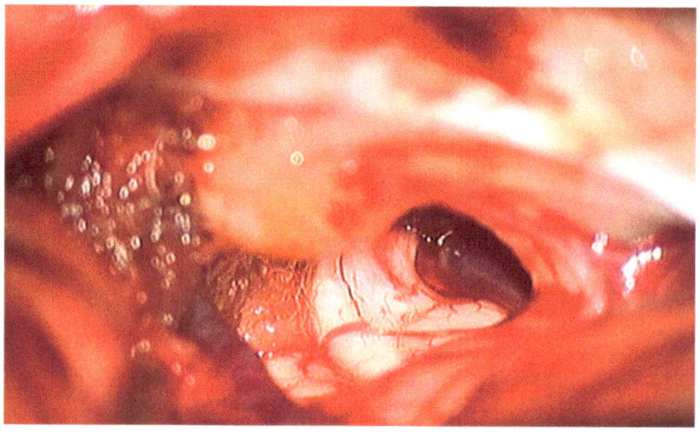

Fig. 8 AICA accompanied by a small pontotrigeminal vein at REZ, also causing NVC

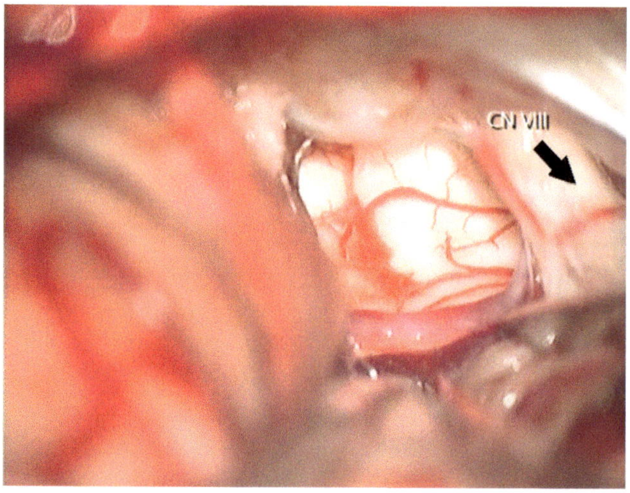

Fig. 9 AICA dissected free off REZ

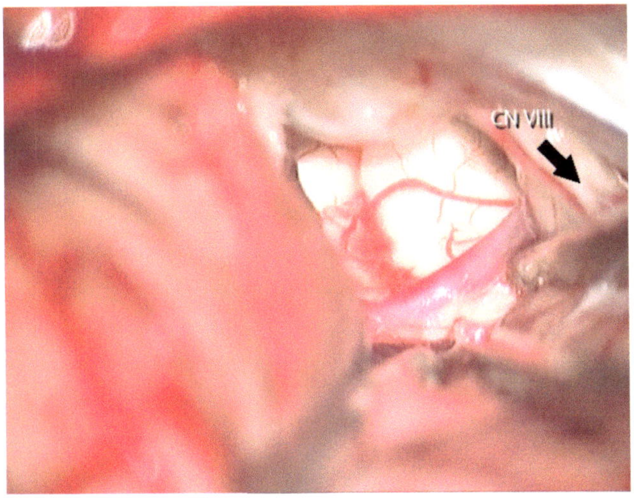

Fig. 10 The overhanging and enlarged SMT that was drilled to gain visibility and access to the conflicting vein crossing VN

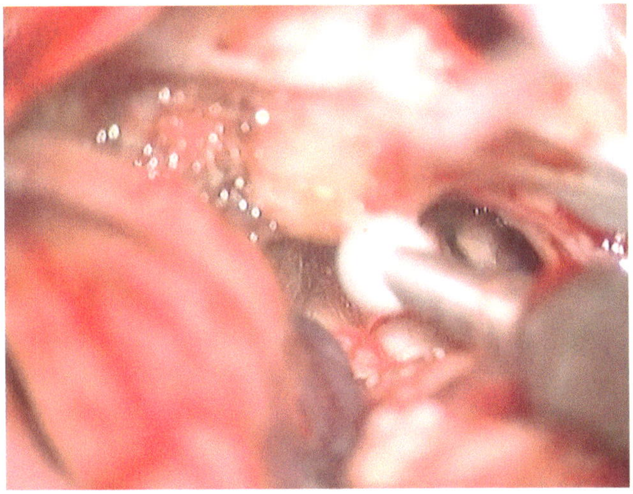

Fig. 11 SMT drilled away

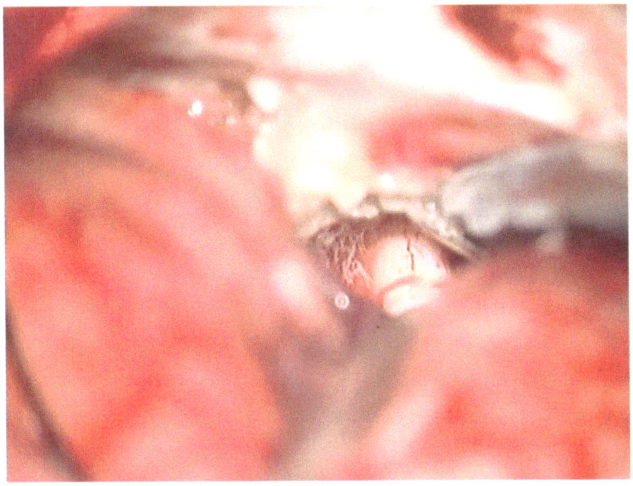

Fig. 12 Teflon inserted between transverse pontine vein and VN

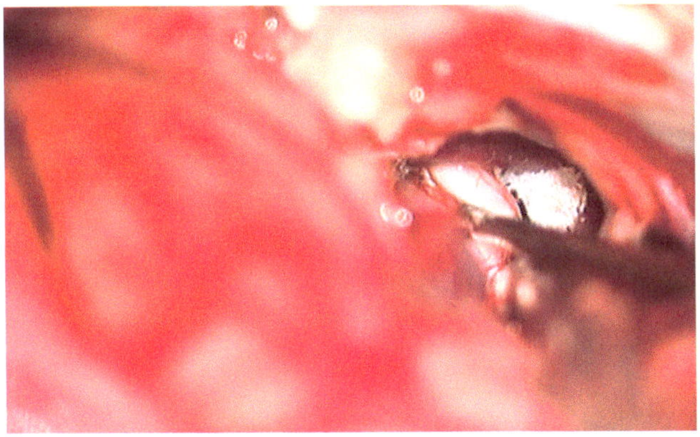

Fig. 13 Teflon inserted between AICA and VN; Teflon at the site of venous conflict

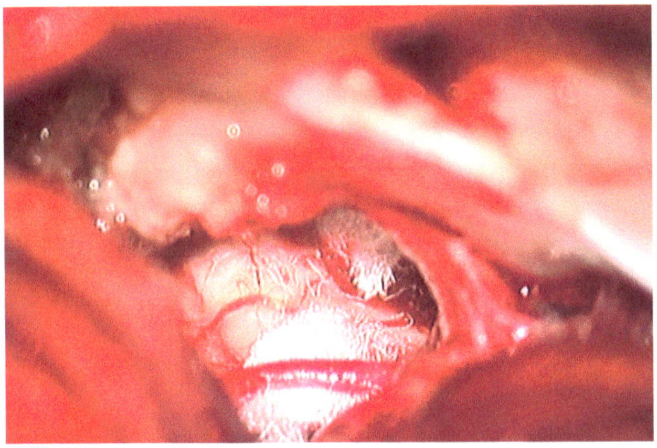

Fig. 14 Six-month postoperative audiometry (19 July 2019) showing full recovery of hearing

Follow-Up

Her dizziness and vertigo settled within a few days, but she was upset by hearing loss, which started to improve after 2 weeks but normalised only after 6 months (Fig. 15). However, her relief from TN was total and gratifying, as per her last communication, 5 years after MVD.

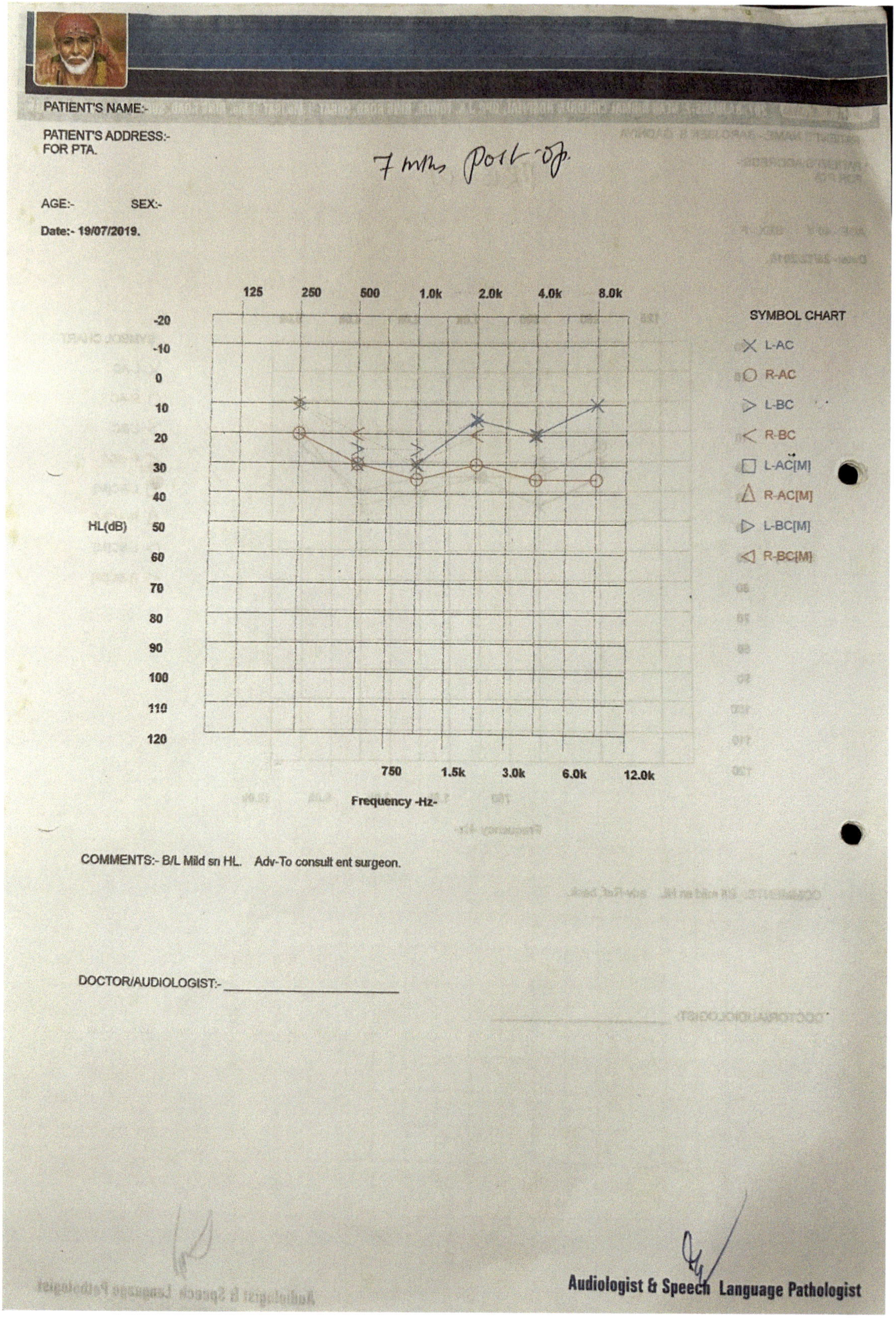

Fig. 15 Seven-month postoperative audiometry

Learning Points

- Detailed and precise clinical and MRI investigations are needed before deciding upon MVD for TN.
- T2-weighted 3D imaging (3D CISS/FIESTA) and TOF MRA are important for predicting NVC and identifying the often-overlooked roles of veins.
- Enlarged suprameatal tubercle (SMT) may sometimes present with difficulty in visual confirmation of NVC and execution of MVD. Although it can be seen on MRI, one tends to overlook it. Observing it on imaging helps us prepare for tackling it.
- Performing preoperative audiometry is important in all cases: It establishes the baseline hearing that can be useful for postoperative comparison, especially when a patient complains of impaired hearing.
- Excessive brain retraction may also cause transient or permanent injury to the cerebellum and some cranial nerves (especially VII and VIII)—more so when the CPA is "smaller" than usual and when the space is cramped—while performing safe and effective MVD. This is also a strong argument in favour of performing endoscopic MVD.
- Most complications are transient or temporary and resolve over time.
- Apart from handling the disease, surgeons must also be adept at handling the patient and family in the face of an unforeseen complication, such as the one presented.
- In view of the liable cranial nerve disturbances, would performing intraoperative neuromonitoring be wise at least in "selected cases"? (Performing it routinely in all cases of MVD for TN may result in wasting time and resources). "Selected cases" are those (a) where one envisages difficulty during surgery (e.g. multiple vessels causing NVC or basilar dolichoectasia); (b) featuring patients who are elderly, have obesity, have a high body mass index (BMI), or have comorbidities; (c) featuring patients with a very short neck; (d) featuring patients with poor or absent hearing or facial function on the contralateral side; and (e) featuring patients with atypical neuralgia or doubtful NVC on MRI.

Reference

1. Andersen, et al. Microvascular decompression in trigeminal neuralgia—a prospective study of 115 patients. J Headache Pain. 2022;23:145. https://doi.org/10.1186/s10194-022-01520-x.